Keep Healthy after

Lifestyle facts for a stronger longer life

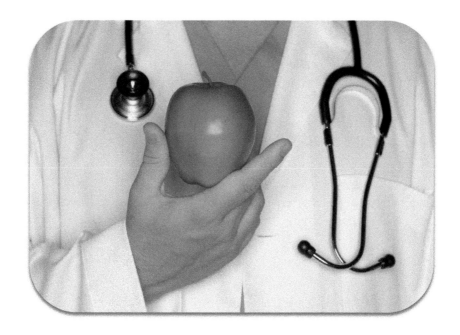

2020 Version

Published by   Health Education Publications
Email: Health-education@clara.co.uk
Websites: Cancernet.co.uk | Keep-healthy.com
Twitter: @cancernetUK
Facebook: @cancernetUK
Lifestyle blog: blog.cancernet.co.uk
Newsletter: Sign up via cancernet.co.uk
ISBN: 978-0-9558212-5-7

Papers used by Health Education Publications are natural, recyclable products made from wood grown in sustainable forests.

Graphics by Erika Silling
Photographs have been taken by the authors are royalty free or the royalties have been paid via shutterstock.com

For more information or to order more books please refer to our website:

Printed and bound by CPI Group (UK) Ltd, Croydon, CR0 4YY

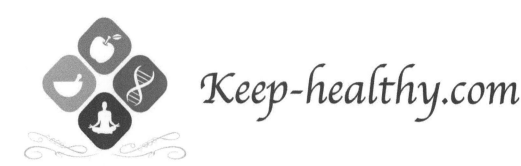

Keep-healthy.com

Foreword

Paula Radcliffe World champion marathon runner

My mum, exceptional in many ways, is, I'm sure, similar to thousands of people who have had the trauma of cancer thrust upon them. As well as wanting to make sure she had the best possible medical care and fully understand her treatment options, she had a strong desire to know the best ways to help herself. Day to day lifestyle activities that were straight forward before her cancer suddenly had an added complexity, especially after the side effects of surgery, radiotherapy, chemotherapy and Herceptin started to become a burden.

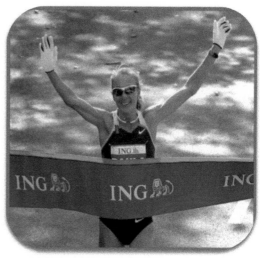

As a cancer expert who has worked closely with patients for many years, Professor Thomas is very aware of the concerns which many patients have, not only with conventional treatments but with dietary, exercise and lifestyle issues after cancer. I know, from my mum's contact with him during her treatment, that he is sensitive to the fact that patients like her need to feel in control and have a strong positive desire to help themselves. As a scientist and a doctor, he has an exceptional knowledge of the important topics around lifestyle and cancer, not only from his own research but from regular scrutiny of the world literature. This book, therefore, provides just what people need to empower themselves - a reliable tool based only on the best available evidence, containing relevant practical guidance sensitive to the psychological, cultural and physical needs of people with and recovering from cancer.

We, as a family, have always striven to win, most obviously in sport and careers, but now also in fighting cancer. To do this, as well as determination, effort and dedication, we needed, and continue to need, accurate advice and help. For my mum, this book has been fundamental in providing this well-needed support and arming her with the tools to win her own personal marathon. I know she cannot thank Professor Thomas enough for his dedication, professional expertise and commitment.

Contents

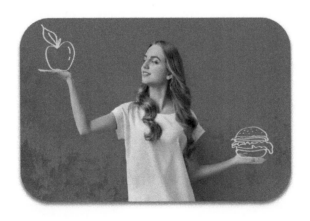

Chapter 1

Introduction

In the past twenty years the chance of surviving cancer has substantially improved. Breast cancer cure, for instance, has increased from 50% to 80%, while for prostate this has increased from 30% to 80%. Exciting new biological treatments are emerging every year, developed as a result of complex scientific endeavour which mankind should be very proud of. As well as increasing cure rates, these are helping to keep people with

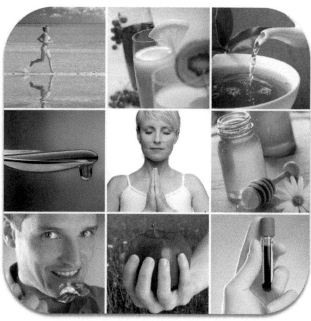

metastatic disease alive for decades rather than months. It is expected that, with good care most men with prostate cancer, who even have disease spread to their bones can live for up to 10 years. Metastatic melanoma used to mean imminent demise but dramatic response are now being seen with new immunotherapies. A diagnosis of chronic myeloid leukaemia is now reduces life expectancy by 3 years as opposed to 25 years previously.

To achieve these better outcomes, however, patients often have to endure complex and arduous therapies, often leaving them beleaguered with physical and psychological adverse effects. In addition to being unpleasant, these toxicities result in greater usage of health resources which have financial implications for patients and their families. Studies have estimated that cancer survivors incur thousands of pounds in added medical costs a year, compared to individuals without a cancer history. Additionally, survivors of cancer have many more general health concerns than people of similar age and sex. They are twice as likely to be hospitalised, attend accident and emergency, and visit their GP. Their ongoing symptoms can lead to feelings of loneliness and isolation, financial burdens and twice the risk of other chronic degenerative illnesses, starting at a much younger age. In fact, a study from Oxford University, presented at the UK's National Cancer conference in 2019 reported that of the £16 billion spend on cancer care each year in the UK, £2 was on drugs £5 on diagnosis, monitoring surgery and radiotherapy and £9 billion was the economic cost to the country and the management of aftercare including, drugs for heart disease, diabetes, weight gain, depression, dementia, hot flushes, arthritis, bowel and urinary problems.

With the increasing total numbers of cancers, alongside better survival rates and improved chances of living longer with active disease, the total number of people living with and beyond cancer, at any one time, is growing by 3% per annum. By 2040, in the UK and USA there will be over 3 million and 18 million people respectively living with the consequences of cancer and its therapies. This all sounds gloomy, but the good news is that many of these toxicities can be alleviated or prevented with the sensible lifestyle, exercise and nutritional strategies highlighted in this book, especially if they are initiated as soon after diagnosis and continued long term

The World Cancer Research Fund (WCRF), Cancer Research UK (CRUK) and the USA National Cancer Institute have all agreed that lifestyle provides enormous benefits in reducing side effects of treatments. Evidence from robust academic research suggests that a healthy, physically active lifestyle could reduce the risk of relapse by between 30-40% for common tumours such as breast, prostate and bowel. Lifestyle has been shown to slow progression of some slow growing tumours, prolong the medical control of metastatic disease as well as help prevent relapse after initial treatments and improve the chances of a long and healthy life.

Fortunately, academic interest in lifestyle and survivorship research is increasing day by day. The positive results of well-conducted trials have given rise to a proliferation of medical publications in traditional journals which have been an eye opener for many doctors. It's also refreshing to see that pharmaceutical companies are waking up to the importance of 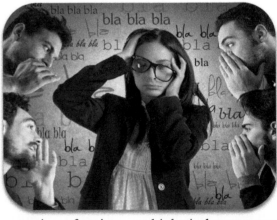 lifestyle initiatives. Many of the new generation of anti-cancer biological treatments work by recruiting the body's own immunity to fight the cancer cells, so it's not a surprise that studies are showing increased response rates if patients have a heathy lifestyle and stronger immunity. The momentum for change is so marked that CRUK and other scientific bodies have announced major funding programmes to investigate the effect of lifestyle on cancer.

Although knowledge is generally empowering, too much information from multiple sources can lead to confusion, especially as it often appears that published trials and their interpretation by the media are frequently conflicting. This lack of clarity does not just apply to patients. It's a sad reality that many doctors still lack the understanding, skills, knowledge, or even worse, enthusiasm to embrace lifestyle and functional medicine. Even if patients ask their doctors about lifestyle issues, they may receive misleading and sometimes patronising answers. Other pitfalls confronting patients, especially online, are the numerous reports of wonder cures and miraculous recoveries. Some of these are written in good faith but are frankly misleading, even lacking a solid diagnosis of cancer in the first place, or failing to mention the contribution of simultaneous conventional or alternative therapies. Others are more sinister, preying on vulnerable patients and persuading them to spend their hard-earned money on *cure-alls* that are unproven, don't work and may even cause harm.

Reassuringly, as this book only refers to original information from genuine, reputable sources, it's accuracy will help resolve myths and unsubstantiated claims. Making the lifestyle changes advocated in the following chapters is no mean feat after the trauma of cancer. Hopefully, this level of robust information will empower readers with confidence, so if they decide to starve themselves overnight, exercise in the rain before breakfast, ditch their favourite beef burger and eat food previously thought only fit for the birds, they will be absolutely convinced that their efforts are worthwhile. For the same reason, this book doesn't just offer advice, it explains in detail, the underlying biochemical pathways of how lifestyle changes work. Although heavy reading at times, with this depth of knowledge, readers can genuinely understand the reasons why these measures are needed.

About this new edition

By Simon Blackburn

Apart from the change of title, every page has been substantially re-written and expanded, in order to provide up-to-date information sensitive to the changing needs of people living beyond cancer like myself. Since the last edition, five years ago, countless studies have been published, across the world of varying degrees of quality and this book does well to summarise and prioritise the best of them.

Because of the enormous expanse in the literature, the new title was chosen to reflect improved understanding of formal self-help or supervised programmes as opposed to just lifestyle. It was also necessary as the book has actually now been split into two. The other version "Rules to live by" provides lifestyle and nutritional advice for overall health with an emphasis on disease prevention. This version targets people specifically living with and beyond cancer especially emphasising advice on reducing long term toxicities as well as improving outcomes.

In order to understand and interpret the results of increasingly complex studies, it is important to be part of the research process itself. Professor Thomas, as head of a lifestyle and cancer research unit which has produced as steady stream of internationally recognised, scientific studies, is in a strong position to critically review other published work as designing studies requires a thorough

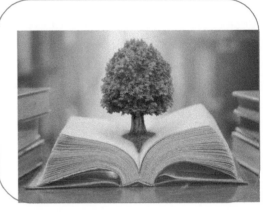

knowledge of the background evidence, and an understanding of the relevant questions and how to best answer them. Only the highest quality studies on nutrition, exercise and physical and psychological wellbeing have been included in this book.

Redundant sections have been removed, and further chapters have been added in response to emerging scientific evidence Although chemotherapy, radiotherapy and hormone therapies still have a major role in cancer management, the era of biological and immune therapies has arrived, so it now includes a description of the unique profiles of toxicities from biological agents and practical tips to alleviate them.

I have undergone the ordeal of surgery, chemotherapy, radiotherapy and biological treatments for a small cell lung cancer, meaning I am writing from a position of some authority. My disease is fortunately still in remission after five years, and I am convinced, in addition to the excellent medical treatment I received from the Royal Marsden and Royal Brompton hospitals, that the lifestyle measures I have adopted have significantly contributed to my rare recovery from this type of cancer. I have been proud to offer editorial advice for this edition which makes it significantly more readable and relevant to the needs and concern future readers.

<table>
<tr><td>**Chapter 2**</td><td></td></tr>
</table>

Mind and brain

with Dr Ashwin Mehta

Fatigue and tiredness

In a survey of 800 patients published in Adelaide 2015, fatigue was reported is the single most troublesome symptom both during acute cancer treatments and in the long term. This is why this has been chosen first in this book, to highlight its significance. In fact, fatigue has overtaken nausea and pain as a concern for patients during chemotherapy yet it is often regarded

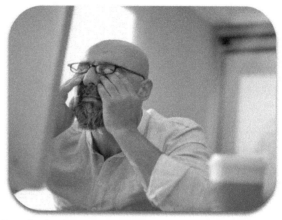

as a rather trivial by health care professionals during consultations. It is characterised by tiredness, exhaustion, depression, feeling unwell, loss of motivation and limitation of mental state. Over 75% of patients complain of fatigue, and in up to a third of cases this impacts on quality of life. Fatigue can have a negative impact on treatment by reducing compliance to drugs, reducing mobility and delaying the recovery from chemotherapy for several months. Post-treatment fatigue, as well as being distressing, can have a considerable bearing on an individuals' ability to return to work or care for dependants. Clinician awareness of the impact of fatigue is improving, but strategies to manage it have not been forthcoming. Fatigue is common, not just with chemotherapy, but with other treatments such as radiotherapy, hormone therapy and new biological therapies.

The management of fatigue

Associated medical conditions which can aggravate fatigue should be addressed initially. Anaemia can be remedied by treating the underlying cause such as stopping blood loss or correcting any underlying iron, folate or vitamin B12 deficiencies, and if these fail, administering blood transfusions or erythropoietin (epo) injections. It may be possible to stop using sedating drugs such as opiates, antihistamines, cyclizine and anxiolytics. Electrolyte imbalance, liver failure, steroid withdrawal, thyroid or adrenal insufficiency can cause correctable fatigue. Sleep can be disturbed by anxiety, depression, passing urine at night, pain, night sweats and itching, most of which can be helped by specific medical treatments. If fatigue continues after these associated conditions have been corrected it is given the general term of cancer-related fatigue

11

(CRF), the underlying cause of which is not exactly known and usually gets worse as the disease progresses or during active treatments.

Anxiolytics (sedatives) may provide short-term relief and help sleep initially. Unfortunately, as time goes on, the length of sedated sleep time diminishes and natural sleep is lost, making the situation worse. Psycho-stimulants such as dextroamphetamine and levoamphetamine (Adderall), or methylphenidate (Ritalin), licensed for deficit hyperactivity disorder and narcolepsy, have been shown to improve fatigue and concentration in the short term but can induce insomnia and agitation with long-term use, aggravating chronic fatigue syndromes.

In men, low testosterone can cause fatigue, demotivation, erectile dysfunction and depression. The use of hormone replacement therapy is effective and certainly under utilised among cancer survivors. Several studies have shown that it's safe to correct subnormal levels of testosterone in cancer survivors and this significantly reduces fatigue. There are even studies which indicate that HRT in men is safe for those who have had early prostate cancer, although most doctors are uncomfortable prescribing them in this situation. Among women, HRT can reduce fatigue as well as other menopausal symptoms.

What can you do to help?

While it is important to discuss fatigue with your doctor, the following lifestyle measures can be easily adopted at home and have been shown to help CRF.

Sleep hygiene
Getting enough sleep at night is vital in helping maintain a regular circadian rhythm and reduce fatigue. Sleep hygiene tips are described in the next section.

Exercise
The role of exercise in helping reduce CRF was reviewed in two comprehensive analyses which summarised 38 RCTs involving over 3000 participants within a variety of exercise programmes. The benefit of programmes which involve unsupervised exercises such as walking, jogging or cycling was small, as their success was hampered by lack of compliance or the intermittent, short-lived nature of the interventions. On the other hand, supervised programmes such as aerobics, resistance exercises and dance classes,

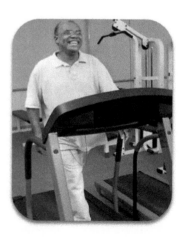

significantly reduced fatigue as trainers were better at ensuring both enjoyment and motivation, ensuring long-term success. Along with reducing CRF, successful regular supervised resistance and aerobic muscle regimens improved strength, stamina, mood and overall quality of life. If you are a member of a gym, a suitably qualified exercise professional should be able to help you. Otherwise, you can ask your oncology team to refer you to a formal exercise rehabilitation programme.

When to exercise: This often depends on pre-diagnosis fitness levels, abilities, preferences and the needs of each individual. In terms of timing, waiting until initial treatments are completed is certainly too late. Although it's not easy to exercise during tough treatments, it is worth trying. In one study, patients with acute leukaemia receiving bone marrow transplantation who undertook a three week supervised 12-minute walking programme had a significant improvement in fatigue compared to those allowed to rest in bed. Another Michigan-based study highlighted how women receiving radiotherapy who jogged or walked briskly daily had significantly higher haemoglobin levels and experienced less fatigue. Another study in men with prostate cancer receiving radiotherapy demonstrated a benefit from 15-minutes of aerobic exercise daily. The PACES study from the Netherlands showed that women on chemotherapy, randomised to undergo an intense 5 hours per week supervised exercise programme, had significantly less fatigue and more rapid recovery than women taking only light or no exercise.

Type of exercise: One study demonstrated that aerobic exercise for 15-30 minutes per day, such as dancing, jogging or brisk walking, was more effective at reducing fatigue than weight lifting or using resistance bands alone. Another study reported that a programme combining both aerobics and supervised gentle resistance training 2-3 times a week for at least 30 minutes was particularly effective, with benefits lasting up to a year after chemotherapy. It was noted that in the first few weeks, fatigue was slow to improve, but benefits were seen as the individual gradually became fitter.

Intensity of exercise: Sports scientists have found that regular light to moderate exercise, defined as a level in which the person has to breathe at a rate of between 40-50% of their peak oxygen consumption (VO2 max which is measured in ml/kg/min at peak exercise), was better than irregular high intensity exercise, defined as >50-70% of VO2 max which is usually above the anaerobic threshold (i.e. you are breathless even after the exercise finishes). The issue with irregular high-intensity exercise is that it draws heavily on energy reserves and can lead to post-exertion malaise, while operating at this level also means that the aerobic system struggles to keep up with the body's oxygen need, creating an oxygen debt which has to be paid back with continued post-exercise breathlessness. The best results came from supervised exercise programmes involving Graduated Exercise Therapy, which entails a progressive build-up of intensity over several weeks and helps avoid the drawbacks associated with sudden, high-intensity exercise.

Relaxation strategies

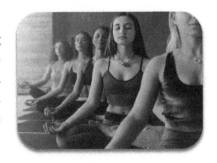

Techniques aimed at reducing stress, including relaxation classes, yoga and massage, improve fatigue i by improving sleep patterns. Regular Tai Chi and Qigong activity, therapist-delivered acupuncture and Cognitive Behavior Therapy have also been shown to help manage fatigue.

Caffeine in tea and coffee

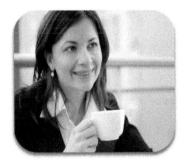

Regular drinkers are all too aware of the immediate 'lift' after their morning brew. Researchers have confirmed that caffeine has an immediate ability to enhance mood, mental and physical performance, and to foster a sense of well-being, happiness, energy, alertness and sociability. The trouble is that, like all additive drugs, there is an upside and a downside. When the positive 'lift effect' wears off there may be a drop in "energy levels", caused by the withdrawal of caffeine from the bloodstream, leading to more fatigue. Those suffering from fatigue may be advised not to drink strong tea or coffee as this withdrawal may cause more problems over the course of the day. For those who have trouble sleeping, remember that caffeine can stay in the bloodstream for 6-7 hours so should be avoided from mid-afternoon.

Sugar and refined carbohydrates

Studies have reported that avoiding sugar and refined carbohydrates, can prevent sudden rises in blood sugar which prompt high insulin release and subsequent periods of low sugars. This period of low sugar can significantly lower energy levels. Slow release more complex carbohydrates provide more steady (and lower) blood sugar levels. Processed sugar also damages gut health and increased chronic inflammation which both contribute to lethargy and fatigue.

Identifying food intolerances

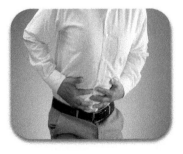

As we get older, it is more common to develop an intolerance to gluten found in wheat and other grains, while our ability to metabolise lactose in milk also falls. Both of these situations can increase gut inflammation, leading to Irritable Bowel Symptoms

(IBS) such as bloating, unsatisfactory bowel movements and fatigue. Keeping a food diary can help identify which foods trigger these symptoms. If gluten is found to be problematic, reduce the intake of bread, pasta and cereals. If milk is suspected, change to fermented products which have already had the lactose broken down and are easier to digest. Probiotic supplements such as Lactobacillus acidophilus help with the digestion and absorption of lactose by producing lactase.

Dark chocolate

A few small studies have suggested cocoa helps functional disability caused by fatigue. Scientists from York Medical School randomly gave either milk chocolate with added dark pigment (placebo) or 45g/day of dark chocolate to people with Chronic Fatigue. There was a significant reduction in fatigue among those who ate dark chocolate, with some patients even able to return to work. Chocolate 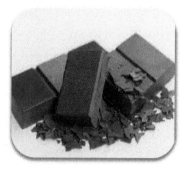 contains many polyphenols but also theobromine, a vasodilator which increases heart rate, lowers blood pressure and boosts brain levels of serotonin (a mood-enhancing chemical). Most trials have used chocolate with sugar which can contribute to fatigue, so trials using sugar-free chocolate may be even better.

Nutritional supplements

In addition to healthy dietary changes, specific wholefood nutritional supplements have been investigated.

Ginseng (Panax quinquefolius) has long been used in traditional Chinese medicine as a natural energy enhancer. Ginseng's active ingredients, ginsenosides, have been shown in animal studies to reduce inflammation and to help regulate cortisol levels, two factors which contribute to the aetiology of fatigue. Ginseng was investigated in a double-blind RCT which 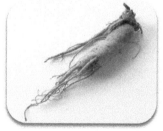 randomised 364 patients to either a capsule containing 2000mg of ginseng (standardised to 3% ginsenosides) or a placebo. By 8 weeks, there was a statistically significant reduction in fatigue in the ginseng group. It must be noted that this study used a whole root product, not ginseng methanolic extract which is commonly used in over-the-counter supplements and has a number of concerns including possible estrogenic effects.

Guarana (Paullinia cupana) is a plant in the maple family that grows along the Amazon and is common in Brazil. It is commonly used as a stimulant and contains about twice the caffeine of the coffee bean. It also contains theobromine and theophylline, other stimulants that affect the central nervous system. Well-conducted RCTs have not been published evaluating Guarana, so it would be best to avoid it until more evidence is published.

Probiotics have been evaluated in a number of interesting studies on chronic fatigue. In one study, Lactobacillus and Bifidobacterium were given to patients with high fatigue severity scores and high disability scores. After 4 weeks, health and physical activity had improved. In another small randomised study, bowel symptoms and emotional well-being improved among sufferers of chronic fatigue taking pro-biotics. Given the

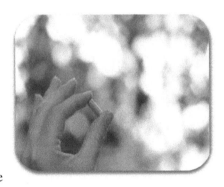

other benefits offered by probiotics for people after cancer, it is certainly worth giving them a try if you suffer chronic fatigue. Other food extracts such as vitamins and minerals are likely only to help if correcting a known deficiency. The later section on gut health emphasizes the importance of buying them from reputable sources such as keep-healthy.com

Other supplements: CBD oils can reduce anxiety and help people sleep. The benefit of organic varieties at small doses will be covered in more detail in the specific section later. While taking melatonin five hours before bedtime has been shown to improve fatigue symptoms by improving sleep patterns, it has not been investigated in people with cancer. Acetyl-l-carnitine has been investigated in small studies, but the evidence of a benefit is not robust. The supplement with the most potential contains green tea, chocolate, probiotics bacteria and American ginseng. These ingredients on their own have credible scientific evidence, and the Vitali-T trial is underway to determine the benefit of using them in combination. If other measures fail to improve fatigue it may be worth having a nutritional test to exclude an underlying deficiency of an essential vitamin, mineral, polyphenol or fat.

Houseplants: The later chapter describes the multiple benefits of placing plants in the house, including alleviating fatigue. A study from Sydney, reported lower fatigue and better efficiency after plants were added to a work environment.

Poor sleep pattern

Several confounding factors conspire to keep you awake after a cancer diagnosis. Firstly, pondering over the diagnosis and worrying about forthcoming treatments is often worst in the early hours. A number of physical conditions can also make night times uncomfortable such as pain, indigestion, breathlessness or having to pass water frequently. Steroids can keep you alert and agitated, as can hormones for

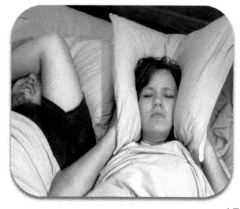

breast cancer which can also cause night sweats and hot flushes. Aromatase inhibitors can cause joint pains and itchy skin which contribute to a restless night.

Consequences of disrupted sleep

Fatigue is the obvious result of sleep deprivation and, in the longer term, this can contribute to a lack of motivation to exercise, lack of desire to commit to other healthy living behaviours and depression. Chronic insomnia is known to be a carcinogen. Interestingly, however, an evaluation of the large UK biobank dataset suggested that women who awoke early and did not have more than 8 hours' sleep had a lower risk of cancer compared to women who went to bed late and rose later – this suggests that it's the disruption to the circadian rhythm rather than lack of sleep itself which adds to the risk.

What can you do to help yourself?

It is helpful to try and accept that it is normal to have sleepless nights from time to time. Being paranoid about not sleeping just makes it worse. The most important advice is to try and maintain a regular light-dark cycle as this affects the production of melatonin, cortisol and other regulatory hormones.

Disruption of the sleep pattern: Try to avoid travelling across time zones and working at night if possible. Try to avoid going to bed very late during the weekends which disrupts the circadian rhythm at the start of the week.

Bright (blue) light exposure during the day: One of the best ways to set your circadian clock is to be exposed to bright light (ideally sunlight) during the day, preferably mornings. The component of sunlight that tells your circadian clock that it's daytime is blue light, which triggers sensitive photoreceptors in the eyes and, to a lesser extent, skin. This is one explanation why you feel in a good mood looking at a blue sea. In general, try to get as 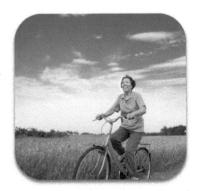 much natural light as possible in the day. If there is no opportunity to get natural light in the day, a biological alternative would be to put your head into a light box for at least 15 minutes at roughly the same time every morning or mid-day. Another option is to make many small changes to brighten your environment by using sunlight spectrum light bulbs in your house (but you'll want to avoid using these light bulbs in the evening), keeping curtains open during the day and trying to face a window. Exercise in the morning, with accompanying bright sunlight exposure, is part of a healthy routine that improves sleep quality by stabilising our circadian rhythm.

Avoid bright and blue light in the evening or at night: Just as it's important for your body to get the signal that it's daytime during the day, it's important to signal it's nighttime. This means avoiding blue light and sticking with red and yellow wavelengths. You can help your circadian clock by keeping your indoor lighting as dim as possible in the evenings with dimmer switches, or just turning on fewer lights in conjunction with investing in red 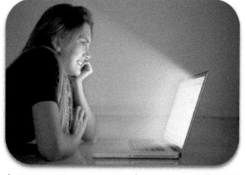 or yellow light bulbs for the evening. If using a computer monitor or watch TV, there are two options. The first is to install *a flux application* on your computer, phones or tablets and set the screen brightness to the lowest setting. The second is to wear amber-tinted glasses for the last 2-3 hours of your day. Several scientific studies show that wearing these glasses in the evening improves sleep quality and supports melatonin production. Be careful with using electronic devices that have screens in the evening, because the content (not just the brightness) is designed to stimulate the arousal centres of the brain. A more sophisticated option is to use programmable light bulbs where you can set the colour spectrum and the brightness for the time of day. Once you get to bed, sleep in a completely dark room, cover up any LED lights on phones, toothbrushes, baby monitors, or whatever other gadgets you have plugged in in your room. Blackout curtains help as can white noise generators, especially if there are high frequency/pitch noises in or outside your home. If you need to use the loo at night, either learn to navigate in the dark or use as little light as possible.

Reduce and manage stress: You probably recognise cortisol as being the master stress hormone but, it's also a very important circadian rhythm hormone. This means that if you're under stress, not only do you have all the effects of elevated and dysregulated cortisol to deal with, but you also experience sleep disruption. The section relating to psychological morbidity later on in the book will cover this in more detail, but salient tips would include making changes to the structure of your work and social life, asking for help or making time for regular exercise life.

Aim for regular bedtimes and try to get enough sleep: Your melatonin starts increasing about 2 hours before bed to prepare your body for sleep. If you're muscling through a sugary snack, a scary movie or whatever else you do to keep yourself awake at night, you are affecting your circadian rhythm. Aim for 7-8 hours of sleep every night. This means shifting your bedtime earlier, so you aren't struggling through that fatigue to get a second wind.

Stay cool at night: The temperature `t night is also a cue to your circadian clock. Ideally, at night the temperature should be lower than in the day. In the room.

Ditch the alarm clock: Waking up to a jarring noise is very stressful. If you don't have the luxury of sleeping until your body naturally wants to wake every morning (which is the best option for protecting your circadian rhythm and overall health), use a light alarm which gradually gets louder and can be set on most mobile devices.

Physical activity: Getting some kind of activity during the day has been shown to support melatonin production. Intense activity in the evening, however, especially in the really bright environment of many gyms, potentially delaying your melatonin production (basically keep you revved up longer in the evening) unless it's routine and your body has adjusted. Other than that, any kind of activity any time of day will help you sleep easier at night.

Manage your blood sugars: Eating a big meal just before bedtime will not only increase the risk of heartburn and indigestion but will also increase cortisol and sugar, just when we do not need it. Instead, of sugary foods, concentrate on complex carbohydrates and healthy fats, as these will help you avoid hunger pangs overnight. In recent studies, it has been found that increasing our overnight fasting intervals to 13 or more hours, improves prognosis after a breast cancer diagnosis. This effect is thought to be related to better blood sugar metabolism.

Eat melatonin-rich foods: Melatonin is made from serotonin, which in turn is made from tryptophan. Seafood has high levels of tryptophan, while also having less of the other amino acids which compete with tryptophan to cross the blood-brain barrier. Montmorency and Morello cherries walnuts and bananas are also rich in plant precursors of melatonin (known as phytomelatonins). Therefore, 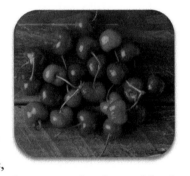 eating more seafood and cherries is a good way to boost production of both serotonin and melatonin. Seafood also contributes long-chain omega-3 fats to your diet that help support circadian rhythms by improving general brain health. Ginger also has phytomelatonin, so a good nightcap would be some grated ginger with hot water, a little lemon and mint. However, avoid drinking too much liquid prior to bed as it fills the stomach and makes you need the bathroom at night.

Alcohol, caffeine and cigarettes: Discontinue or reduce the use of caffeine (tea, coffee, energy drinks) after 4 pm. Alcohol may make you initially sleepy, but often you then have a restless night because alcohol disrupts our ability to enjoy the benefits of deep sleep (alpha-wave intrusion during stage III sleep). Nicotine is a stimulant which can keep you awake so avoid smoking at night. Heavy smokers suffer withdrawal of nicotine at night, so they wake up anxious and alert.

Dietary melatonin supplements: Melatonin is licensed in the UK for adults who are aged 55 or over, but is not recommended to take for more than a 13-week course. It can be obtained with a prescription and comes in the form of a 'prolonged-release' tablet. In the USA and many countries, it is freely available over the counter. Double-blind RCT 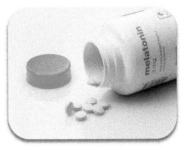 have shown that this hormone helps people sleep, shortens the number of awakenings in the night and improves the quality of sleep. However, it is not a viable long-term solution. It is most useful in treating jet lag, as it promotes quicker recovery from that muzzy stage one may experience after extended periods of flight. The ideal time to use melatonin is 60 minutes prior to bedtime.

Summary - Advice to help you sleep

- Establish a regular pattern of sleeping. Set a time to retire and get up
- Avoid temperature extremes and noise when in bed
- Ensure your bedroom is dark. Consider blackout curtains
- Avoid being uncomfortable or in pain. Consider taking painkillers
- Try not to watch TV or read exciting books in bed
- Exercise routinely but try not to exercise within two hours of bedtime
- Reduce the intake of caffeine, alcohol and nicotine after mid-afternoon
- Avoid drinking large amounts of liquids prior to bedtime
- Avoid food colourings and preservatives which can act as stimulants
- Avoid hunger or excessive eating prior to bedtime
- Avoid taking daytime naps
- Avoid sleeping tablets unless you are getting over a short-term issue
- If awakening to pass water, discuss medication with your doctor
- Engage in a quiet, relaxing activity before bedtime
- Consider a short term melatonin supplement
- Consider a low dose of CBD oil
- If awake for >30 minutes, leave bed, walk around, cool then return

---

Mood, anxiety and depression

With Simon Maguire

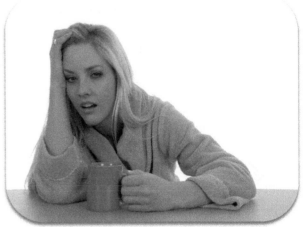

When specifically looked for, up to 30% of people with cancer are found to have anxiety or depression. As well as being distressing for the patient and carers, depression has also been linked with reduced outcomes. The best example of this was highlighted in an observational trial from California which evaluated the records of 41,275 men with prostate cancer. They found a 40% higher prostate cancer death rate among men with a proven diagnosis of depressive illness compared to non-depressed men. Interestingly, the greater difference was seen in the men with the less aggressive forms of the disease. An Ohio State University study found that mice living in a happy environment had a slower rate of progression of their implanted tumours, compared to those in a more confined stressful environment. Happy mice also had lower levels of a protein called leptin which is known to stimulate tumour growth.

Long-standing psychological stresses in the workplace, an unhappy marriage or even a poorly performing football team can also reduce immune function and leave people more prone to infection. Chronic stress produces a stress hormone called cortisol, released by the adrenal glands, that lowers immune function. Initially, it reduces inflammation, which at first glance appears good, but chronically high cortisol also disrupts blood sugar balance, often leading to high insulin, obesity and sometimes diabetes, all of which increase the wrong type of inflammatory markers, creating a situation involving both increased infection and increased inflammation.

Being told you have a life-threatening illness is enough to trigger anxiety and depression in even the most level-headed of individuals. Other factors, however, can specifically contribute to anxiety after diagnosis, such as steroid agitation, allergy to drugs and withdrawal from sedatives. Anxiety is common before a scan and in the period waiting for results, and doctors should consider "scanxiety" and try to shorten the time before results are given. Low mood or depression can be aggravated by steroid withdrawal, as well as treatments that put women into menopause or reduce testosterone in me, such as after chemotherapy, surgery or hormone therapy. Unless lower testosterone levels are needed, such as in the treatment of prostate cancer, testosterone replacement therapy can play a major role in helping improve mood and motivation in men. As already mentioned, the use of testosterone is often underappreciated and certainly underused among cancer survivors. In post-menopausal women with breast cancer, Aromatase inhibitors can lower mood, but our own research has shown that different brands of breast cancer drugs, even within the same category, are tolerated differently from one person to another, so it may help to ask for a change of drug.

Ideally, psychological health should be routinely screened at all stages of the cancer journey. A particularly risky period is shortly after the end of the initial intensive therapies, such as after the last cycle of adjuvant chemotherapy for breast or bowel cancer, where the sudden end to hospital support may make people feel at their most vulnerable. Clinical psychologists and psychological counsellors who can offer interventions and treatments are now available in most cancer units, but in the UK most GP's are more than capable of offering help to individuals with uncomplicated anxiety and depression.

What can you do to help?

In the first instance, vocalise your anxiety or depression with your clinical nurse specialists, oncologist or GP, as therapeutic interventions can be considered such as appropriate counselling. Self-help strategies, including support groups, relaxation classes and mindfulness, help re-channel negative energy and fear into positive enthusiasm for lifestyle and exercise.

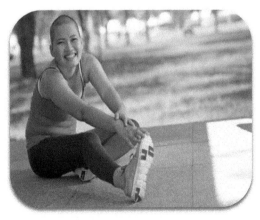

Exercise programmes have a significant impact on psychological health and improve self-esteem, feelings of hopelessness and loneliness, especially if they entail group activities. Recent summaries of several RCTs involving women with breast cancer reported a 15% reduction in depression following group or supervised exercise classes. Another study, involving nearly 2000 patients with colorectal cancer, found that those achieving at least 150 minutes of physical activity per week had better mood scores and an 18% higher quality of life. Another study highlighted similar benefits for patients who had recently completed surgery, radiotherapy or chemotherapy. Interestingly, this study outlined how improvements in oxygen consumption correlated directly with changes in mood, suggesting a dose-response relationship - the more exercise, the better the mood. A summary of 40 further studies involving 3,000 participants with a range of health problems, including cancer, found that exercise in sessions of at least 30 minutes, three times a week, leads to a 20% reduction in anxiety and depressive symptoms. The underlying reason for the benefit may lie in the release of positive brain chemicals (neurokins) that make people euphoric. Exercise also significantly reduces inflammatory cytokines (chemicals) which are can help reduce brain fogginess as well as a number of other general symptoms such as joint pains, nausea and fatigue. Exercise is usually generally fun and gets people out of the house, enabling them to socialise and interact with others.

Yoga was investigated in a RCT involving women with breast cancer which demonstrated a significant decrease in anxiety and improvement in QoL after surgery. Other data suggested meditation and yoga altered the body's protein expression, potentially leading to better immunity.

Processed sugar: An analyses of data from the substantial Whitehall cohort reported that participants with a high consumption of sugary drinks, sweetened desserts, had a 58% increased odds of depression. That said, it's hard to delineate the cause and effect as low mood may make people reach for sugar and have other unfavourable lifestyle habits, so more research on sugar and depression is needed.

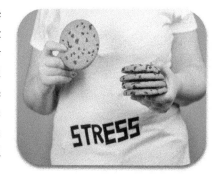

Mindfulness is a well-established practice that is drawn from Buddhist teachings which focus attention on the present experience. It sounds remarkably easy, yet during a cancer experience the mind likes to wander into a dark future. However, with practice and dedication, mindfulness can offer emotional direction and reassurance that the present moment is a good place to spend time. Many people find mindfulness to be an extremely rewarding and self-compassionate endeavour.

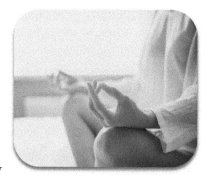

One of the most notable examples of mindfulness helping during a physically and psychologically stressful situation was Viktor Frankl, an Austrian Psychotherapist interned at the Auschwitz concentration camp. He survived and published an influential book, *Man's Search for Meaning*. His main assertion was that individuals who still felt that they had to make a profound contribution during their life were more likely to withstand the atrocious environment and hold onto hope. Finding meaning can come from many outlets including publishing a book, parenting, a career, a hobby or a charitable cause. Mindfulness done properly elicits a relaxation response (RR) that is characterised by decreased oxygen consumption, increased exhaled nitric oxide and reduced psychological distress. A form called Mindfulness Based Stress Reduction (MBSR) therapy was investigated in a controlled study involving women with breast cancer. The half randomised to a 6-week MBSR programme experienced significantly enhanced mood compared to those on standard care. Researchers from the Benson-Henry Institute for Mind Body Medicine went a step further with another fascinating study which looked at the difference in expression of over 2000 genes within three groups - a group offered no intervention, a group given a short 8-week MSBR intervention and a group given a long-term MBSR intervention. The short and, to an even greater extent, long-term interventions had favourable (epigenetic) alterations in gene expression.

A healthy diet combined with exercise was investigated in a trial of 252 younger women with breast cancer. Women randomised to a high vegetable, low fat diet (prudent diet), low sugar had lower intrusive depressive thoughts, reduced concerns regarding cancer recurrence and mortality, better self-concept perceptions and enhanced self-efficacy expectations. There is also some evidence that suboptimal levels of minerals such as zinc and magnesium could contribute to lower mood and higher anxiety. As well as following the guidelines later in this book, an online nutritional test may be advisable if ongoing mood changes.

Probiotic, healthy bacteria has been the subject of much attention recently as more and more evidence emerges suggesting a link between gut health and a healthy mind. Studies involving mice, conducted at the University of Cork, demonstrated that those fed with Lactobacillus had significantly fewer stress, anxiety and depression-related behaviours than those fed with standard feed. Moreover, bacteria-fed mice had lower levels of the stress-induced hormone corticosterone and had altered expression of receptors for the neurotransmitter GABA in the brain. In humans, a study

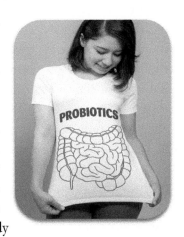

from California showed that women consuming live yoghurt had improved brain function and less environmentally induced markers of stress.

Most of us have experienced feeling "down" when we have a cold or flu. Taking regular hot and cold showers have been shown to reduce the frequency of colds as well as eating lots of polyphenol rich fruit, vegetables, herbs and spices. A randomised study from Australia gave athletes either a probiotic twice daily or a placebo. After one year, the probiotic group had contracted fewer colds and, as a

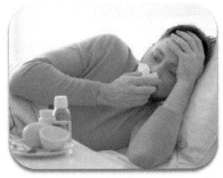

consequence, had experienced less disruption to their training. Athletes across the world now take probiotics regularly. Several other studies have highlighted how regular intake of live Lactobacilli and Bifidobacteria, shortened the duration and severity of upper respiratory tract infections. In 2011, a summary of all international studies was published in the prestigious Cochrane Database and concluded that probiotics also reduced the incidence of upper respiratory tract infections in non-athletes. The economic implications of these findings are enormous, with the impact of colds alone estimated to cost the US economy some $40 billion each year!

Massage, especially those combined with exercises such as yoga or Pilates, are excellent remedies for anxiety and the muscle tension associated with it. Fairly robust analyses have also shown hands-on complementary therapies such as massage, reflexology and acupuncture to be helpful in improving anxiety. Note that despite common folk-lore, gentle massage is safe and there is absolutely no evidence that it "spreads cancer cells around the body".

Smoking, alcohol and recreational drugs: Contrary to popular opinion, cigarettes greatly increase anxiety, and it is a complete myth that smoking calms the nerves. Although there is an immediate sense of relief, even a few minutes after finishing a cigarette the body begins to 'withdraw', leading to tremors, sweating and anxiety which can only be relieved, momentarily, by another cigarette. This leads to an escalating

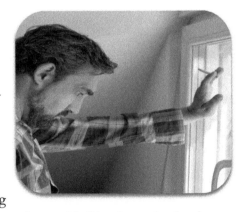

spiral of anxiety. Although a small glass of wine or beer with friends can lead to better social interaction, excess alcohol, as well as other illegal recreational drugs such as cocaine and heroin, lead to anxiety. When the initial euphoric effect wears off, users feel irritable, depressed and experience withdrawal anxiety. This explains why suicide rates are considerably higher among heavy smokers, alcoholics and illegal drug users.

Houseplants have been linked to reduced stress and increased mood. The aforementioned study from Sydney highlighted significant reductions in stress among workers when plants were introduced to their workspace and home. They provide colour, reduce toxins from the air and produce oxygen. They bright colours and fragrances also contribute to subliminal sensations of well-being

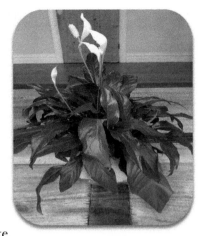

Cannabis is often re smoked with tobacco which increases anxiety. The psychotropic effects of THC within Cannabis can exaggerate mood, so can make you happier or sadder depending on your starting position. After cancer, it's usually the latter. Withdrawal from cannabis can aggravate anxiety. Some studies have suggested that CBD oils which does not have the psychotropic effects of THC can help reduce anxiety but more robust medical trials are needed to confirm their benefits. Remember to use organic verities which substantially reduces pesticide contaminants and buy from reputable sources. Such as the keep-healthy.com website.

Summary - Advice to improve anxiety and mood

- Take regular light exercise
- Take part in regular social activities
- Maintain an interest or hobby
- Eat a healthy diet
- Eat healthy bacteria and consider a probiotic supplement
- In men without prostate cancer, consider androgen replacement therapy
- Try to maintain good sleep hygiene habits
- Consider investing in a psychological counsellor
- Avoid excess alcohol, coffee and strong tea
- Stop smoking and recreational drug use
- Improve gut health consider a quality probiotic supplement
- Consider a trial of CBD oils
- Review medications with your doctor

Chemo Brain (Treatment brain)

The term 'chemo brain' describes a feeling of increasing forgetfulness, alongside a loss of concentration and interest in complex tasks. Other terms include mental fogginess, loss of alertness and treatment brain, but the medical term is cognitive impairment which, in its worse form, can lead to dementia. Although forgetting where you left the car keys can be frustrating, it does not usually interfere with the activities of daily living. On the other hand, if not 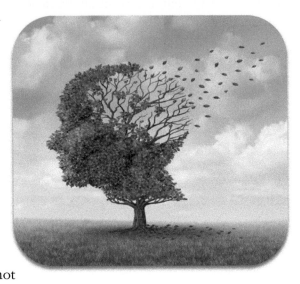 managed early on, this condition can reduce self-confidence and prevent some people from going back to their jobs during or after treatments.

Post-treatment mental fogginess is more pronounced after chemotherapy, particularly in the first year. It usually resolves itself, but in a minority can be an ongoing problem. A number of studies have reported a reduction in intellectual ability after bowel cancer surgery, even without chemotherapy. Recent research has demonstarted a link between long-term anti-androgen therapies and an increased risk of irreversible dementia among men. Formal tests demonstrated that after a year of taking tamoxifen or aromatase inhibitors (e.g Arimidex), women scored lower on verbal memory functioning and other cognitive skills than before they started their treatment. Recent studies have confirmed that androgen deprivation (e.g. Zoladex) in men with prostate cancer can trigger dementia after only 6 months of use. Painkillers, sedatives and antidepressants can exacerbate the loss of brain power independently of the fatigue they also cause. Radiotherapy to the head initially causes a 'muzzy head', and in the longer term, it can lead to brain cells being directly damaged and a loss of intellect. It's also important to exclude other medical problems which could be contributing to reduced brain power such as anaemia, renal and liver disfunction and an underactive thyroid.

Medical interventions: Your medical team will look for aggravated medical conditions or other causes of memory loss, such as an underactive thyroid or electrolyte and vitamin impairments (e.g. B1, B12). Your doctor may investigate for other underlying causes or adjust your regular medications to ones which don't affect the brain. Most hospitals have a memory loss clinic, run by a specialised neurologist who can prescribe drugs such as cholinesterase inhibitors (Aricept, Exelon, Razadyne) or memantine (Namenda), all of which have been approved to treat cognitive symptoms (memory loss, confusion and impaired reasoning).

What can you do to help?

General measures: Regular daily physical activity increases oxygen to the brain and also gets you out of the house, giving you a change of environment and providing visual, social and intellectual stimulation. Numerous studies have shown exercise to be one of the most successful interventions when it comes to delaying the progression of vascular dementia and accelerating recovery from

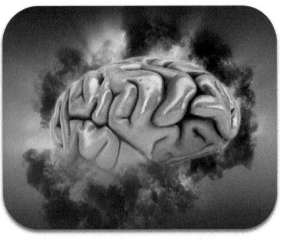

temporary chemo-brain. It's also best to stop smoking and adopt an anti-inflammatory lifestyle including a low sugar and high polyphenol-rich diet.

Brain exercise: Social interactions help stimulate the mind, especially when engaging in interesting conversation. Learning something new or writing in a diary will enable you to think more creatively, help your memory and enhance your ability to make logical connections. Various brain exercise tools are now available commercially, ranging from crossword and Su Doku books to electronic brain-teaser

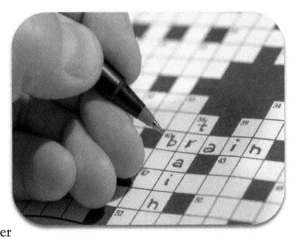

gadgets. Imagination exercises have been shown to improve brain power and can be performed anywhere. Imagine different rooms of the house and how they would look if decorated differently or, while looking out of the window, try to imagine how it would look during different seasons or when covered with snow. You can do this while taking a walk or running on a treadmill – you will be exercising your mind and body at the same time.

Intermittent fasting: One laboratory study, involving mice that had been genetically engineered to develop changes in brain tissue similar to those seen in people with Alzheimer's disease, saw those which were given the 5:2 diet experience a slower rate of cognitive decline than those on a normal diet. While certainly intriguing, we can never be sure that the results are applicable to humans. For individuals who are also overweight this many be worth a try to see if memory improves

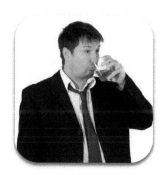

Alcohol, even in moderation, best avoided if you have chemo-brain. We are all aware of the 'thick head' that occurs with even the mildest of hangovers. When meeting up with friends, if they really want to help, suggest the gym or going for a walk rather than the pub. The advice, in the previous sections on mood and sleep are also very relevant advice to improve vitality, mental alertness in order to cope with the intellectual challenges of everyday life

---

Summary - Advice to improve your brain power

- Take regular exercise, stop smoking and reduce alcohol intake
- Eat a healthy, balanced diet with plenty of polyphenols and fibre
- Look after your gut health and reduce inflammation
- Take a fish oil regularly unless there is a contraindication
- Review your medication with your doctors
- Use your brain - engage in conversation, socialise, visit friends
- Stimulate your brain - learn something new, read, listen to audio books
- Exercise your brain - puzzles, singing, brain teasers, imagination
- Use brain exercise gadgets - electronic challenges, chess
- Identify negative thoughts which may be sapping your concentration
- Try to establish a regular sleep pattern
- If you have memory loss from medication, discuss with your doctor

Chapter 3

Weight gain after cancer

With Dr Rob Lawson

A recent study reported that >60% of patients with early cancer who had undergone cancer treatments gained a significant amount of weight, making it one of the commonest side effects. Being curvy is regarded as attractive by many individuals and a sign of prosperity in many cultures. However, the reality is, obesity aggravates many day-to-day problems and is linked to an increased risk of many medical conditions:

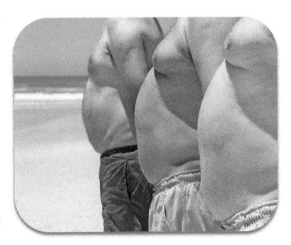

Day to day problems:
- Breathlessness on exertion
- Hot flushes
- Sweating
- Snoring / sleep apnoea
- Low physical activity
- Fatigue
- Low self-esteem
- Feeling isolated
- Higher daily costs of food
- Higher medical costs
- Depression

Medical conditions:
- Type 2 diabetes
- High blood pressure
- Heart disease and strokes
- Thromboembolic disease
- Surgical complications
- Indigestion
- Osteoarthritis
- Urinary & kidney problems
- Impotence
- Skin infections, candida
- Lymphoedema

Why weight is gained after cancer treatments

If not associated with cancer, obesity doesn't happen overnight but develops gradually over time as a result of environmental, genetic, lifestyle and dietary choices. The bottom-line is an consumption of calories in excess of the body's needs for metabolism and level of physical activity. An average physically active man needs about 2,500 calories a day to maintain a healthy weight, and an average physically active woman needs about 2,000 calories a day. This amount can be easy to reach, especially with common types of calorie-rich food. For example, eating a large takeaway hamburger, fries and a milkshake can total 1,500 calories – and that's just one meal. After cancer, there may be a tendency to snack between meals or comfort eat. Some people are also told not to worry about weight gain by well-meaning doctors and nurses, but this is not good advice as people who had previously controlled their weight would very rapidly pack on extra pounds, which would then be very difficult to lose. These factors are still an issue after cancer but are compounded by problems which create barriers to exercise.

Disability either from the disease itself or the treatments. Some disabilities can be overcome with retraining, support and education, such as exercising with a stoma or while suffering peripheral neuropathy which can occur after some chemotherapy. Fatigue, particularly when associated with a low mood, can have a considerable demotivating influence on the decision to exercise. Arthritis affects over 55% of men and women on hormone therapies. A study from Bedford presented at the Adelaide cancer conference reported that arthritis was one of the main barriers to exercise after prostate or breast cancer.

Steroids are usually given with chemo drugs. They encourage a strong appetite and tend to cause increased fat deposition. Underactivity of the thyroid can be caused by radiotherapy to the neck. Some chemotherapy regimens can also damage the thyroid so if fatigue is associated with weight gain, feeling cold and dry skin (classic symptoms) then you should ask for a thyroid function test from your doctor. Hormone therapies, tamoxifen, aromatase inhibitors and testosterone-reducing drugs cause weight gain. These are now recommended for 10 years after surgery.

Obesity affects cancer outcomes

The National Surgical Adjuvant Breast and Bowel Project evaluated 4,310 patients who had successfully been treated and found that obese patients with colon cancer had worse overall survival than patients of normal weight. On a cautionary note, however, patients who were very underweight (BMI <19 kg/m^2) also had a worse outcome. Another study from Los Angeles evaluated 1,069 men treated with prostate cancer after surgery or radiotherapy and found that obese men had a significantly higher rate of early disease recurrence.

An evaluation of 365 women with estrogen receptor positive (ER^{+ve}) breast cancer found that obese women, those who consumed more than 7 alcoholic beverages a week or those who smoked, had double the risk of developing a new breast cancer. A further analysis of 5,204 registered nurses within the Nurses' Health Study reported that high BMI at diagnosis correlated with overall worse survival and breast cancer relapse in non-smokers. Of more clinical relevance was that weight gain of more than $0.5kg/m^2$ at 1 year correlated with both worse outcomes. This effect was strongest in women who gained the most weight (>$2kg/m^2$).

The underlying causes of the harm linked to obesity are multifactorial and strongly influenced by other lifestyle and genetic factors. The most dangerous situation is called sarcopenic obesity, which is the combination of muscle wasting with obesity. This can affect people at any stage in the cancer journey, but particularly those in the later more advanced stages. The European consensus on the definition of sarcopenic obesity is a BMI greater than 30 kg/m^2 combined with low skeletal muscle mass, low grip strength and slow gait speed. People with sarcopenic obesity have particularly high levels of inflammation and reduced immunity. They have higher risks of cancer, poorer surgical outcomes and more complications such as infection and blood clots. They also have poor tolerance to chemotherapy, leading to dose delays and dose reduction. Ultimately, this will lead to worsening of both short and long-term cancer outcomes. Scientists are still discovering how obesity and sarcopenic obesity influences the expression of genes which promote cancer, but the most likely mechanisms can be summarised into the following:

Direct mechanisms:
- Oestrogen higher / Progesterone lower
- Insulin resistance / Insulin-like growth factor receptor (IGF-1)
- Higher leptin / lower adiponectin
- Chronic inflammation / poor immunity

Indirect mechanisms:
- Low mood
- Abnormal gut microflora
- Lower Vitamin D

Oestrogen and progesterone levels

Adiposity influences the production and availability of the body's sex hormones including oestrogen, androgens and progesterone. In post-menopausal women, oestrogen is made in the peripheral body fat, while in pre-menopausal women it is produced primarily in the ovaries. Therefore, overweight post-menopausal women have higher levels of oestrogen. This may explain a higher risk of breast and endometrial cancer for overweight post-menopausal women but not for pre-menopausal women.

Another important hormone affecting women who are overweight is progesterone. Compared to women with pre-menopausal 'normal' weight, obese women have reduced serum progesterone. There is a significant body of evidence demonstrating that progesterone plays a role in preventing or slowing cancer progression, particularly in the ovaries. Progesterone increases during pregnancy, which may be why women who have had children have a lower incidence of breast and ovarian cancer. In a study of post-menopausal women with breast cancer from Boston, no such correlation was found with progesterone. Breast cancer, in another large study from Sweden, was actually slightly higher in post-menopausal women taking progesterone containing HRT. It is likely, therefore, that the protective effect of progesterone is only in pre-menopausal women.

Insulin and Insulin-like growth factor receptor (IGF-1)

The increased risk of cancer, or its rate of progression, is not just hormone-related. We know this because overweight women have a worse prognosis after cancer, regardless of whether their cancers were sensitive to oestrogen (ER positive) or not (ER negative). One mechanism for a non-hormone-related increased risk of cancer progression is via IGF-1, which is higher in overweight people. Higher levels have also been associated with breast, ovary and prostate cancer. This protein, also higher in sedentary individuals, has been shown to promote cancer cell division, to inhibit cancer death and encourage cancer cells to spread. Fortunately, this cancer-promoting protein level drops if individuals lose weight or exercise.

Leptin and adiponectin

Leptin is a multifunctional neuro-endocrine hormone generated primarily from fat cells, so overweight, particularly post-menopausal women, have higher levels. Leptin is known to promote breast cancer directly and independently, through involvement with the oestrogen and insulin signalling pathways, which explains the links between higher levels of leptin and hormone-related cancers such as breast and uterus. Conversely, serum concentration of another hormone, called adiponectin, is lower in people who are overweight. Unlike leptin, which is pro-inflammatory, adiponectin has significant anti-inflammatory properties which may explain why levels tend to be lower in people diagnosed with breast and prostate cancer. Furthermore, adiponectin, via a pathway which involves nitric oxide, reduces platelet aggregation (platelets sticking together in the blood). Tumour cells tend to induce platelet aggregation, and this is thought to encourage metastasis by 'cloaking' tumour cells with platelets which stick onto them. This hides them from natural killer immune cells. Studies have shown that weight reduction results in lower platelet aggregation, lower leptin levels and increased adipokine levels – clearly a good thing.

Chronic inflammation and metabolic syndrome

Several factors contribute to the activation of inflammation among individuals who are overweight, especially those with established metabolic syndrome (insulin resistance, glucose intolerance, central obesity, abnormal fats, high cholesterol and hypertension). People living with this syndrome have a significantly increased risk of heart attacks, strokes and cancer, and have particularly high levels of inflammation.

Cells too full of fat are more fragile to physical trauma, and cell rupture evokes the accumulation of macrophages in fat stores. Organs such as the liver and pancreas, when heavily infiltrated with fat, suffer from reduced functioning which contributes to impaired insulin regulation. Increased metabolism to deal with greater amounts of food increases free radical production and oxidative stress, particularly when poor dietary choices lead to deficiencies in essential micronutrients and anti-inflammatory polyphenol-rich foods. Moreover, overweight individuals tend to have a 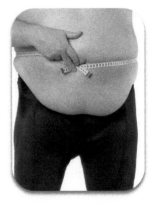 suboptimal microbiota; have an increased risk of chronic infections, such as those of the urinary tract or candida in the skin folds; and are at greater risk of psychological disturbances, all of which affect inflammatory regulation.

Poor gut microflora

There is a tendency for overweight individuals to have a suboptimal microbiota. Research is underway to establish whether it's the abnormal gut flora which causes obesity or the obesity which causes poor gut health. One reason as to why these bad (*Firmicutes*) bacteria affect our weight is because they regulate how much fat we absorb. In one experiment a prebiotic (inulin) given to mice, was capable of maintaining gut wall health and lowering obesity levels without changing the amount of fat or calories the mice consumed. Another study involving obese rats discovered that Lactobacillus and Bifidobacterium prevented the accumulation of fat in the liver. In another animal study, mice which were fed a high-fat diet and then given a probiotic had far lower insulin levels, body fat and fatty liver deposits than rats given just a placebo. Another theory is that chronic inflammation, caused by poor gut health, eads to low mood and fatigue which demotivates individuals from pursuing exercise. Another is that in response to inflammatory stress, the body will also store more energy, preparing for famine which of course never happens. A study from Cornell University showed that the weight of mice could be changed by just by shifting their intestinal bacteria. Transplanting bacteria from the gut of obese humans has even been shown to trigger obesity in mice.

Low vitamin D levels

The link between obesity and lower vitamin D deficiency has been established by the Genetic Investigation of Anthropometric Traits (GIANT) study which evaluated some 123,864 individuals. The authors hypothesised that as vitamin D is stored in fatty tissue, obese people store more vitamin D in their fat, so have less vitamin D circulating in their blood. Additionally, obese people are less likely to exercise in the sunshine, and when they do venture outside, they are more likely to cover up due to body image issues. The mechanism by which vitamin D influences cancer is thought to be due to calcitriol's effect on cellular proliferation, differentiation and apoptosis. The vitamin D receptor is highly expressed in epithelial cells known to be at risk of carcinogenesis, such as the breast, skin and prostate. Other studies have found that suboptimal vitamin D levels are associated with higher colorectal, breast and prostate cancer mortality, while higher sunlight exposure, independent of vitamin D levels, has been linked to a lower incidence of prostate and bowel cancer.

Low mood

Several studies have linked obesity with low self-esteem, lower mood status and subclinical depression. The RAINBOW study from the USA published in 2019 showed that an intervention which helped weight loss also improved mood. As well as being distressing, low mood and depression have been linked to a reduced survival following cancer treatments. Low mood contributes to an unhealthy oxidative and inflammatory status, while also reducing the incentive to change to more weight controlling behaviours such as eating less and being more active.

Tips to lose weight

It is hard enough to lose weight at the best of times, but it is even harder after cancer, both physically and emotionally. Although it is rarely talked about at the start of medical treatments, awareness of the risk of weight gain and its causes is imperative because weight gain can be avoided. Several studies of interventional strategies confirm prevention of weight gain after starting hormones is readily achievable, but few oncology units in the UK offer organised weight gain prevention programmes. Once weight has been assimilated, it's much harder to lose and weight reduction programmes have to continue for several months in order to make any difference to body stores. Faddy diets may seem initially successful, but they seldom lead to a sustained long-term change of behaviour and often leave people feeling hungry and uncomfortable. Once the weight has been lost, the energy intake then has to match the energy requirement, so people cannot relax and start overeating again. The more successful weight control programmes include:

Improving daily exercise levels?

Following cancer therapies, it may be more difficult to exercise so a more flexible and innovative approach to exercise strategies is required as most people, even those who had exercised regularly before their diagnosis, may not have the same motivation or abilities afterwards. The cancer itself, surgery or the anticancer treatments may have caused physical disability, fatigue, weight gain, reduced self-esteem and body-image concerns. When contemplating exercise, many see it as an insurmountable hurdle, but those who recognise the barriers and are able to ask for help are more likely to succeed. Support and encouragement from doctors, friends, relatives and physicians play a vital role in promoting exercise.

In terms of weight loss after cancer, it is often quoted that exercise has no impact, but that is simply not true. Several interventional studies show that exercise programmes have a significant impact. For example, the ENERGY Study, involving 690 women with breast cancer, reported that those randomised to a group aerobic exercise intervention such as dance had a 6% reduction in weight as opposed to the 1.5% reduction among those randomised to standard care. Likewise, the American Society of Sports Medicine concluded that weight reduction, resulted in a 10% reduction in weight if >150-250 min moderate exercise / week was maintained for over 6 months. If participants did <150 mins / week there was no change in weight. A combination of resistance and endurance exercises seem to be most effective, but the important thing is that it is sustained and combined with calorie reduction and fasting. Ideally, try to do some of the exercise first thing in the morning, before breakfast, even if only for 20 mins. This means the stomach is empty, so the body has to use energy from stores in the liver and fat tissues. It also extends the period of overnight fasting which also significantly helps weight loss and prevents diabetes.

Regular physical activity is particularly beneficial for obese individuals, even though it is much harder to sustain regular levels. Even before weight reduction, oestrogen and leptin levels decrease, and adiponectin levels increase. Exercise also mitigates many of the adverse risks of obesity, particular thrombo-embolism, indigestion and low mood. Moreover, the positive biochemical changes which occur when exercising, counter-balance the negative factors caused by obesity, particularly raised levels of IGF, increased insulin resistance and also blood markers of chronic inflammation.

Unfortunately, in western societies the vast majority of people are not physically active enough, so most of the calories people consume end up being stored in the body as fat. It particularly important to avoid long periods of sedentary behaviour both at work or at home as this is when the eight piles on, try to move around as much as possible. For the general population, The Department of Health recommends that adults do at least two-and-a-half hours of moderate-intensity aerobic activity, such as cycling or fast walking, every week. This doesn't need to be done all in one go, but can be broken down into smaller periods. For example, you could exercise for 30 minutes a day for five days a week. The trouble is, if trying to lose weight, you have to eat <2500 calories a day and exercise >2.5 hours / week to even start burning up energy stores. What's more, this has to be sustained for many months to have any long-term benefit.

The first step is to go shopping! It is important to buy a comfortable pair of training shoes and suitable sports clothing. Next, aim to go for a walk every morning, even if just for 10-20 minutes, preferably before breakfast. Repeat before lunch and your evening meal. This is great for your circulation and digestion, and will help with weight reduction. Although this is a relatively low level of exercise, the trick is to

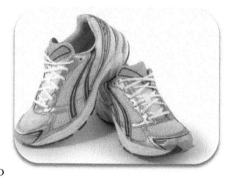

perform it regularly. If a walk or alternative exercise session is missed out, consider going for an extra walk the following day to catch up. All too often, people who say that they exercise regularly have excuses, often legitimate, for missing sessions. It may be worth keeping a wall chart or an exercise diary as an aide memoire or tracking your activity using a smartphone app or a wearable device.

Prioritise exercise: In many communities, exercise is regarded as an after-thought and not important in its own right. If work colleagues see you are going for a walk or jog in your lunch break, they may make comments that you have too much time on your hands. Even at home, family members may start complaining that you are not helping around the house because you have gone to the gym or an exercise class. You may say to yourself, I can't exercise today, there are important tasks to do such as shopping or catching up on social media. If this is the case, you will need to find ways to build exercise into your daily routine.

Within the normal activities of daily living: Throughout the day we are confronted by several choices which require different levels of exertion. Time allowing, it would be better to take the more active option. For example:

- Walking instead of using the car for short journeys
- Getting off the bus one stop earlier
- Using the stairs instead of the lift
- Walking rather than standing on the escalator
- Parking your car further away from the shop entrance
- Cycling to the shops – invest in a bike with a basket
- Stretching and taking short walks regularly

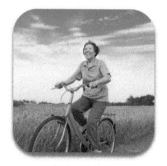

Around the house: The advantage of exercising at home is that it is time efficient and convenient. It doesn't, however, have the social interaction of group activities unless a friend is invited round for a joint exercise session. Cycling in a park or exercising with someone else can be more fun and usually ensures a higher level of activity. Most people are keen to offer help after a diagnosis of cancer – and what better way to do so? If you have decided to start exercising at home, it is worth having a semi-formal programme to follow. There are many useful gadgets available to make it more feasible (bikes, treadmills, rowing machines, dumbbells). Alternatively, you could follow an exercise video or an application on a tablet or phone – there are literally thousands to choose from. Always remember to perform some gentle stretches before and after exercise, and try to get make yourself breathe harder and get warmer during exercise. If you can afford an exercise professional to come to your home, this could be a good investment as they can help plan your programme and motivate you.

At the office or workplace: After a cancer diagnosis, it is important not to remain sedentary for long periods of time. This can happen in the workplace, particularly during long meetings or sitting at a desk. Commuting to work by car or train, especially in a confined space, can also be disadvantageous. Walking as much as possible is encouraged. Use the stairs instead of the lift and walk on escalators. It may be better to commute wearing training shoes and change to more professional attire on arrival. Getting up from your desk every 30 minutes or so and walking for two to 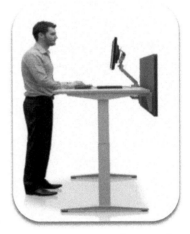 five minutes is a good habit. You could walk to speak to a colleague face-to-face instead of emailing, get yourself a drink more often or even just use toilets that are further away from your desk. Walking or some other exercise at lunchtime is a great thing to do. If walking is not feasible, desk exercises could keep you alert, especially when getting tired or sleepy. Ignore any negative comments – people will secretly admire your enthusiasm. If you think your boss has the budget, ask for a desk which adjusts into a standing position.

Within your social life: There are alternatives to the pub or watching TV. It's a question of changing your frame of mind and adopting a fresh approach to socialising. The majority of recreational and sports activities have a strong social aspect to them. Exercise can and should be sociable and enjoyable – try to find something that is fun and which can be 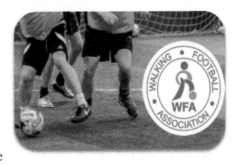 integrated into your social life. Dance, aqua aerobics and fitness classes are very cordial places and, particularly if you go regularly, are somewhere to form new acquaintances and even friendships. Golf and bowls are great ways to meet people and concentrate during exercise. Walking football is emerging as a particularly attractive social sport for both men and women, and Football Association affiliated clubs are popping up all over the UK. Watching sport while running on a treadmill or cycling on a fixed bike is a fantastic alternative to sitting on a couch. Consider asking a friend to watch the game at the gym instead of in the pub.

Find something for you: Numerous walking groups exist around the country, meeting once or twice a week. Walking for health has an excellent website (walk4life.info) indicating times and locations of walks for different levels of ability within any post code area. Many swimming pools offer lessons on how to swim and water aerobics. Swimming is particularly good for building up stamina while 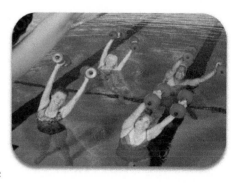 protecting most of the weight-bearing joints. There are numerous dance classes available in most towns, either in gyms or dance studios. The most common choices include conventional ballroom, line dancing, Indian, Latin American, ceroc and salsa. Some traditional studios offer ballet and the trendier ones, jazz, funk and even street dance. Yoga and Pilates are particularly recommended for balance and core strength, both of which are often impaired by cancer treatments. They are also recommended for joint and muscle suppleness and posture. Don't worry if even touching your toes is impossible – yoga and Pilates are not about the lotus position anymore. Individuals with any level of flexibility can benefit if the stretches are conducted regularly.

Eat less high calorific foods

It sounds obvious, but overweight people have eaten more than their body's energy requirements. Caloric requirements change on a daily basis, so on sedentary days, it's vital to eat much less. Fast food outlets generally offer foods high in unhealthy fat and sugar, yet people often regard these as a snack between meals. Sometimes, it's not clear 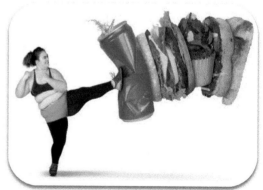 which foods are high in calories, but the usual culprits include cakes, biscuits, muffins, pasties, pies, fatty chips, crisps, pakoras, samosas and bhajis. Alcohol contains a lot of calories and also stimulates the appetite. The urge to go for a curry on the way back from the pub or raid the fridge after getting home is often strong. Dining out may be a danger zone as you are often offered three courses and food can be higher in unhealthy fat and sugar.

Less processed sugar

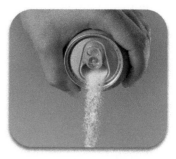

Quenching your thirst with sugary drinks and processed fruit juices is not a good idea. They have a lot of calories, are not satiating (don't fill you up), and their high glycaemic index (GI) means there will be peaks and troughs in blood sugar levels, triggering hunger an hour later. This usually results in an urge to snack which ultimately increases caloric intake further. Many low-calorie ready meals have the fat removed but still contain sugar, adding to GI issues. Particularly avoid sweets and cakes particularly on an empty stomach.

More whole foods

Breaking down foods reduces the need for chewing and allows foods to be absorbed quicker. Chewing sends signals to the brain that a substantial meal is being eaten. Whole foods have more bulk and fibre, making them slower to eat and more satiating without increasing the calorie content. A good example is whole, wild rice which has the same number of calories as plain white rice, but is more filling as it also includes the germ and husk. Both of these add to the bulk, the taste and overall nutritional value. Likewise, whole grain bread is less likely to contribute to weight gain than highly processed white bread, while it also contains vitamins and fibre.

Enhance the gut flora

For the reasons mentioned above it's a good idea to improve gut health by, increasing dietary intake of fermented foods such as live unsweetened yoghurt, miso, kimchi, kefir or sauerkraut, as well as including a good probiotic supplement would be a very sensible option.

Stop snacking

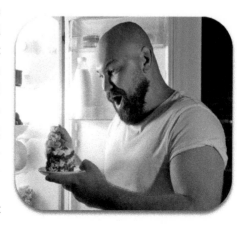

Hunger has become an unacceptable sensation in Western societies, but it should be embraced because this is when weight starts falling. The fall in blood sugar triggers the breakdown of glycogen in the liver and conversion of triglyceride fats to fatty acids and glycerol for energy. Instead of grazing throughout the day, it's best to have a meal and allow it to digest completely before the next one. This also allows the digestive mechanisms and stomach acids to rest before the next meal. If you do feel distressing hungry pangs then drinking a glass of water or going for a brief walk may help take your mind off food.

More chilli and spicy foods

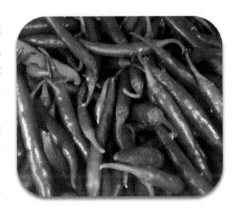

Laboratory research conducted by the University of Wyoming showed that mice fed a high-fat diet, but also given chilli extract (capsaicin) which increased their metabolic activity, burned more energy and gained less weight. A study from Adelaide found that receptors in the stomach interacted with capsaicin, signalling a feeling of fullness which may help weight loss. Formal studies in humans have yet to be performed.

Fasting

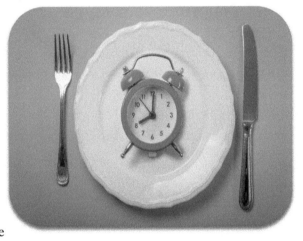

One interesting laboratory experiment gave one group of mice as much food as they wanted all the time, and the other group had their food withdrawn for a few days every fortnight. The group that endured a modest degree of regular fasting maintained a normal weight and lived almost twice as long as the others. It is not clear how this relates to humans, but maybe the fasting practices in some religions are based on a fundamental wish to improve the health of their followers, rather than a penance to demonstrate their faith.

The most sustainable way of fasting is to extend the gaps between meals and avoid snacking. The best evidence of sensible effective fasting comes from a study which evaluated a large cohort of overweight women who completed their initial treatments. They discovered that initially overweight women who adopted early dinners or late breakfasts, leaving 13 hours between the meals (without intermediate snacking), lost significantly more weight, had lower levels of glycated Hb (a marker of glucose control over time) and lower inflammatory markers. What's more, after 5 years there was a 36% lower risk of breast cancer recurrence. The chapter on diets explains energy modifying diets in more detail.

Intermittent fasting diets

Intermittent fasting is gaining popularity as a way to improve health, lose weight, and even reverse T2D. There is strong evidence that fasting reduces blood glucose, IGF levels and markers of chronic inflammation. One lab experiment in which a healthy colony of mice was split into two groups and kept in a safe, comfortable, stimulating and warm environment, underlines the apparent benefits of fasting. While one group had as much food as they wanted at all times, the other group had their food withdrawn for a few days every fortnight. The group that endured a modest degree of regular fasting maintained a normal weight and lived almost twice as long as the others.

Several diets advocate intermittent fasting in humans, but despite their popularity in the media, they are not particularly practical or sustainable for the large majority of people. The 5:2 is the most widely broadcast. This entails five days of normal eating, with calorie control almost a complete afterthought, alongside two days where calorie intake is reduced to 500 calories for women and 600 calories for men. Since participants are only fasting for two days of their choice each week, while eating normally on the other five days, there is always something to look forward to on the near horizon. Anecdotal reports of negative effects during fasting days include:

- Difficulties sleeping
- Bad breath
- Irritability and anxiety
- Dehydration

While evidence directly assessing the 5:2 model of intermittent fasting is limited, largely because very few formal human trials have been performed, some information regarding its impact on a number of conditions has been published.

One study, carried out in 2010, found that women placed on a 5:2 diet achieved similar levels of weight loss as women placed on a calorie-controlled diet. They also experienced reductions in a number of biological indicators (biomarkers) that suggest a reduction in the risk of developing chronic diseases such as type 2 diabetes.

The 5:2 is somewhat similar to the 16:8 diet, another form of intermittent fasting which received media attention after the publication of its apparent benefits following a small RCT. Individuals fasted for 16 hours a day and then ate whatever they wanted in the 8 hours between 10am and 6pm. On average, this diet resulted in 341 fewer calories a day. After 12 weeks, people on the diet had an overall average reduction in body weight of about 3% compared to a control group. This meant their average BMI decreased from 35 to 34, while their blood pressure was also lowered by 7mmHg (±2mmHg). Despite the excitement following the encouraging nature of the diet's results, it should be remembered that most supervised weight reduction programmes, including exercise, would have achieved better results over a similar time-frame.

Summary – Tips for losing weight

- Avoid 'faddy' diets and instead, aim for a long-term plan
- Extend time between the evening meal and breakfast to 13 hours
- Don't worry about feeling hungry and drink plenty of water
- Avoid sugary drinks
- Distract yourself from thinking about food – get up and take a walk
- Avoid processed food (unhealthy fat, sugar, high GI foods)
- Eat less food cooked in fat e.g. deep-fried batter, chips, crisps
- Avoid pastries and pies
- Avoid biscuits and cakes.
- Avoid muffins which have more fat than a bacon sandwich!
- Trim the excess fat off meat
- Stew, boil or broil rather than grill, roast or fry
- Eat less meat and more oily fish
- Eat a large 'rainbow-of-colours' i.e. fresh salad with every meal
- Reduce alcohol intake (alcohol is liquid sugar)
- Try not to snack between meals, especially sweet snacks
- Avoid snacking between meals
- Increase exercise levels (see exercise)
- If convenient try a 20min walk before breakfast
- Consider having no more than 2 meals a day with no snacking
- Eat real, minimally processed food if possible
- Try to make your meals yourself– you know what's in them

Chapter 4

Abdominal symptoms

Poor appetite, nausea and vomiting

Comments such as "Gone off your food?" or "Don't feel like eating?" tend to trivialise the seriousness of poor appetite, a symptom which can have serious consequences including weight loss, fatigue, malnutrition and even cachexia. For the majority of patients, poor appetite is linked to chemotherapy-induced nausea and vomiting (CINV), a dreaded side effects which can severely disrupt a patient's quality of life and undermine patient compliance, both of which diminish the overall chances of therapy being successful and place a significant burden on the patient, carers and supervising healthcare team.

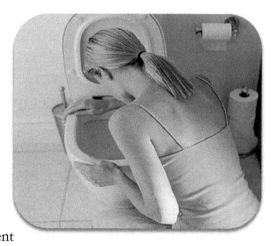

Although chemotherapy is usually the cause, many other factors should be considered, investigated and treated:

- Gastric outflow obstruction from a tumour mass or surgery
- Metastasis to the liver or brain or deranged function
- Fluid and electrolyte imbalances e.g. high calcium
- Severe constipation, depression or anxiety
- Opioid painkillers - tramadol, morphine, oxycodone, codeine
- Some antibiotics - ciprofloxacin, metronidazole and tetracycline
- Excess alcohol, excess sweet food or overeating
- Food intolerances, food poisoning
- Travel sickness, particularly after a long car journey
- Chemicals released from the disease itself

Types of CINV: It is usually organised into the following categories:

- Acute (within 24 hours), delayed (24 hours to five days)
- Anticipatory (before, during or after treatment)
- Breakthrough (despite optimal preventative treatment)
- Refractory (recurring when previous treatments have failed)

Management of nausea and vomiting

Drug therapies target the underlying pathways which cause CINV, either in the brain via the neurotransmitter 5-HT3 (ondansetron), or in the gut via substance P receptors (aprepitant). Steroids are often used to enhance the effect of these drugs. Other antiemetics include metoclopramide, domperidone, and cyclizine. Sedatives such as lorazepam are useful in reducing anticipatory nausea. Synthetic cannabis is licenced for CINV but often causes sedation, dizziness and altered mood. Chemotherapy agents with a high risk of nausea include anthracyclines, alkylating agents and platinum compounds. The medical team look for other causes of nausea such as for salt and calcium disturbances, dehydration liver, brain or gut issues. It is a good idea to increase the antiemetics for individuals who are likely to be sensitive to CINV. This includes women who have a history of nausea during pregnancy; a history of motion sickness; being teetotal (don't drink alcohol) or have a history of anxiety

What can you do to help?

Acupuncture: The role of acupuncture, electroacupuncture and acupressure has been extensively investigated as a potential aide to conventional drugs when treating CINV. These practices, based on traditional Chinese medicine, usually involve the stimulation of the Neiguan (P-6) pressure point near the wrist. A summary of the most robust RCTs has concluded that acupuncture and electroacupuncture do offer a small but significant benefit. Acupressure, while slightly less effective, is particularly convenient for patients because it can be learnt and self-administered.

Exercise: A major RCT from the Netherland (The PACES study) showed that women in a moderate to intense exercise programme had significantly reduced CINV. Yoga programmes and progressive muscle relaxation classes have demonstrated improvements, especially if there is associated anxiety.

Nutritional interventions: Avoid overeating pre and during chemotherapy. One study highlighted how fasting, before and during chemotherapy administration, led to some reduction in nausea and vomiting. Although it's important to drink water regularly to prevent dehydration, avoid strong coffee and fizzy sugary drinks.

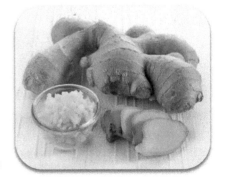

Ginger (Zingiber officinale) has a long history in many cultures as a remedy for nausea, and there is increasing scientific evidence to support its use. Ginger has multiple active constituents

including gingerols, shogaols, zingiberene, zingerone and paradol. Lab studies suggest that they stimulate oral and gastric secretions, regulate gastrointestinal motility and interact with 5-HT$_3$ receptors (similar to ondansetron). In humans, ginger has been found to be useful for treating NV associated with motion sickness, surgery and pregnancy. In terms of CINV, a major review of the 8 early RCTs found variable mild benefits and one study found that higher doses (2 g) of ginger made CINV slightly worse in participants also prescribed the strong anti-sickness drug aprepitant. The largest and most statistically vigorous RCT was a multi-site, randomised, placebo-controlled, double-blind trial involving 576 patients who had experienced nausea following a prior chemotherapy cycle. They received at least three further chemotherapy cycles, during which different doses of ginger were investigated. The ginger was prepared as a purified liquid extract dispensed as a 250mg ginger root capsule. They reported decreases in CINV, with an optimal amount being between 0.5 - 1g.

Other supplements: Glutamine has been investigated in one small RCT but its effect was minimal so it cannot be recommended. Some patients are reporting that CBD oils can help reduce nausea and the anxiety associated with it.

Summary - Lifestyle advice if feeling sick or nauseous

- When feeling sick, it is not a good idea to 'insist' on eating
- It is important to keep fluid intake up to avoid dehydration
- Cool water may be better tolerated, voiding strong coffee or sweet drinks
- Drink warm water mixed with grated whole ginger root
- Consider a quality ginger supplement if more convenient
- Food should be eaten slowly, followed by relaxation. Avoid lying flat
- Drinks should be taken 30 minutes after a meal, rather than with it
- A short walk and some fresh air before eating helps reduce nausea
- Tight-fitting clothes are best avoided
- Fatty foods can make nausea worse
- Cold foods are better if the smell of cooking causes nausea
- Avoid the kitchen if it triggers nausea
- If cooking is a chore, cold meals can be as nutritious as hot ones
- Experiment with different foods which you don't usually eat
- A small glass of wine or beer may boost your appetite before a meal
- Accept support from friends with cooking or shopping

Exercises after abdominal surgery

Although many operations are now via a laparoscope, open surgery to the abdomen requires cutting through muscles and fibrous bands in the abdominal wall. This leads to an inherent weakness that not only creates a lax and less toned stomach but also increases the risk of hernia, either through the scar or elsewhere. Advice in the days after the operation is best sought from your surgical team.

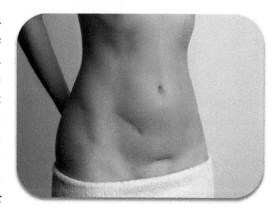

After the acute period of recovery, abdominal exercises are helpful. The aim of exercise after abdominal surgery is to tone up the muscles and prevent a hernia. It would, therefore, be counter-productive to increase the pressure inside the abdomen during exercise, as this is would encourage herniation of tissues through the scar. The two most important rules when performing abdominal exercises are to breathe correctly and keep the mouth and lungs open when straining. That means no red-faced squeezing or holding breath.

Performing abdominal strengthening exercises, in addition to getting generally fitter, will aid recovery, improve local symptoms and help prevent long-term complications. For optimal recovery, it is important to perform these exercises regularly, 2-3 times a day for more than 5 minutes. If you miss a day, try to make up for it the next day. The exercises include:

Pelvic tilting: Lie on your back, on a soft but level surface (exercise mat, towel or a carpet). Relax with the knees bent. Take a breath in and then push the lower back against the floor, tightening the stomach 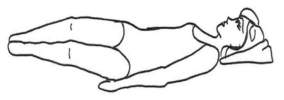 muscles while breathing out slowly. Repeat 5-10 times. To help prevent backache, tighten your stomach muscles and pull them in, pressing your back down into the bed. Repeat 2 or 3 times a day.

Knee Rolling: Hands by your sides, draw in your stomach muscles and roll your knees over to one side. Slowly bring them up again and roll them the other way.

Bottom lift: Draw in stomach muscles. Lift your bottom up off the bed, lower slowly and relax. After 10-14 days, provided recovery is going well, try some gentle sit-ups. Lift your head and shoulders off the ground, hold for 2-3 seconds, and then repeat 10-20 times, three times per day. 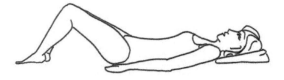 Keep your elbows back, with your hand behind your head, looking forward. Keep your lower back flat against the ground. It is most important to keep your mouth open and breathe out slightly every time the head is lifted. This will prevent the pressure inside your abdomen increasing, while at the same time strengthening your abdominal muscles. Repeat the sit-ups with your legs twisted to the right, and then to the left.

Abdominal surgery may also affect the pelvic structures and the muscles which support the bladder and rectum. It would also be wise to start pelvic floor exercises regularly in order to prevent incontinence.

Heartburn

Indigestion and heartburn are common complaints during chemotherapy or after surgery. The cause of pain is usually gastric acid irritating the lining of the stomach or oesophagus. If there is too much acid, or if the sphincter doesn't work properly, it refluxes up into the oesophagus, causing heartburn. It is aggravated by steroids and anti-inflammatory drugs.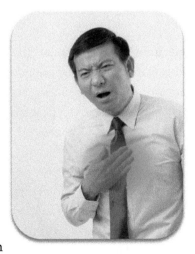

In terms of diet, people often say – "I can't eat fruit because I get heartburn". Although it's true that fruit can cause a little irritation in vulnerable individuals, it is not the root cause of the problem and, in the long term, fruit will improve the health of the stomach and oesophagus (gullet). The underlying cause is usually an unhealthy balance of fat, meats and sugar which the stomach has to work harder to digest – i.e. produce more of its own hydrochloric acid. To make matters worse, sufferers often turn to antacids for immediate relief. The stomach then senses a more alkaline environment and responds by producing yet more acid, perpetuating the problem. On the other hand, consumption of mildly acidic fruit sends signals to the stomach lining to produce less of its own acid. After a while, with perseverance, eating fruit and other less gastric-irritating foods will reduce acid levels and improve the health of the gastric lining, thus preventing indigestion.

You may be prescribed antacid medication after an endoscopy in order to rule out an ulcer. Indigestion and heartburn can also be helped by avoiding some foods individual to you so keeping a food journal could identify foods that trigger heartburn or indigestion. In general avoid large meals late at night, drinking large amounts of liquids with the meal and eat slowly, chew your food properly and try not to overeat A good trick is to raise the head of the bed slightly, so the chest is higher than the feet – putting two bricks under head of the bed will help.

Diarrhoea

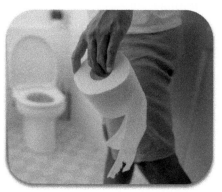

Diarrhoea can be a troubling side effect of radiotherapy, chemotherapy biological agents, a complication of graft versus host disease, or a consequence of hospital-acquired pathogenic infections. Chemo-induced diarrhoea (CID) can occur in up to 50% of patients receiving agents such as irinotecan, Taxotere, 5FU or capecitabine. The impact of these agents is often worse when they are given in combination with other chemotherapy drugs or biological agents such as cetuximab, pertuzumab or lapatinib. CID can cause dehydration and loss of electrolytes, problems which can lead to treatment delays. Some people have a genetically reduced ability to metabolise capecitabine (which can be measured), causing life-threatening CID which requires hospitalisation.

Medical treatment usually involves reducing the dose reduction or delaying the next cycle of chemotherapy, in tandem with fluid and electrolyte correction and administration of loperamide, codeine and octreotide. Prophylactic neomycin gained some popularity but is now rarely used due to concerns over antibiotic resistance.

What can you do to help?

Nutrition: Dietary advice consists of good food hygiene and avoidance of foods that can loosen the stool. Patients with pre-existing, diarrhoea may have underlying food intolerances such as gluten and lactose which may be improved with dietary interventions. Nutmeg has natural anti-diarrhoea properties.

Probiotic bacteria supplementation has been shown to prevent CID in laboratory animal experiments. In the clinical setting, a probiotic powder reduced grade 3–4 CID, flatulence and borborygmi by 41% in an RCT involving patients with colorectal cancer receiving 5FU chemo. Another study showed probiotics to have a protective effect on patients taking irinotecan. Both studies showed no increased risk of infection following regular intake of probiotics, even when patients had a low white cell count (low immunity). The chapter on microbiota has already highlighted how probiotics can have numerous benefits, including reducing the risk of urogenital, intestinal and respiratory tract infections, as well as limiting the severity of radiation-induced diarrhoea by preserving the integrity of the gut mucosa.

Other supplements: One lab study involving rodents suggests that glutamine stimulates intestinal mucosa growth, reducing gut toxicity. A small study involving humans showed a small benefit, but another trial involving patients receiving high-dose chemotherapy was linked with more relapses and deaths so cannot be recommended. Activated charcoal reduced irinotecan-induced diarrhoea in one small study involving children, by 25% reduction and discontinuation rate of irinotecan was much lower. Another study showed no benefit so it should be further investigated in robust studies before it can be recommended.

Summary - Dietary advice for diarrhoea

- Eat small, frequent meals rather than binging on larger meals
- Drink plenty of caffeine-free fluids throughout the day
- Note which foods make you worse and consider avoiding:
  — Alcohol, strong tea, coffee, cola, fruit juice and malted drinks
  — Spicy or highly seasoned foods e.g. chilli, curry and pickles
  — Very 'fatty' foods e.g. fried foods
  — Unripe fruit, pips, seeds, skins, nuts, raw vegetables and salads
  — High fibre breakfast cereals and large amounts of dried fruit
  — Foods labelled as 'Low sugar' or 'diet'
- Foods to consider trying if you have diarrhoea:
  — Sipping high energy drinks between meals
  — Probiotic 'live' yoghurts or a good quality supplement
  — Grilled, steamed or boiled potatoes, white bread, pasta and rice

Constipation

By disrupting dietary routines and preventing people from being more active, cancer therapies often leave many patients with constipation. Similarly, anti-sickness medication such as ondansetron, and opiate pain-killers such as codeine, tramadol morphine and iron, can often disrupt the normal function of the bowel. Other non-medical contributory factors include not eating enough fibre, inactivity, bowel muscle weakness, recent abdominal surgery, haemorrhoids or an anal fissure.

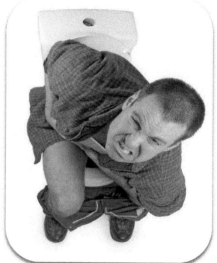

We are all familiar with the common symptoms of constipation - discomfort, bloating and abdominal cramps - but people can be affected in other ways:

- Fatigue, apprehension, irritability and being argumentative
- Reduced mood even contributing to depression
- Cancelling or leaving social engagements early
- Diminished sexuality - either sufferers feel unattractive or are in pain
- Embarrassment due to the associated flatulence

What can be done to help?

Despite the frequency of this complaint it is often only addressed when it becomes a significant problem. Lifestyle prevention strategies are always better than waiting until constipation has set in and having to resort to suppositories and laxatives. With some foresight, constipation can be anticipated. If drugs such as opiates have been prescribed, it is better to change your diet before the stools harden. Likewise, if a previous cycle of chemotherapy caused constipation, eating some ground linseeds, dried prunes or figs the evening before and the morning of chemotherapy will certainly help.

Exercise:
Non-sedentary activity is very important. A brief walk or cycle ride in the evening after chemotherapy treatment is a good tactic. This may seem hard work but will help keep your bowels moving and also help reduce nausea and fatigue. At other times regular exercise, particularly jogging, walking, cycling and dancing all have a positive effect on the bowels.

Fibre and whole foods:

While unlike other components of food such as carbohydrates, proteins and fats, humans cannot digest fibre, it still has incredible health benefits. Dietary fibre increases the weight and size of your stool and softens it. A bulky stool is easier to pass, decreasing your chance of constipation lowering the risk of developing haemorrhoids and diverticular

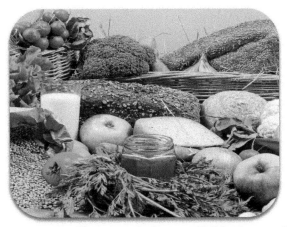

disease. Even if you have loose, watery stools, fibre may help to solidify the stool because it absorbs water and adds bulk. A summary of over 25 studies reported that people who regularly eat more than 10g a day within with whole foods had a 10% lower risk of bowel, breast and other cancers cancer compared to people with low fibre diets. One mechanism for this Is that soluble fibre is fermented in the colon and acts as a prebiotic, promoting healthy bacteria which helps to reduce inflammation and improving immunity. High-fibre foods also tend to be more filling, so individuals are likely to eat less and stay satisfied longer. High-fibre foods tend to take longer to eat and are less "energy dense," meaning they have fewer calories for the same volume of food.

It's a good idea to stock up with wholegrain staples such as oats, bran, and cereals. The only caveat to this is that a higher intake of wheat and gluten can cause bloating, especially in wheat intolerant individuals. Quinoa, chia seed and linseed porridge is available from

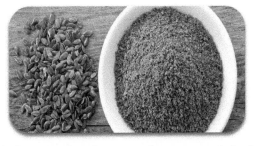

health food stores and easy to make – mix in some berries, nuts, bananas and fresh fruit and that will set you up for the day.

In general, the more refined or processed the food, the less fibre it contains. White rice, for example, has had its fibre-rich outer coating removed. Brown rice is marginally better as it usually still contains the germ which is rich in vitamins, protein and minerals. Wild rice is the best, as it contains both the bran and the germ. The king of all rice, albeit a bit pricey, is sprouting organic wild rice. It has everything, including higher amounts of polyphenols brought on by the sprouting process. Linseed (flaxseed) is an excellent source of both soluble and insoluble fibre, as well as healthy polyphenols and omega fats, and helps to lubricate and soften the stool without bulking. It is particularly helpful for those with gluten intolerance.

Summary - Measures that can be taken to avoid constipation

- Whole fruits: apples, pears, pineapples, plums, bananas and prunes
- Dried fruits: prunes, raisins, dates, apricots, goji berries and figs
- Juices and smoothies: a good source of soluble fibre
- Whole berries: cherries and grapes
- Legumes: beans, lentils, linseeds, chickpeas and peas
- Cereals: whole grains, bran and wholemeal oat or quinoa porridge
- Seeds: dried pumpkin, sunflower and linseed
- Nuts: any nut has fibre, particularly hazelnuts and almonds
- Salads: lettuce, watercress, radish and peppers
- Leafy green vegetables: cabbage, sprouts, spinach and hemp
- Vegetables: squashes, carrots, broccoli, cauliflower (better raw)
- Have a tea spoon of crushed flaxseeds everyday
- Ready crushed flaxseed are readily available in many shops or
- Linseed: soak overnight, or better still, crush in a food blender
- Drink plenty of water
- Have a regular routine in the morning e.g. after breakfast
- Try not to ignore the call to go. If you need to go - go!
- Take your time and try to stay until you have a good result
- Exercise regularly - it reduces gut transit time, softening the stool
- Activity softens the stool and makes it easier to pass
- Avoid constipating medications if possible e.g. codeine
- Take a note of which activities constipate you
- Take a note of which foods work for you and keep these in stock
- Prevention is better - anticipate constipation and change diet first
- If starting constipating medications, increase fibre intake
- If necessary, use ointments or suppositories to relieve a painful anus
- Change your diet before chemotherapy to avoid constipation

Mouth care

Chemotherapy and radiotherapy can affect the rapidly dividing normal cells of the lining of the mouth. The most common and understated result is an alteration in taste - many describe a sudden metallic taste which interferes with the enjoyment of food and drink. As well as being disconcerting, this symptom can contribute to poor appetite and weight loss. In more severe cases, inflammation and ulceration (mucositis) can cause pain

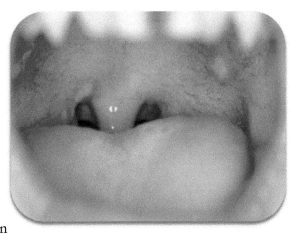

and discomfort. In this instance, or if your white cell count is low after treatment, you will be susceptible to oral infections such as thrush (candida). Oral mucositis can often be painful, and this, in turn, can make it difficult to eat and drink. Chemotherapy can increase the risk of dental caries and gum disease, so it's a good idea to get the teeth checked and cleaned before the start of treatment.

Radiotherapy around the area of your mouth can cause very troublesome mucositis. If the field includes the major salivary glands, there is a risk of a permanent an distressing dry mouth Opiate pain killers, Anti-cholinergic drugs including amitriptyline and some of the newer targeted biological agents including Kadkyla.

Dry mouth or xerostomia can leads to a higher risk of tooth decay and ulcers. To treat xerostomia different approach should be followed at the same time: to increase existing saliva flow or replace lost secretions, to control the state of oral health, to control dental caries and to treat secondary infections. When residual secretory capacity is present, it is advisable to regularly stimulate the salivary glands by mechanical or gustatory stimuli as

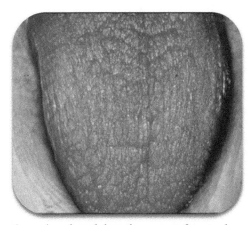

supportive oral care. The salivary flow can be stimulated by the use of sugarless chewing gum or xylitol/sorbitol candy or through parasympathomimetic drug such as pilocarpine. Pilocarpine is a natural alkaloid that activates cholinergic receptors, authorized to treat xerostomia. It can cause vomiting, sweating, headache, increased urinary frequency, wheezing, watery eyes, nausea and gastrointestinal intolerance, hypotension, rhinitis, diarrhoea, and visual disturbances.

Acupuncture, in a few trials has been shown to alleviate radio-induced xerostomia but it mechanism of action is not totally clear and systematic reviews indicate its efficacy as doubtful. Aqualief® is a food supplement based on carnosine and hibiscus. These two ingredients are mixed in specific proportions to form a pH buffering system which maintains the pH of the oral cavity at the proper value which is required for the regular secretion of saliva. In a RCT on 70 subjects with grade 1-2 xerostomia enrolled at the Dental Clinic of the University of Insubria, it demonstrated significant benefits over placebo.

Mouth Ulcers As well as dryness, many of the new biological drugs can cause troublesome mouth ulcers. If marked, a reduction in the dose should be considered. Bone hardening drugs, frequently given to people with bone metastasises. Although they do not cause mouth ulcers, they can cause necrosis of the jaw. If users get a progressive deep painful ulcer in the mouth over a jaw area, this should be reported to the medical team. Coating agents such as Gelclair coat the lining of the mouth with a protective film that can prevent further irritations, contributing to pain relief. Several studies have shown that, if used regularly, they can help soothe mouth lesions caused by disease, radiotherapy, chemotherapy and oral surgery. In many oncology centres, Gelclair is now prescribed routinely with medications which are more likely to cause ulcers.

Dental caries and gum disease: Chemotherapy can increase the risk of gum disease and dental caries by upsetting the mouth flora and altering immunity. It's really important to reduce sugar intake as it is also a major cause of tooth decay, especially boiled sweets, toffies and sugary drinks. Dental caries, as well as being painful and a source of chronic inflammation also increases the risk of jaw damage (avascular necrosis) associated with bone hardening drugs which are now commonly given after breast and prostate cancer. In addition, what is less well known is that dental caries may also be an increased factor for bowel cancer. Two studies, between them looked at more than 100 samples of healthy and cancerous bowel tissue – one from Canada and another from Boston USA and published in the journal Genome. They both found that DNA codes from bacteria, commonly found in dental caries (Fusobacterium) was present in the bowel cancer genes but not normal genes – this raises a strong suspicion that the bacterial DNA traveling through the body interacts with and gets absorbed into gut cells causing them to become cancerous. Dental caries is also prominent source of chronic inflammation.

Mouth microflora:

Hundreds of oral bacteria live in harmony within the mouth, especially between the teeth and gums. When the balance of healthy to unhealthy bacteria is upset, a number of conditions can ensue including inflammation of the gums, periodontal disease, dental caries, overgrowth of candida (Thrush), abscesses and mouth ulcers. Additionally, research has found that infection in the mouth, caused by poor oral health and gut flora, leads to increased chronic inflammation in the rest of the body, increasing the risk of reduced cardiac health and cognitive functioning, as well as elevating bowel cancer risk. Research conducted at the University of Glasgow Dental School evaluated the oral health of 2,000 people with throat and mouth cancers, finding that, even when taking smoking, drinking and poor economic status into account, there was still a connection between poor oral health and higher incidences of oral cancer.

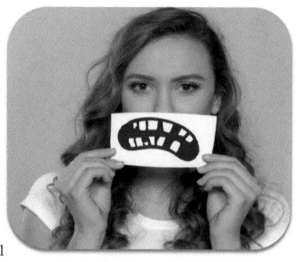

As well as bad breath, poor oral hygiene triggers excess sensitivity to temperature and a low PH. The normal pH of saliva is typically between 6.7 and 7.4, but as bacteria break down the carbohydrates, they release lactic acid, butyric acid, and aspartic acid, bringing down the pH of saliva. When the pH level in the mouth goes below 5.5 (a critical pH value), the acids begin to break down the enamel on teeth. The longer the teeth are exposed to a low salivary pH, the more likely the development of dental caries. Some people measure their salivary PH using strips bought from a chemist or online. When using them, it's important not to eat or drink for a minimum of two hours before testing. The PH of the saliva and urine can reflect the effectiveness of an alkaline diet but does not correlate with the PH of the blood which is strictly controlled by vital biological processes.

What can be done to help?

See a dentist before treatment starts and keep your teeth and mouth clean. Inform the medical team if a sore mouth develops, particularly if it is associated with red areas, blisters, white spots, coated tongue or bleeding.

Avoid trauma: Be careful eating foods which could cause small cuts in the mouth and gum mucosa such as crisps, hard bread and dried snacks, as this could trigger the start of an ulcer. Avoiding overbrushing with a hard toothbrush. Stop smoking if you do and try not to breathe excessively through your mouth as this causes dryness.

Anti-fungal treatments: Although thrush can cause a sore mouth and throat, it can also aggravate mouth ulcers as the breach in the normal mucosa allows them to take hold. This will aggravate the ulcer and delay its healing. Anti-fungals are often prescribed routinely during chemo to prevent an infection, but if ulcers have occurred, it would be wise to take them for a longer duration.

Mouthwashes: Swill the mouth with a salt water mouthwash after every meal (a heaped teaspoon of salt in 500 ml of tepid water) for 1-2 minutes but do not swallow. Antiseptic and alcohol-based mouthwashes pose something of a problem because they often kill healthy bacteria as well as pathogenic bacteria. Although the mouth may seem clean immediately after use, as the bacteria race to re-colonise, pathogenic bacteria usually grow back first and in greater numbers, especially if acid or sugary foods have been eaten prior to cleaning. Ironically, these mouthwashes may actually promote bad breath and increase the risk of caries. A further study from the University of Glasgow found that using mouthwash containing alcohol could contribute to the development of oral cancer, a finding attributed to the overgrowth of pathogenic bacteria. However, the American Dental Association has yet to conclude whether mouthwashes containing alcohol are good or bad. For people who eat and drink a lot of sugary food, and don't brush or floss regularly, they can be helpful at reducing caries risk. Otherwise, they are an unnecessary risk. Mouthwashes containing probiotic bacteria instead of alcohol have now become commercially available. Studies comparing them with chlorhexidine and sodium fluoride have been shown them to be just as effective at reducing plaque bacteria levels. Their regular use seems very sensible as they help to maintain a lower PH. It is certainly worth giving one a try or, if you can't get hold of one, order some

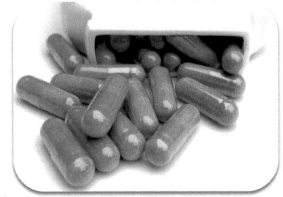

good quality oral probiotic capsules (see keep-healthy.com) and break 1 open, dissolve in water and swill 2 times a day.

Summary - Advice for mouth care

- Clean teeth thoroughly but gently after each meal and before bed
- If the gums are delicate, use a soft toothbrush (baby/infant)
- Suck ice/sugar-free ice-lollies prior to and during chemotherapy
- Swill the mouth for two to three minutes but do not swallow
- Strong antibacterial mouthwashes can damage the lining of your mouth
- Some mouthwashes can also stain teeth (read the label)
- Try a probiotic mouthwash
- If the mouth is dry, try sugar-free sweets (too many cause diarrhoea)
- Be careful of boiled sweets as they can cut your mouth, leading to ulcers
- Spicy foods are not harmful but can be uncomfortable
- Use plenty of fluids to keep foods moist e.g. gravy, yoghurt, sauces
- Avoid tobacco and alcohol
- Avoid sugary soft drinks
- Avoid boiled sweets and chewable soft candies or mints.
- If you eat or drink something sweet, follow up with a drink of water
- Avoid black coffee. Adding dairy can help counteract the acidity
- Brush your teeth at least twice a day, floss once a day
- A water jet can also help to remove debris and bacterial build up
- After acidic fruit juices, cider, wine, or beer, swill the mouth with water
- Avoid brushing your teeth after drinking high-acidity beverages
- Chewing gum can help maintain salivary flow
- Stay hydrated by drinking adequate amounts of water
- Consider a probiotic mouthwash

Bloating, colicky pains, excess gas

Food intolerances

Gluten: As we get older it is more common to develop an intolerance to gluten, leading to bloating, wind and colicky pains often referred to as Irritable Bowel Syndrome (IBS). If gluten intake persists and symptoms continue inflammation of the gut can occur, which damages the villi impairing the body's ability to effectively digest and absorb nutrients from the small intestine is 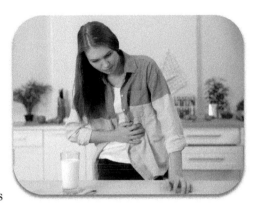 compromised leading to leaky gut syndrome. Initially, the best move is to reduce the intake of bread, pasta and cereals, but a number of studies have demonstrated how these efforts can be augmented with increased probiotic intake.

Milk and lactose: One of the main problems with milk intake is the reduced ability to digest lactose - commonly known as lactose intolerance. Many believe this is because trough evolution humans only eat milk in early infancy so need to make the lactase enzyme in adults diminished. Undigested lactose results in abdominal symptoms such as intermittent diarrhoea and constipation, excessive intestinal gas, cramps, and bloating after drinking milk. If chronic and unrecognised, this leads to symptoms such as fatigue, low mood and even depression. It is estimated that up to a third of white Europeans and Americans are lactose intolerant, but it can affect up to 50% of Mexicans and 75% of those of African and Asian ancestry. This condition is not an allergy; most people with lactose intolerance can consume some milk, so it is important to know your limit. A small amount of milk in a cup of tea is usually not a problem, but a large latte coffee often is. Live yoghurts and many cheeses have already had the lactose partially broken down by the fermentation process, so are better tolerated. There are many alternatives to milk on breakfast cereals such as soy, almond or rice milk, but obviously, avoid the brands with added sugar. Lactose-free has a higher GI so is not recommended on an empty stomach in the morning. The probiotic Lactobacillus acidophilus helps with the digestion and absorption of lactose by producing lactase and can counteract intolerance.

Lectins and phytic acid: These are carbohydrate binding proteins that are present in both plants and animals. Limited studies have suggested, in excess, are in people who have sensitivities, they can bind with and damage the intestinal lining and in particular the villi of the small intestine, causing IBS symptoms. People intolerant of lectin have increased release of a gut protein called zonulin which open gaps in the villi causing leaky gut syndrome. This increased permeability, opens the doorway to increased absorption of carcinogenic chemicals, inflammation and autoimmune diseases such as Crohn's and ulcerative colitis. Included in the list of undesirable chemicals, which could enter the blood stream is lectin itself. Lectins that are free floating in the bloodstream have an affinity for the insulin and leptin receptors and are believed to desensitize these receptors contributing to insulin and leptin resistance. Lectins are ubiquitous foods particularly those which actually help to reduce cholesterols levels. In some foods such as red kidney beans their levels are so excessive they need to be cooked or fermented to reduce their lectin content.

Phytic acid also has important functions in the body as an antioxidant. Some studies suggest it may have a protective against kidney stones and cancer. Scientists have even suggested that phytic acid may be part of the reason whole grains been linked with a reduced risk of colon cancer. Phytic acid, however, also impairs the absorption of iron, zinc and calcium, leading some people to refer to it, perhaps unfairly, as an anti-nutrient. If you do eat a lot of these foods, it would be a good idea to supplement the diet with foods rich in zinc, iron and calcium. Some people are sensitive to these two proteins even when cooked, so if removing gluten and lactose from the diet does not improve IBS symptoms it's worth keeping a food diary then reducing these foods. There are also specific techniques which can reduce phytic acid levels in these foods which include

- Soaking cereals and legumes overnight reduce phytates by >50%
- Sprouting or germination of the seeds causes phytate degradation
- Fermentation, such as in the making of sourdough bread

Abnormal bacterial growth

Trillions of bacteria, fungi and viruses live on our bodies, particularly in our gut, skin, and lungs, and collectively form our microbiota. Incredibly, just over half the genetic material from cells in our body is derived from these micro-organisms. Healthy bacteria play a fundamental role in ensuring our gut functions properly, yet it is becoming clear in the UK and other western

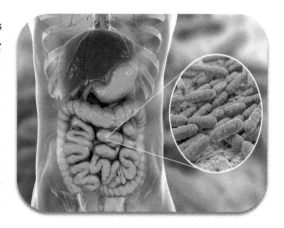

countries that our diets are woefully deficient in levels of these crucial bacteria.

Numerous clinical studies have established that a healthy, diverse population of bacteria strengthens immunity and helps regulate inflammatory reactions both in the gut and around the body. In turn, a poor gut flora leads to dysregulation of the immune system, leading to increased susceptibility to infection and excess chronic inflammation. By competing for space and nutrients and preventing the colonisation of unhealthy (bad) bacteria, good bacteria also form an important additional physical barrier for the oral and gut mucosa against pathogenic bacterial invasion.

Bad bacteria can be categorised as pathogenic or pro-inflammatory. Pathogenic bacteria can have a range of serious effects including life-threatening infections such as cholera and typhoid; food poisoning such as E.coli, salmonella, campylobacter or botulinum; and chronic infections such as heliobacteria. Pro-inflammatory bacteria, 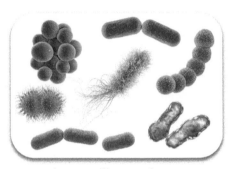 often referred to as the *Firmicutes* group, don't cause such acute illnesses but can cause long term health issues if they colonise the gut in excess. More common strains include the gram-negative bacteria E.coli and Shigella, and the gram-positive bacteria Bacillus, Listeria, Staphylococcus, Enterococcus and Clostridium.

Good bacteria interfere with the growth or survival of pathogenic microorganisms in the gut lumen, while also improving the mucosal barrier and the mucosal immunity. Beyond the gut, they improve overall immunity and help reduce chronic inflammation. They are also responsible for the formation of butyrate from soluble fibre and polyphenols. The prominent health benefits of Butyrate are described in detail below. Good bacteria are generally referred to as probiotic bacteria and include the gram-negative anaerobic *Bacteroidetes* group which are linked with numerous positive health benefits.

Despite an elevated risk of parasites and worms, people living in rural regions of Africa and South America actually have a more diverse and healthy *Bacteroidetes* gut flora than those living in the US and Europe. Western populations commonly have lower *Bacteroidetes* and higher *Firmicutes* ratios. As well as IBS like symptoms this results in and increased risk of food intolerances, inflammatory bowel disease and diarrhoea when travelling of visiting hospitals.

Chronic suboptimal gut flora and leaky gut syndrome also leads to an interference in the general immune system, leading to both a reduced ability to fight infections and inappropriate chronic inflammation. In this case, pro-inflammatory cytokines (

Interleukin 1,2,8, c-reactive protein, gamma interferon) are increased and the anti-inflammatory cytokines (interleukin 4, 6, 10, 11, 13 and 22) are reduced. This leads to an increased risk of a number of degenerative chronic diseases including:

- Fatigue
- Joint pains
- Low mood & depression
- Joint pains leading to arthritis
- Weight gain or obesity
- Poor muscle recovery

- Diabetes
- Cancer & cancer growth
- High cholesterol & heart disease
- Multiple sclerosis
- Fibromyalgia
- Dementia & Parkinson's

How does gut health effect cancer

The underlying cancer protecting mechanisms of a healthy gut are complex but the most important known so far include:

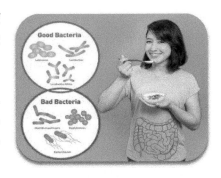

Chronic inflammation: Excess inflammation increases oxidative stress, impairs DNA repair, lowers immune surveillance, drives cancer growth and spread.

Inhibits carcinogenesis: Animal experiments have found that Bacteroidetes growth in the colon leads to the inhibition of carcinogens in the colon and a lower rate of polyp formation. This was attributed to the pH-lowering effect of Bifidobacteria in the colon, which subsequently inhibited the growth of pathogenic (bad) bacteria. A decrease in pathogenic microorganisms also modulated enzymes that convert pro-carcinogens such as nitrates to carcinogens such as nitrosamines.

Butyrate and glycan production: Healthy bacteria produce butyrate and glycans from polyphenols, an acid which stimulates an immune attack on cancer cells. They are also food for the normal cells lining the colon and prevents these cells from undergoing self-digestion, or worse, sustaining genetic damage and growing abnormally, causing hyperplasia and dysplasia which can lead to cancer. They improves the colon's integrity, preventing "leaky gut syndrome" which allows toxins to pass into the bloodstream and nutrients to escape. Butyrate can also exert a direct effect on established colon cancer cells by deactivating genes involved in cell growth and activating genes that trigger cell suicide (apoptosis). Butyrate production can be enhanced by dietary intake of probiotics, especially if and prebiotic fibres.

Improving polyphenol absorption: Healthy bacteria break down larger polyphenols into more biologically active, healthy and absorbable versions.

Reduce cancer spread: There is also some suggestion that gut health influences colon cancer metastasis. Bad, Fusobacterium are not only found in cancer in the gut but in the metastasise which spread from the gut to other parts of the body. It is thus thought that they have an influence on the rate of metastasis. Research is now investigating whether targeting these bacteria could reduce metastatic pathways.

Enhance anti-cancer immunotherapies: Strong immunity plays an essential role in ensuring modern immunotherapies work. There is no point uncloaking a cancer cell to be killed by the immune system if this system is not functioning efficiently. Recent laboratory and clinical studies have revealed important roles for gut bacteria in determining the body's response to immunotherapies, with healthy gut bacteria 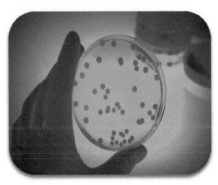 known to increase the therapeutic benefit of immune drugs in animals with melanoma. A clinical study conducted at the MD Anderson Cancer Hospital in Texas has further underlined the impact healthy bacteria have in facilitating effective immunotherapy treatment. It discovered that men and women taking PD1-inhibitor drugs to treat metastatic melanoma, had a 40% better response and lower side effects if they had a diverse and optimal gut flora with low levels of bad gut bacteria.

Major institutions are now racing to improve our understanding of the human microbiome and how it varies between people. A one-size-fits-all approach is unlikely to succeed when it comes to improving an individual's microbiome but taking extra probiotic supplements can certainly play a role in helping. It's envisioned that a tailored probiotic regimen could help maintain or restore a person's unique microbial "fingerprint", and, in doing so, could substantially improve responses to targeted biological treatments.

Factors which promote gut health

Bacteria-rich foods

Probiotic bacteria occur naturally in many fruits and vegetables, as well as in a range of fermented foods. Matured cheeses are an excellent source of healthy bacteria and fungi, yet its high-cholesterol content can prove problematic. A good way to circumvent this issue would be to eat smaller quantities of good quality cheese. In general, bacteria-rich foods include:

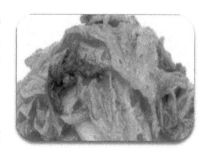

- Live yoghurt, kefir, aged cheeses
- Miso, kimchi and tempeh, sauerkraut pickled veg

Prebiotics

These stimulate the growth of healthy bacteroidetes and impair the growth of bad firmicutes. The two main groups are polyphenols and soluble fibres, and the main mechanisms of action are:

- Prevent adhesion of bad bacteria, providing more space for good bacteria
- Protection of good bacteria from enzymes in the saliva and stomach,
- Their natural antibiotics kill frmicutes but not bacteroidetes

Polyphenol prebiotics: It has been estimated that only 5–10% of total polyphenol intake is absorbed in the small intestine. The rest accumulates in the large intestinal lumen where they are subjected to the enzymatic activities of the gut microbiome. Healthy probiotic bacteria are therefore responsible for the extensive breakdown of the original polyphenolic

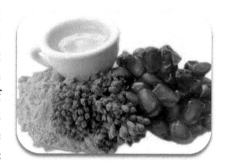

structures into biologically more active phenols, which can then be absorbed more efficiently. Polyphenols also help preferentially feed healthy gut bacteria, thus improving the composition of the microflora. This is because the metabolism of polyphenols produces glycans such as butyrate, which are used as energy by the intestinal bacteria. *Firmicutes (bad bacteria)* have less of the enzyme required to digest glycans than *Bacteroidetes,* so are less able to use them as food. Moreover, *Firmicutes* are more repressed than *Bacteroidetes* by the natural antibiotic properties of many polyphenols. The polyphenols and other phytochemicals which have the most notable effect on gut health include plant lignans found in nuts, bananas and cranberries, resveratrol in red wine, ellagic acid into ellagitannin found in tea, pomegranate and chocolate.

Soluble fibres: These occur naturally in gums and pectins which are found in citrus fruit, pears, apples, peas, guar gum, chicory root, garlic, onions, asparagus, Jerusalem

artichoke, as well as grains such as oats, barley and psyllium. They also include; fermentable soluble fibres such as inulin, resistant starches such as oligosaccharides, including fructooligosaccharide (FOS); and the polysaccharide beta-glucans most commonly found in mushrooms. They provide a substrate for the microbiota within the large gut. In addition, they increase faecal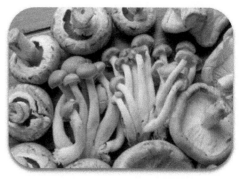
bulk and their fermentation produces short-chain fatty acids. This fermentation impacts the expression of a number of genes within the large intestine which enhance digestive function, cholesterol and glucose metabolism, as well as the immune and systemic metabolic functions in the body. They are also rich in natural antibiotics including penicillin, streptomycin, and tetracycline, which promote a healthy gut flora and, reassuringly, have not been shown to pose any risk of antibiotic resistance.

Physical activity: Higher fitness levels have been associated with both a greater abundance of butyrate, a short-chain fatty acid that's important for overall health, and butyrate-producing bacteria. One particular study found that professional rugby players from Ireland had a more diverse gut flora and twice the number of bacterial families than control groups matched for body size, age and gender. It was unclear whether having a healthy gut made them able to train to become ultra-fit, or rather that the training process itself actually improved gut health [Clarke].

Sugar and artificial sweeteners: *Firmicutes* thrive on ingested sugar whereas *Bacteroidetes* prefer to utilise on glycans produced by the breakdown of polyphenols. So, a high-sugar, low-polyphenol diet will encourage the growth of bad bacteria and lead to poor gut health. Many people are turning to artificial sweeteners as low calorie and potentially healthier alternatives to sugar, however, rats fed aspartame were shown to have increased blood sugar and increase the colonisation of proinflammatory clostridium and enetrobacterteria.

Other lifestyle factors: As mentioned above The proportion of *Firmicutes* increase while *Bacteroidetes* decrease with increasing BMI. It remains unclear whether it is the bad gut profile which causes obesity or vice versa [ref]. In excess, alcohol can adversely affect long-term gut health with spirits and beer being worse than red wine due to the protective effect of resveratrol. Binge drinking causes transient dysbiosis, which may responsible for many of the symptoms of a hangover [ref]. Cigarette smoking have recently been confirmed as an important risk factors for inflammatory bowel disease, and smoking cessation has been linked to increased gut flora diversity. Mice exposed to stresses such as isolation, crowding and heat, developing higher levels of bad bacteria. A human study, monitoring the effect of stress on the composition of gut bacteria in 23 college students before and after studying for their end-of-term final examinations, found that the high stress associated with exams caused a reduction in several bacteria, including Lactobacilli. A diet high in saturated animal fat can increase firmicutes growth. Likewise, people eating a high-protein, low-carbohydrate diet have reduced fermentation in the gut, leading to increased levels of harmful nitrosamines, decreased levels of butyrate and a reduced metabolism of polyphenols into the absorbable and biologically active phenols.

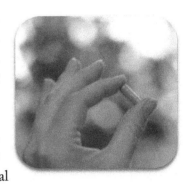

Probiotic supplements: Studies so far suggest that young active people with a good diet, and therefore a healthy gut already, are unlikely to benefit from probiotic supplementation. Unfortunately, most studies have been conducted in healthy volunteers. People with poor gut health may benefit and there is evidence for a short course in people with irritable Bowel Syndrome (IBS) summarised in a 2010 Cochrane review. As a consequence, the National Institute for Health and Care Excellence (NICE) recommends taking them for at least four weeks. Likewise, they appear to benefit with hospital acquired, antibiotic induced or travellers diarrhoea. One study suggested they reduced chemotherapy induced diarrhoea. The main risk posed by a probiotic supplement is a contaminated supply, so it's very important to buy probiotics from a reputable source. Be sure the ingredients are clearly marked on the label. Look for probiotic blends produced by a long established, reputable manufacturer with a high-quality assurance track record compliant with EU, UK and USA standards (more information can be found on keep-healthy.com).

Factors which negatively affect gut health

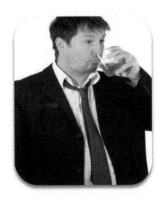

Age: The biodiversity of the gut and skin bacteria deteriorates over time unless extra dietary measures are undertaken. Anti-inflammatory microbiota tend to diminish with age, whereas inflammatory and pathogenic microbiota increase.

Medical treatments: Abnormal gut bacterial growth can be caused by a recent illness, antibiotics, antacids, chemotherapy and radiotherapy.

Alcohol: In excess, alcohol can adversely affect long-term gut health. Binge drinking causes transient dysbiosis, which some nutritionists pinpoint as being responsible for many of the symptoms of a hangover. This has prompted some to suggest that if a period of heavy alcohol intake is anticipated, it may be better to take a course of probiotics. One study examined the gut flora of 41 alcoholics and compared them to 10 healthy individuals who consumed little-to-no alcohol. A poor bacterial profile was present in nearly a third of the alcoholic population. The type of alcohol may be relevant as well. An analysis has been made of the effects of three different types of alcohol on gut health. For twenty days, a group was randomised to consume either a couple of glasses of red wine, the equivalent amount of de-alcoholised red wine or two gin-based drinks each day. Gin decreased the number of good bacteria, whereas both types of red wine actually increased the abundance of bacteria known to promote gut health, while also decreasing harmful gut bacteria. The beneficial effect of moderate red wine consumption appears to be due to its polyphenol content.

Smoking: Cigarettes have recently been confirmed to be one of the most important risk factors for inflammatory bowel disease. Fortunately, in several stud, smoking cessation increased gut flora diversity.

Psychological imbalance: Stress hormones such as cortisol and adrenaline act, via the vagus nerve, to increase acidity in the stomach, reducing the blood flow needed to properly digest foods and manage the balance of bacteria in the gut. This has been demonstrated in animal studies, with mice exposed to stresses such as isolation, crowding and heat, developing higher levels of bad bacteria. A human study, monitoring the effect of stress on the composition of gut bacteria in 23 college students before and after studying for their end-of-term final examinations, found that the high stress associated with exams caused a reduction in several friendly bacteria, including Lactobacilli.

Sugar and artificial sweeteners: Firmicutes thrive on sugar whereas Bacteroidetes prefer to feast on glycans produced by the breakdown of polyphenols. It is therefore abundantly clear that a high-sugar, low-polyphenol diet will encourage the growth of bad bacteria and lead to poor gut health. Many people are turning to artificial sweeteners as low calorie and potentially healthier alternatives to sugar. It may come as a surprise then that studies have shown that they can also negatively affect gut microbiota. In a recent study, rats fed aspartame were shown to have increased blood sugar, impaired insulin response and higher clostridium and enetrobacterteria, both of which are associated with inflammation when present in high numbers.

High saturated animal fats and protein: A diet high in saturated animal fat can increase Firmicutes growth, in turn promoting colon and oesophageal cancers.

Likewise, people eating a high-protein, low-carbohydrate diet have reduced fermentation in the gut, leading to increased levels of harmful nitrosamines, decreased levels of butyrate and a reduced metabolism of polyphenols into the absorbable and biologically active phenols.

Obesity: The section above has already highlighted the links between obesity and poor gut health. It is well established that with increasing body mass index (BMI), the proportion of Firmicutes increases while Bacteroidetes decrease.

Summary – improving gut health

Factors which promoting gut health
- Identify food intolerances and avoid responsible foods
- Increased intake of healthy bacteria rich foods:
    - Live yoghurt, kefir, aged and blue veined cheeses
    - Miso, kimchi, tempeh, sauerkraut, pickled vegetables
- Increased prebiotics
    - Nuts, flaxseeds, sesame seeds
    - Pulses such as beans, lentils and peas
    - Peanuts, mushrooms, chocolate, banana, cranberries
- Increase polyphenols
    - Resveratrol, Pomegranates, tea, turmeric, broccoli
- Increase intake of soluble fibre
    - β-Glucans, Inulin & Fructooligosaccharide (FOS)
- Taking a good quality probiotic supplement
- Regular physical activity

Factors which damage gut health Obesity
- Being overweight
- Medical treatments such as antacids, chemotherapy and antibiotic
- Alcoholic binges
- Excess meat and saturated fats
- Sugar and artificial sweeteners
- Psychological stress

Rectal damage (Radiation proctitis)

Despite advances in radiotherapy, damage to the bowel can still occur after treatment to the pelvis for prostate, rectal, bladder and cervical cancer, especially when larger fields are needed. Highly targeted radiotherapy techniques are reducing the risk of damage, while procedures which insert spacers, pushing the rectum away from the prostate, further reduce the volume and dose of radiotherapy to the rectum.

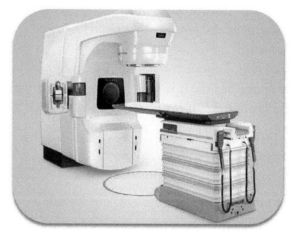

Radiotherapy damage is broadly split into either acute (within 3 months) or chronic (occurs later and could be permanent). Acute symptoms include diarrhoea, nausea, cramps, tenesmus, urgency, mucus discharge and minor bleeding. Symptoms of chronic proctitis may include those in the acute phase but could also include severe bleeding, urgency to open the bowel, faecal incontinence and, in extreme cases, strictures, fistula and bowel obstruction.

Prevention: The best way to avoid rectal damage (proctitis) is to use the most sophisticated radiotherapy equipment operated by an experienced radiotherapist. Inflammatory bowel disease, diverticular disease and diabetes can increase the risk of post radiotherapy symptoms, so alternatives to radiotherapy such as surgery may be better. A study of over 400 men who had had radiotherapy at the Cambridge University Hospital found that smoking increased the risk, so it's strongly encouraged to give up before radiotherapy or at least stop for its duration. The same trial found that those who exercised regularly during and after their radiotherapy had a reduced risk of damage.

Make the diagnosis of proctitis: Once symptoms develop, it is important to get referred for an endoscope to confirm the diagnosis but, just as importantly, exclude another disease, especially bowel cancer. Sometimes the endoscopist can identify a localised bleed point from a prominent vessel which is amenable to ablation with formalin, coagulation or an argon laser.

Medical treatments: In the acute phase, steroid suppositories can help, as does loperamide if diarrhoea is an associated feature. Drugs such as metronidazole, anti-inflammatory drugs and sucralfate are used with variable success. In refractory cases, hyperbaric oxygen has some evidence of success.

Lifestyle measures: It's important to avoid constipation as the straining can increase the damage to the rectum and anal canal. Crushed linseeds can help, provided they do not soften the stool too much. Exercise increases the blood flow through all tissues and can encourage new vessel formation, especially if combined with pelvic floor exercises.

Short-chain fatty acids and probiotic bacteria: Short-chain fatty acids such as butyrate are produced when prebiotic soluble fibres are fermented in the colon by healthy bacteria. Butyrate is important for colon health because it is the primary energy source for colonic cells, enabling them to grow and repair. It can be taken as a supplement, or enhanced production can be achieved naturally from a combination of prebiotic oligosaccharides, polyphenols and probiotic bacteria. Studies on probiotic bacteria have shown they can reduce the severity of radiation proctitis. Their effect is likely to be further enhanced with simultaneous intake of polyphenols and studies are ongoing.

Lignan polyphenols: Oxidative stress is a major mechanism in the development of radiation proctitis. The earlier chapter describes the factors which help reduce oxidative stress, particularly phytochemicals and vitamins, so it's important to maintain a healthy diet. An animal study of lignin-rich flaxseeds revealed a significant reduction in the risk of radiation damage. As flaxseed does not bulk the stool or produce gas, it can be used with the diets recommended during radiotherapy to the prostate. Some trials have already suggested that these prebiotic foods improve the severity of proctitis symptoms, especially in combination with a probiotic supplement.

Summary – Tips for radiation proctitis

- Get referred to a specialist gastroenterologist
- Exercise - Walking, running, aerobics, dancing, cycling
- If you smoke, stop!
- Increase soluble fibre intake, keep the stool soft but not bulked
- Try crushed flaxseeds in moderation
- Avoid foods which may cause intolerance or infection
- Try a probiotic supplement with a fructooligosaccharide prebiotic
- If this fails, try a polyphenol and probiotic supplement combination

---

Urinary dysfunction

Urinary function usually deteriorates as men and women get older. Radiotherapy and, more commonly, surgery to the pelvis can impair the ability to hold a full bladder. Fortunately, although urinary symptoms associated with prostate cancer are common, new precision radiotherapy techniques avoid the risk of permanent urinary dysfunction, in most cases. For up to two months after radiotherapy to the prostate or bladder, there are usually marked symptoms. These can be broadly divided into 'stress incontinence', where urine leaks out when coughing, sneezing or laughing, and 'urgency incontinence', where there is a strong desire to rush to find a toilet. This symptom is more common in women, and it is particularly prevalent after pelvic surgery, if the uterus is enlarged or prolapsed, or if the person is overweight. It is common in men with prostatic enlargement and particularly following prostatectomy.

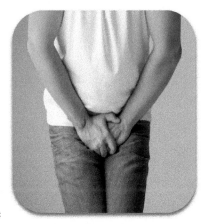

What can be done to help?

If there is a sudden onset of incontinence, particularly if associated with a burning pain (cystitis) on passing water, a raised temperature or needing to pass water frequently, this could indicate an infection. In this case, a sample of the urine should be tested and the appropriate antibiotics taken for treatment. For men with prostate problems who have a poor flow and get up a lot at night, tablets can be given such as alpha blockers (e.g. tamsulosin). These relax the muscles at the entrance to the bladder, allowing the bladder to empty correctly. If there is a severe problem with flow, or not emptying your bladder an operation to open up the tube from the bladder (urethra) may be required. Make sure you drink enough liquid so the urine is light yellow. A concentrated urine can irritate the bladder and is more favourable environment for pathogenic bacteria. If you are overweight, try to slim down. Try to keep your stools soft, as constipation can aggravate incontinence and reduce the capacity of the bladder. Too much tea and coffee, especially in cold weather, can cause urgency and sometimes incontinence.

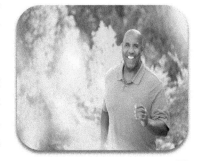

Exercise has been shown to help, not only by aiding weight loss but also by toning the abdominal and pelvic muscles. It is important to remember, however, that when exercising the abdominal muscles, you should breathe out slowly when tensing, for example, during a 'sit up'. This avoids increasing the pressure inside your abdomen (intra-abdominal pressure), which can aggravate incontinence by putting pressure on the pelvic muscles.

The most important and relevant exercises to improve incontinence are those which strengthen the pelvic floor – pelvic floor exercises. It's a good idea to include pelvic floor exercises as a routine part of your regular exercise programme, especially because, as we get older, our pelvic muscles and ligaments generally become lax. The earlier after cancer treatment they are started, and the longer people continue with them, the more effective they are. A general rule is to attempt some form of exercise at least once or twice every day and to keep it going regularly. Benefits usually appear within two to three weeks, but may take several months to peak. These exercises are particularly helpful if you are overweight, have had abdominal or pelvic surgery, or radiotherapy to the pelvis. Studies have shown that, if performed regularly, they can improve pelvic tone and muscle strength, which can benefit a number of urinary, sexual and bowel functions such as helping piles, bowel urgency, rectal prolapse. Some advocate pelvic floor exercises to improve sexual performance. In men, it can help to control orgasm and improve the local blood supply, helping reduce erectile dysfunction if performed over many months. In women, it is reported to increase sensitivity as it generally increases blood supply to the area.

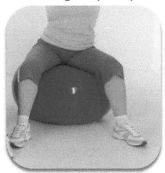

How to perform pelvic floor exercises

First of all, locate the pelvic floor muscles. Imagine trying to stop passing wind and urine at the same time. Tighten the muscles around the back and front passages, and lift them up. When doing this, you should be able to feel the pelvic floor muscles tightening. If you really concentrate, it is possible to tighten and contract different parts of the pelvic floor. Try the left side then the right side, then the front and back – this may seem hard at first but gets easier with practice. Avoid the following when performing pelvic floor exercises:

-   Do not pull in your stomach
-   Do not squeeze your legs together
-   Do not tighten your buttocks
-   Do not hold your breath

Exercise 1 – The slow exercise: Tighten your pelvic floor and count to five, then relax. Repeat this at least ten times. Perform this exercise five times daily. When feeling confident with this regime, increase the tightening time to ten seconds and include exercise 2 as well. Another way to do this is to tighten the muscles slightly, hold for 3 seconds, tighten further, hold for 3 seconds, really tighten (maximum force) for 3 seconds, then relax and repeat.

Exercise 2 – The quick exercise: This exercise works the muscles quickly to help them react to sudden stresses like coughing, laughing or exercise. Draw in your pelvic floor, and hold it for just one count before letting go. Repeat this up to ten times, five times a day.

Pelvic floor exercises can be performed whenever you are feeling relaxed – you could be lying down, standing up, in the supermarket or in a bus queue. The level of exercise depends on your fitness level. As an extra form of discipline, some men and women keep an exercise diary and tick off each day. If you miss a day, you can make up for it the following day, ensuring that at the end of each week sufficient time has been spent on the pelvic floor exercises. Be aware that the benefits which were shown in the clinical studies only appeared after a minimum of six weeks, with progress potentially taking months to peak. Most people give up after a week or so, thinking the exercises are not working. It is important to keep going for at least six weeks – even if you are not initially seeing a benefit. Likewise, when a benefit does occur, don't stop; keep going as otherwise progress may be lost.

Cranberries contain a class of polyphenols called proanthocyanidins (PAC) which have been shown to diminish pathogenic bacteria within the urinary tract (particularly E.coli) by preventing their ability to stick to the bladder wall, making them more likely to be washed away by the urinary flow. Its effect on urinary tract bacteria 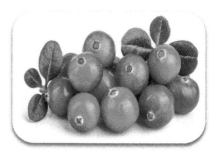 was first reported by two trials in 2004 and 2008 which reported how cranberry extract significantly reduced symptomatic urinary tract infections, particularly among women. However, a further Cochrane meta-analysis of several more trials in 2012 concluded that cranberry juice and standard cranberry supplements did not help. The authors concluded that the pills used in the studies were unlikely to contain enough PAC to be effective. They also pointed out that cranberry juice could increase urinary acidity and their high sugar content could impair bowel and vagina bacterial health, both factors which would increase the risk of infection. They recommended using a dried whole cranberry powder with high PAC levels for further trials, alongside a number of ways to improve absorption such as using enteric-coated capsules which maintained the integrity of the PAC further down the GI tract. A trial observing these recommendations was conducted in Italy in 2013. It used enteric-coated cranberry extract containing at least 30% PAC and reported a 3-fold reduction in urinary infections, as well as improvements in pain and cystitis feeling following radiotherapy to the pelvis and bladder. It is also clear from the microbiota chapter that polyphenol-rich foods and probiotic bacteria work together, so further studies would do well to include both enteric-coated cranberry and probiotic bacteria.

Probiotic supplements: If recurrent urinary tract infections (UTI's) are the cause of intermittent cystitis there is some data to suggest that probiotic supplements can improve the profile of bacteria in the vagina and rectum, reducing the chance of pathogenic (bad) bacteria spreading to the urethra.

Alkalisation: There is some evidence that an alkaline urine can help reduce the incidence of recurrent UTI's. An alkaline urine helps prevent kidney stones and urinary tract infections, as there is medical evidence to suggest that alkaline urine is a less favourable environment for pathogenic bacteria and the development of stones. Some over the counter remedies try to enhance this with agents such as sodium bicarbonate

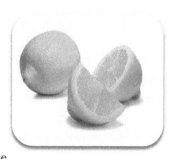

or potassium citrate but there is less evidence to suggest that these work. This is very different to a popular nutritional regimen called The Alkaline Diet

The alkaline diet claims to help your body maintain a higher blood pH. In reality, while urine, skin and saliva pH can change depending on what you eat, food is not going to substantially change the pH of your blood. Human blood is slightly alkaline at a tightly controlled pH between 7.35 and 7.45. If these mechanisms which maintain the PH of the blood fail, symptomatic acidosis

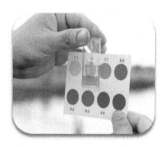

or alkalosis can occur, something which can be life-threatening. Medical conditions which cause changes in blood pH include respiratory acidosis, metabolic acidosis and respiratory alkalosis and these are medical emergencies. Despite the underlying hypothesis being fundamentally flawed the alkaline (or Ash) diet is generally healthy and as it advocates:

- More fruit and vegetables
- More nuts
- More legumes
- More seaweed and garlic

- Less meat, poultry and fish
- Less light beers and lagers
- Less bread and cheese
- Less processed carbs and sugars

It is thought that certain foods leave an acidic trail (or ash) when metabolised. These include animal proteins, as well as phosphorus and sulphur found in meat, grains, dairy, light beers, caffeine and cocoa. Adhering strictly to the diet, however, may create deficiencies in certain proteins unless individuals significantly increase their legume intake. It is also worth remembering that while removing grains may help those with gluten intolerance, it also eliminates a good source of fibre and B-vitamins from a person's diet. Alkaline diet proponents particularly recommend calcium, magnesium and potassium, all of which are alkaline nutrients which can be found in red and white wine, as well as mineral soda waters. Some even drink alkalinised water or bicarbonate (baking soda), a move which has no scientific basis and which a number of advisory bodies, including the Memorial Sloan Kettering Integrative Medicine Panel, strongly advise against. Taking alkaline liquids may actually cause a fall in pH (more acid) as the stomach reacts to alkaline by secreting more hydrochloric acid, some of which ends up being absorbed in the upper gut. This also explains the other potential mechanism for alkalisation which involves using foods which are slightly acidic, such as fruit. After ingestion, the stomach responds to the acid in these fruits by reducing acid production. Moreover, extending the times between meals and overnight fasting reduces acid production because there is no food in the stomach to stimulate acid production. On the other hand, certain foods produce more stomach acid because they stay in the stomach for longer, particularly meat.

Summary – Advice to help incontinence and urgency

- Test urine and treat urinary infection if present
- At the end of urinating try to ensure the bladder is empty
- Avoid aggravating stimulants - strong tea, coffee, alcohol
- Slim down, especially if overweight
- Exercise generally to increase muscle tone
- Perform regular pelvic floor exercises every day
- Avoid holding your breath when lifting
- Avoid straining when opening the bowels
- Avoid constipation
- Try a course of a healthy probiotic bacteria
- Try a course of enteric-coated cranberry (preferably with a probiotic)
- Consider some aspects of an alkaline diet

Chapter 5

Heart and Vascular Health

Cancer treatments can directly damage the heart, increasing the risk of irregular heartbeats, heart failure and heart attacks. Moreover, both cancer and cancer treatments can increase the risk of Venous Thromboembolism (VTE) - blood clotting in the veins. In the long-term, sustained high cholesterol and high blood pressure can lead to vascular disease and further damage the 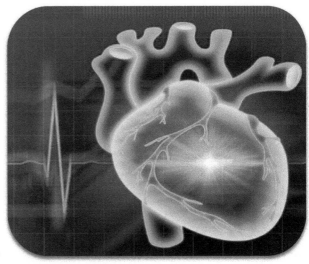 heart and brain after they have already initially been directly weakened by chemotherapy, radiotherapy or surgery.

Heart dysfunction

Heart problems are an uncommon but serious side effect of some cancer treatments. Often referred to as cardiac toxicity, there are a number of ways to prevent, monitor and treat these troubling problems. The three acute (early) heart toxicities are:

- Heart muscle damage (Cardiomyopathy)
- Coronary artery spasm
- Irregular heartbeat (Arrhythmia)

Heart muscle damage impairs the heart's ability to pump blood which, if severe and untreated, leads to eventual failure. The primary chemotherapy drugs which damage heart muscle are anthracyclines, such as adriamycin and epirubicin. Biological drugs, particularly Herceptin, Avastin and pertuzumab, can also damage the heart. Before and during these treatments, the medical team will monitor your heart function with echocardiograms. The risk of cardiac damage is elevated among smokers, those with a pre-existing cardiac history or those using both Herceptin and anthracyclines together. Direct radiotherapy can damage the coronary arteries, as well as the heart muscle, potentially leading to cardiovascular disease later in life. Fortunately, modern radiotherapy techniques exclude heart tissue, avoiding this damage.

Coronary artery spasm can occur, albeit rarely, with oral chemotherapy drugs such as capecitabine. They are thought to make the endothelium (cells which line the interior surface of blood and lymphatic vessels) particularly sensitive, leading to the production of a chemical called endothelin-1 which causes coronary vasospasm and symptoms similar to angina. In terms of lifestyle, some exercise-induced ECG changes have been observed with capecitabine. If you are on this drug, it's still a good idea to exercise.

Irregular heartbeats (Arrhythmias) can occur with the newer biological drugs. Oncologists are now finding themselves routinely measuring something called the QT interval - essentially the time it takes for the ventricles of the heart to contract and relax. Prolongation of the QT interval can trigger arrhythmias (atrial or ventricular fibrillation). Some unfortunate individuals can be born with cardiac defects which cause an increased QT interval and consequently have an increased risk of sudden death with these drugs.

Other causes of increased QT interval which can add to the risk include low levels of potassium, magnesium or calcium, caused by vomiting, diarrhoea or treatment with diuretics, chemotherapy and Erbitux. The anti-sickness drugs domperidone and, to a lesser extent, ondansetron can also prolong the QT interval.

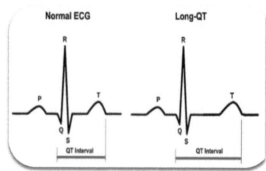

What can you do to help?

Lifestyle measures aimed at looking after the heart are similar to those designed to help fight cancer. The most relevant include:

- Giving up smoking, getting more active, reducing excess weight
- Eating less bad fats and more healthy fats
- Controlling cholesterol, blood sugar and blood pressure

Tips to give up smoking, increase physical activity, increase fibre and manage weight, and blood sugar levels are covered in other specific sections of this book. We will now concentrate on how, why and what to eat and do to improve the profile of fats in the body.

Lowering bad fats and increasing good fats

Fats are crucial for cell wall formation, brain development and a number of important enzymatic functions. Oily foods are a good source of the fat-soluble vitamins (A, D, E and K) and are an ideal slow release energy source, as they have a low glycaemic index which helps avoid peaks and troughs in blood sugar. It's because they are energy rich that too much intake, especially of the wrong type of fats, can lead to obesity, fatty liver and hardened arteries, which in turn cause heart disease, cancer and a host of other debilitating chronic diseases. Before dietary advice is discussed, it is worth describing the different types of fats.

Unsaturated triglycerides fats are categorised into monounsaturated (containing one C=C bond) and polyunsaturated triglycerides (containing more than one C=C bond). Monounsaturated triglycerides have their glycerol's component linked with omega 7 or 9 fatty acids, while polyunsaturated triglycerides are linked with omega 3 or 6 fatty acids. People often refer to triglycerides only by their fatty acid element e.g. 3 omega fats, without mentioning the common glycerol element making them triglycerides. That's why triglycerides containing omega 3 & 6 are often referred to as polyunsaturated fatty acids (PUFA).

Omega 3 fatty acids
These can't be synthesised, have to be ingested regularly and are essential for many important biological pathways. The short and long chain varieties are:

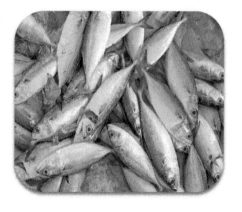

Short chain omega 3 – alpha-linolenic acid (ALA) and eicosatetraenoic acid (ETA) are found in plant oils such as walnuts, avocado, edible seeds, sage, algae oil, flaxseeds, echium and hemp oils.

Long chain omega 3 – eicosapentaenoic acid (EPA) and docosahexaenoic acid (DHA) are more generally more biologically potent. In plants they are found in linseeds (flaxseeds) have tree nuts particularly walnuts, pumpkin, hemp and Chia seeds. Algae and seaweed contain DHA is the primary structural component of the human brain, skin and retina but little ETA. oily fish such as herring, mackerel, salmon, sardine, cod liver, squid, krill oils, muscles, oysters, plankton are excellent sources of both DAH and ETA ,

Countless clinical studies have linked low intake and low serum levels of omega 3 with poorer health. They help to regulate inflammatory processes by producing anti-inflammatory fat products such as resolvins. In children, deficiency is associated with a higher risk of neurological under-development and in adults it is linked to a a higher risk of arthritis, coronary heart disease dementia and cancer. It is well known from serum tests that many people in the UK are deficient in omega 3 and increasing oily fish intake to at least three times a week is certainly recommended. It may be worth measuring your blood levels with a micronutrient test.

The evidence for a benefit of omega 3 supplements is conflicting. Cod liver oil is rich in omega-3, but there are some concerns that the vitamin A content is too high which some trials have linked to an increased cancer risk. A number of prospective trials have not linked their intake with a reduced heart attack risk.

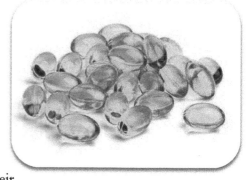

In term of cancer, omega-3 fatty acids have been shown to reduce the growth of tumours in a laboratory studies setting and one interventional study reported the their regular intake may reduce breast cancer risk. However, there is not reported benefits for bowel and ovary and two studies in prostate cancer suggested there may be an increased risk of more aggressive subtypes. This may however be due to the added vitamin E (to prevent oxidation) which is common in these supplements and has been shown separately to increase prostate cancer risk.

Omega-6 fatty acids

Linoleic acid, the shortest-chained omega-6 fatty acid, cannot be made by the body, so has to be consumed via vegetable oils, nuts, grape seed oil, soya, flaxseed and oily vegetables such as avocado. The other omega-6s can be found in smaller amounts in evening primrose oil, borage oil, cannabis oils and black currant seed oil. The long chain varieties, GLA, DGLA and AA, can be made by the body (converted from short chain omega 6) or found in these foods directly.

Health issues related to Omega-6 fatty acids: As well as a useful source of energy, omega-6s are reported to help stimulate skin and hair growth, maintain bone health, regulate metabolism and maintain the reproductive system. Linoleic acid is converted to GLA, which is then metabolised further to either AA or DGLA. AA can be metabolised, by cyclooxygenase 1 & 2, into prostaglandins and eicosanoids inflammatory cytokines. The enzyme 5-lipoxygenase also breaks down AA into leukotrienes, which are powerful local triggers of an inflammatory response which involves the release of histamine and recruitment of mast and killer cells.

The enzymes used to convert short-chain omega-6 (linoleic acid) into long-chain omega-6 (GLA, DGLA and AA), are actually the same as those required to convert short-chain omega-3 (ALA) into long chain omega-3 (EPA). So, too high an intake of short-chain omega-6 and 3, and too little long-chain omega-3 and 6 could, therefore, potentially lead to a deficiency in the enzymes required to form long-chain forms which are regarded as more biologically active and healthier. It is therefore important to consider diets with plenty of both long-chain omega-3 and omega-6.

Because of this competition with enzymes affecting omega-3s, and the importance of omega-6 in the immune process, it is widely quoted that omega 6s are pro-inflammatory. There are some reports among people with hyper-immune syndromes, like asthma and rheumatoid arthritis, that a diet high in omega-6 can exacerbate symptoms. In reality, clinical evidence for omega-6 being pro-inflammatory is, at best, circumstantial. In fact, a well-functioning inflammatory pathway is more efficient at detecting how and when to appropriately respond to trauma and infection and knows when to turn off when the risk has resolved. Moreover, adequate omega-6 is metabolised into both pro-inflammatory and anti-inflammatory eicosanoids. This is why GLA and DGLA actually reduce inflammation, especially when provided there are no deficiencies in essential nutrients required for good enzymatic function (including magnesium, zinc, and vitamins C, B3, and B6).

In support of this, well fed animals in the lab did not demonstrate increased inflammation with omega-6-rich diets. In humans, cohort studies show that omega-6s, including AA, are not carcinogenic. In fact, the two largest studies which measured serum omega-6 (HPFS and SELECT study) both showed that higher serum omega-6 was linked to lower risk of prostate cancer.

Furthermore, arachidonic acid (AA) is one of the most abundant fatty acids in the brain and is present in similar quantities to omega-3 (DHA). The two account for approximately 20% of its fatty acid content. AA activates syntaxin, a protein involved in the growth and repair of neurons, so it's not a surprise that early trials have found an improved intellect in children with adequate intake. Ongoing trials of omega-6 & 3 for dementia are underway. In terms of sport and exercise performance, AA is metabolized to eicosanoids during and after physical activity which promote growth and muscle repair via conversion to prostaglandins. Researchers from the University of Tampa reported that AA enhanced diets increased lean body mass, strength, anaerobic power and exercise performance in a study involving experienced resistance-trained men. Similarly, a meta-analysis from Cambridge University, looking for associations between heart disease risk and individual fatty acids, reported a significantly reduced risk of heart disease with higher levels of both long chain omega-3 and omega-6.

The balance of omega-3 to 6 fatty acids: It is clear from the scientific (rather than the lay) literature that we should not avoid foods rich in omega-6 as they are healthy and beneficial. The American Heart Association recommends individuals follow a diet to maintain sufficient intake levels of both omega-3 and omega-6 fatty acids, which in practical terms means at least 10% of calories coming from omega-6 fats. Most researchers agree that raising long chain omega-3 blood levels is far more important than lowering omega-6 acid levels. The trouble with a typical western diet is that it is becoming increasingly low in long chain omega-3. As a consequence, the ratio of omega-3 to 6 is changing to as much as 10-20:1, when ideally it should be 3-4:1. In Japan, where fish consumption is high, EPA and DHA levels are about twice those of Western populations. The dietary advice below highlights how to increase both omega-3 and 6-rich foods.

Omega-7 and 9 fatty acids

The main omega-7s in nature are mainly palmitoleic acid and vaccenic acid, found in macadamia nuts, sea buckthorn and, to a lesser extent, avocado fruit. They have been shown to increase insulin sensitivity and suppress inflammation. These are found in both animal and vegetable oils. The two most common omega−9 fatty acids are erucic acid, found in rapeseed, wallflower and mustard seeds, and oleic acid, found in avocado, macadamia nuts and most

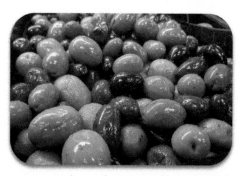

olives. Olive oil has many health benefits; it is an antioxidant and free radical scavenger; it reduces chronic inflammation and has an ability to increase good cholesterol (HDL) and reduce bad LDL cholesterol (LDL), as well as other saturated fats. Environmental studies have shown that higher olive oil use correlates with a lower incidence of atherosclerosis, diabetes, heart disease, inflammatory and autoimmune diseases, skin wrinkling and skin ageing. For centuries, Greeks and Egyptians have used olive oil typically for the treatment of what they termed 'erythema' or redness, while wealthy Romans would rub it on their skin before a steam bath. In laboratory experiments, it has been shown to repair DNA damage caused by excessive sunlight. In mice, massaging olive oil into their skin every evening, after excess exposure to UV light, had a major effect on reducing skin damage and the number of skin cancers. It reduced the formation of 8-hydroxy-deoxyguanosine (8OhdG), a marker of DNA damage. This DNA repair effect is the reason olive oil is being used more frequently in "after sun" skin care products. If you have sunburn, it is certainly worth applying olive oil to the skin before a shower for the next few days. The lignans in olive oil also have direct inhibitory activities on the HER2 gene. Over expression of this gene correlates with more aggressive breast cancers and is the target of the drug Herceptin. Olive oil is, therefore, a natural Herceptin.

Reduce trans-fats

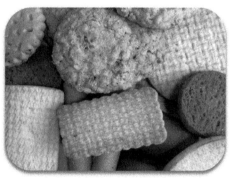

These are man-made in a process where unsaturated vegetable oils are partially hydrogenated to produce saturated fats. This alters the melting point and freezing points, making them useful for margarine, snack foods, packaged baked goods and frying. The trans-fats found in food have no known nutritional benefits, and emerging evidence suggests that they are worse than saturated fats. Studies have consistently shown their intake is associated with increased risk of heart disease, in part by raising levels of LDL and lowering HDL. As a result, Denmark and the USA have started labelling foods with their trans-fat content and pressure on the food industry is reducing their use. In Canada, from the end of 2018, they have been banned.

Reducing cholesterol

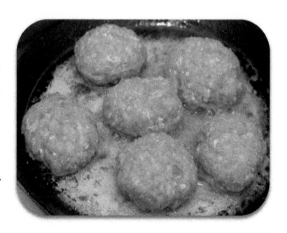

Cholesterol is a sterol (modified steroid) that is an essential structural component of animal cell membranes, maintaining their structural integrity and fluidity. They are not needed by plants. In animals, cholesterol is also a building block for the synthesis of testosterone, bile acids and vitamin D.

Absorption and secretion of cholesterol: Cholesterol can be absorbed directly from the gut, from animal sources, or can be made by many tissues, including the liver, with the help of the enzyme HMG-CoA reductase (the target for statins). To a certain extent, the body compensates for the absorption of excess cholesterol by reducing cholesterol synthesis. In addition, cholesterol is regulated via the gut as it is both absorbed, recycled or excreted in the small intestine. Every day, up to 1g of cholesterol enters the gut. This cholesterol originates from the diet, bile, and desquamated intestinal cells, and can be metabolised into a non-absorbable sterol that is excreted in the faeces by cholesterol-reducing bacteria. The liver also excretes it in a non-esterified form (via bile) into the digestive tract, which can be reabsorbed. Typically, about 50% of the excreted cholesterol is reabsorbed by the gut back into the blood. This balance of absorption or excretion can be affected by the genetic makeup, the health of the gut bacteria, level of stress, chronic inflammation and levels of polyphenols in the diet.

Transport of cholesterol: Cholesterol is transported around the body in lipoproteins. The total level measured in the bloodstream should ideally be less than 5mmol/L for healthy adults, or less than 4mmol/L for people with a higher cardiac risk. A lipoprotein with a low protein: cholesterol ratio is called a low-density lipoprotein (LDL), while one with a high protein: cholesterol ratio is a high-density lipoprotein (HDL).

HDL carries cholesterol away from the cells and back to the liver, where it's either broken down or passed out of the body as bile. For this reason, HDL is referred to as "good cholesterol", and higher levels are better (1mmol/L or more).

LDL carries cholesterol to the cells that need it, but if there's too much cholesterol for the cells to use, it can build up in the artery walls, leading to disease. LDL is known as "bad cholesterol" and it is better to have lower levels (3mmol/L or less).

Although we need normal levels of cholesterol for the production of cell walls and hormones, too much cholesterol is linked with greater risks of heart disease, stroke, dementia, other neurodegenerative disorders, cancer development and its progression after diagnosis. Other evidence on the cancer risk of cholesterol come from studies using statins. These are now commonly used to reduce blood fat levels by reducing absorption from the gut and reducing synthesis in the liver by blocking the enzyme HMG-CoA reductase. Five randomised trials suggested fewer breast, colon and melanoma cancers in long-term users of statins compared to controls. The data for prostate cancer, however, is inconclusive, as 2 of 3 large clinical studies did not demonstrate a reduced risk with statin intake. The consensus opinion from these studies was that it was the lifestyle which people follow to reduce their fat levels which confers the anticancer benefit, rather than just reducing the levels with a statin.

There are also concerns that statins may restrict the absorption of the healthy fats as well as the unhealthy ones, actually increasing the risk of some chronic illnesses such as dementia, although this is not completely established.

Lowers cholesterol levels. Soluble fibre found in beans, oats, flaxseed and oat bran may help lower total blood cholesterol levels by lowering low-density lipoprotein, or "bad cholesterol" levels.

Other factors which influence cholesterol and fat levels

In terms of cholesterol levels, the type and amount of fats we eat are very important, but the energy-in / energy-out hypothesis is a gross oversimplification. Several other factors influence how much cholesterol the body chooses to absorb, synthesise, excrete and reabsorb from the gut:

- Excess energy intake from eating too much food
- High cholesterol and fat intake
- Low unsaturated fatty acid intake
- Low physical activity
- High processed sugar intake
- Chronic inflammation
- Poor gut microflora
- Low polyphenol-rich food intake
- Low dietary intake of plant sterols

Physical activity: Exercise lowers serum triglycerides, total cholesterol and improves the ratio of HDL to LDL even before weight reduction occurs. It also directly lowers excess serum testosterone, oestrogen and leptin levels and raises adiponectin levels independent of weight loss, all of which have a favourable effect on inflammation and cholesterol absorption.

Fasting: Overnight fasting in overweight women after breast cancer treatments reduces cholesterol levels, alongside weight and breast cancer relapse rates.

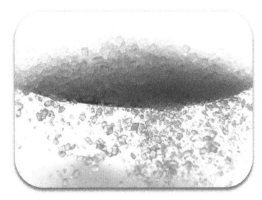

Processed sugar: People do not normally associate sugar with cholesterol, but a number of well-conducted studies have strongly linked higher processed sugar intake with higher serum cholesterol and heart disease. Notwithstanding the influence of sugars on obesity (see next chapter), the increased insulin levels caused by repeated sugar intake signal the metabolism into believing it needs to store more energy, thus decreasing excretion of cholesterol. Moreover, sugar leads to increased expression of inflammatory markers including 12-lipoxygenase (12-LOX). The body, in times of perceived inflammatory stress, reacts by storing more energy and consequently absorbs more cholesterol from the gut. The most convincing study, published in the Journal of the American Medical Association, analysed the dietary habits of a cohort of 6,110 Americans and showed that, after several years, those who eat more than 10% of their daily calories as sugar had significantly raised triglyceride levels, lower HDL and higher LDL cholesterol levels.

Unsaturated fatty acid intake: Numerous studies have highlighted that individuals who have higher plant unsaturated fatty acid intake, even if the calories consumed are the same, tended to have lower LDL cholesterol levels and certainly lower incidence of high cholesterol-related disease. This is thought to be due to their anti-inflammatory properties.

Abnormal gut bacteria: Cholesterol in the gut, originating from bile and desquamated intestinal cells, can be metabolized into a non-absorbable sterol by a cholesterol-reducing bacterium, allowing it to be then excreted in the faeces. Typically, about 50% of excreted cholesterol is reabsorbed by the small intestine back into the bloodstream. Research, presented by the American Heart Association, reported that abnormal gut bacteria reduce the natural excretion of cholesterol and increase serum levels. They also reported that a formulation of *Lactobacillus* contained in a supplement helped reduce blood LDL.

Chronic inflammation: Inflammation increases cholesterol levels because it makes the body think that it is under attack. This triggers stress, flight and fight pathways which preserve as much energy as possible (blocking excretion in the gut). To recap, the factors that increase chronic inflammation in the body include sedentary behaviour, obesity, sugar intake and exposure to environmental toxins. Factors that reduce inflammation in the body include regular exercise, higher PUFA intake, a polyphenol-rich diet, healthy bacteria intake or even a good probiotic supplement.

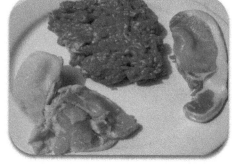

Meat: Most meat is high in cholesterol and saturated fats but are also a good source of vitamin B12, and can also be a reasonable source of omega-3. Grass-fed animals, particularly game, have more omega-3 than grain-fed animals. In most countries, commercially available lamb is typically grass-fed, and thus higher in omega-3 than other grain-fed or grain-finished meat sources. Chickens which roam around eating grass, worms and insects, as well as grain, generally have much higher omega-3. Cholesterol and animal saturated fats have the highest energy storing potential. This is good when we need it, but too much intake compared to what we require leads to serious long-term problems. Eating far too many high calorific fats combined with low requirements (inactivity) is the usual way to cause obesity as the body simply cannot use it fast enough. When the body absorbs or makes too much cholesterol, LDL levels increase in the bloodstream, forcing the body to have to find places to dump its cholesterol load, such as the liver, skin, soft tissues or walls of arteries. As a general rule, in Western societies we need to reduce animal saturated fats and cholesterol, eliminate trans fats and increase polyunsaturated (Omega-3 & 6) and monounsaturated (omega 7 & 9) fat intake within the limits of our energy needs. The following section provides dietary and other lifestyle tips to help achieve this.

Eggs: They can be a good source of omega-3 (mostly ALA) and protein, but only if produced by chickens fed a diet of greens and insects rather than chickens fed corn or soybeans. The addition of fish oils, flax, chia and canola seeds to the diet of chickens, both good sources of alpha-linolenic acid, increases the omega-3 content of the eggs. They contain good quantities of vitamins A, B2, 5, 12, folate, selenium and phosphorous.

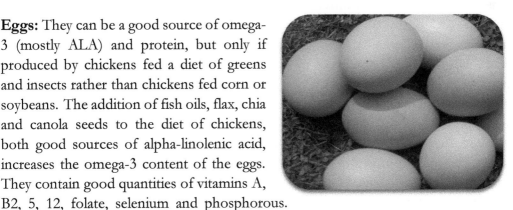

Eggs also contain decent amounts of vitamin D, vitamin E, vitamin K, vitamin B6, calcium and zinc. One large egg has 77 calories, 6 grams of protein and 5 grams of healthy fats.

More than any other food, the reputation of eggs has swung from wicked to wonderful and back again on a year by year basis, leaving most people bewildered and sometimes quite angry. It is true to say there is a lot of conflicting research regarding their benefits and many experts remain divided. However, please do not be scared of eating eggs in moderation, as they are actually among the most nutritious foods available on the planet. A whole egg contains all the nutrients required to turn a single cell into a baby chicken. The egg yolks are rich in the polyphenols lutein and zeaxanthin that accumulate in the retina of the eye. Studies show that consuming adequate amounts of these nutrients significantly reduce the risk of cataracts and macular degeneration, two common eye disorders. In one controlled study, eating just 1 egg yolks per day for 4.5 weeks increased blood levels of lutein up to 50% and zeaxanthin up to 140%.

On the negative side, yolks are high in cholesterol so eating too many will increase blood levels. However, one study, showed that eating less than two eggs per day for six weeks actually increased HDL (good cholesterol) levels by 10% and lowered LDL (Bad cholesterol). Another study showed that eating just five omega-3 enriched eggs per week for three weeks reduced triglycerides by 18%. Another study showed that people on a low carbohydrate diet, eating eggs led to changes in blood markers linked to lower risks of heart disease. However, one review of 17 studies with a total of 263,938 participants found no association between egg intake and heart disease or stroke. Of more concern, another study found that people with type 2 diabetes who ate eggs had an increased risk of heart disease although it was not clear whether this related to eating eggs or their other unhealthy lifestyle habits.

In terms of cancer, a summary of 13 cohort studies found no association with eggs consumption and bladder cancer, and there was even a protective effect in Japanese societies. Another Australian study found a link between higher egg consumption and colorectal cancer in females. A summary of 8 major studies involving over 30,000 participant published from Nuthetal Germany reported that eating >1.5 eggs a day increased the chance of an earlier death by 10%. They admitted, however, that the statistical power (certainty) was not strong, unlike the increased risk they found from red and processed meat. In fact, when they looked at people had a higher intake of the foods they found most protective; whole grains, fish, nuts, fruit and grains there was no increased risk form eating eggs. The biggest blow to the reputation of eggs came with a major study from Harvard School of Public Health in 2015, which suggested a correlation between egg consumption and prostate cancer. More specifically they reported a correlation between those who eat more than 2.5 eggs a week and a higher risk of progressing to fatal prostate cancer. These results have worried a lot of men living with prostate cancer and those concerned about getting it. There were several caveats however, which suggest that this data should not put you off your omelette: In this study, men who consumed eggs and red meat tended to exercise less, be overweight, smoke and have a family history of prostate cancer; The small number of lethal cancers occurred suggest that this association could easily have occurred by chance; These results are inconsistent with previous research, which found no association between eggs and prostate cancer.

The authors of these studies hypothesise that eggs raise the cancer risk via their higher choline content (also present in milk, and meat). Dietary choline is transformed into trimethylamine (TMAO) in the gut. There is some evidence that TMAO may increase inflammation, and this may the reason why it promotes progression of early prostate cancer to lethal disease. Further evidence pointing to the role of choline in prostate cancer was seen in a Cleveland Clinic study in which participants were fed hard-boiled eggs. This resulted in a significant rise in TMAO, and markers of chronic inflammatory even in individuals with low levels of cholesterol. To confuse matter more, choline is also present in cruciferous vegetables, but presumably the beneficial effects of their polyphenols overrides the effect of TMAO and the net result is still a reduction in inflammation.

Whilst some authors are vilifying choline, others are singing its praises. Choline is needed for the synthesize of two major phospholipids vital for cell membranes. Therefore, all plant and animal cells need choline to preserve their structural integrity. In addition, choline is needed to produce acetylcholine, an important neurotransmitter for memory, mood, muscle control, and other brain and nervous system functions. Choline also plays important roles in modulating gene expression, cell membrane signalling, lipid transport and metabolism, and early brain development. A deficiency of choline may play a role in liver disease, birth defects and dementia.

One study of 2,195 adults from Norway showed that participants with low blood choline had poorer sensorimotor and perceptual speed, executive function, and global brain power than those with higher levels. A second study from Framingham found that those with higher choline intakes had better verbal and visual memory. Studies evaluating heart health and choline are split almost equally into those showing arm an those showing benefit.

It is clear that egg intake needs to be considered alongside other lifestyle factors. Most trials show eggs are a healthy source of protein, vitamins and minerals, and if free range or supplemented they are a reasonable source of omega3 and other healthy fats. Like all foods, if you do not exercise and hence do not require the energy, they will contribute to an energy excess, weight gain and higher cholesterol leading to heart and vascular damage. Then again, if you exercise and do not eat much meat, they are an excellent healthy addition to the diet. The evidence for a cancer risk is weak and is thought to be due to a potential ability to increase chronic inflammation of the gut. It therefore makes sense when eating eggs, to practise lifestyle behaviours that improve gut health and reduce inflammation such as eating friendly bacteria, polyphenol rich food, exercising, and lowering sugar intake.

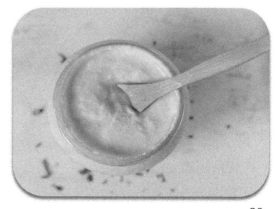

Milk, yogurt and cheese: These are energy-rich so not good if you are struggling to lose weight. Milk from grass-fed cows can also be a good source of omega-3. One UK study showed that half a pint of milk from grass-fed cows provides 10% of the recommended daily intake of ALA, while a piece of organic cheese the size of a matchbox may provide up to 88%.

Human breast milk provides an ideal nutrition for infants and is a good mix of hydration, vitamins, protein and fat. Breastfeeding lowers the risk of infant infections, asthma, eczema and childhood obesity. In adults, provided individuals do not have lactose intolerance, milk from grass-fed animals can be a useful source of vitamin B12, omega fats, energy and protein. It's also a useful source of post exercise nutrition. A study by the University of Connecticut, found that runners who had half a pint of milk after a 45 minute run had better muscle protein repair and glycogen levels than those who had a calorie-matched carbohydrate-only drink.

Milk, butter, cheese, cream, and yogurt are most commonly obtained from cows, but also from other animals including sheep, goats, and even camels. The exact content of milk varies between animal species, what they ate and how they were raised. Cow's milk typically includes 86% water, 5% lactose which is broken to galactose and glucose in the gut; 5% saturated and unsaturated fats and cholesterol; 3% Protein (casein and whey) all contain the full range of essential amino acids; <1% Vitamins A, B_1, B_2, B_{12}, B_5, C, D, E and K; <1% (Calcium, selenium, Cu, Mg, Mn, K^+ and Zn).

The concept that milk and dairy products are carcinogenic remains controversial but the risks of moderate consumption are likely to have been previously over-emphasised. It is often quoted that as Asian cultures have a low cancer rate because they don't drink much milk. This is a weak association because they are not usually overweight, are more physically active and eating foods rich in bacteria and polyphenols to name but a few.

In terms of hard evidence, there are no randomised trials linking milk with cancer but there are a number of population studies appear to suggest that that although moderate intake is safe, excessive milk intake could increase the risk of breast, ovarian and prostate cancer and could influence relapse rates. For example, a pooled analysis of 12 prospective cohort studies showed no excess in ovarian cancer incidence with moderate milk intake but a high intake (>2 glasses/day) increased the risk of breast and ovarian cancer relapse. One study has linked high calcium intake from milk and supplements with an increased risk of prostate cancer while other studies suggest that moderate intake has no effect. Ecological studies have suggested a link between eating animal fat from all sources, and an increased risk of breast cancer. Health journalists and advisory bodies extrapolated these results to say milk, as a source of fats, was the culprit but other studies, which determined which looked more specifically at milk and breast cancer have produced mixed results. Higher dietary calcium intake has actually been found to reduce bowel cancer risk for a number of reasons. First, calcium helps to inhibit the formation of nitroso-compounds from heterocyclic amines. Second, other naturally occurring omega fats in milk include sphingomyelin and butyric acid, which have been shown to directly reduce colon cancer in animals. Other benefits of milk products relate to their Vitamin D content and the lactobacillus bacteria, found in fermented dairy products like yogurt, can help gut health and reduce inflammation provided the individual does not have lactose intolerance.

The reasons excess milk could be harmful are multifactorial. Milk, and particularly cheese and cream, have a lot of calories in view of their saturated fat and cholesterol content, and may contribute to obesity which indirectly increases cancer risk. The lactose in milk is rapidly broken down to glucose and galactose in the gut. Lactose-free milk is even worse because the added lactase breaks lactose down before it's drunk. The rapid absorption of this sugar increase in Insulin-like growth factor and inflammatory markers. Milk naturally contains hormones and growth factors produced within a cow's body. In addition, synthetic hormones are commonly injected into cows to increase their production and these can find their way into milk. Most of the foods produced for humans are grown using PCBs, PBBs, organophosphates dioxins, herbicides and disinfectants which have each been found in milk. It has been estimated that dairy products contribute over a quarter of our dietary intake of dioxins. Fortunately, this level is still typically below the tolerance set by the Environmental Protection Agency (EPA). Nevertheless, very small amounts ingested over long periods of time can eventually build up to concerning levels as these toxins do not readily leave the body. Other contaminants introduced during processing of milk products include melamine, which is often found in plastics, and carcinogenic toxins including aflatoxins. These contaminants are additionally concerning because they are not destroyed by pasteurization and could negatively affect the kidneys and urinary tract due to their high nitrogen content. Needless to say, grass-fed animals have lower levels of contaminants, as does organic milk. The treatment of mastitis and other infections using oral, intravenous or intra-mammary antimicrobial drugs are important to keep the cow healthy. As a result, low levels of fungicides, anti-helminths, antibiotic and sulphonamide drugs can be found in milk. The risks of this low-level exposure are not certain, but some researchers hypothesise that they may lead to alteration of gut bacteria and antibiotic resistance in humans.

Skimmed milk: The trend for consumers to switch to low-fat versions of milk such as semi-skimmed or skimmed milk is unsupported by science. Most of the good stuff in milk is in the fats such as the soluble vitamins A, D, E, and K as well as trans-palmitoleic acid, and polyunsaturated omega fats such as pentadecanoic acid, *linoleic acid and* linolenic acid which have associated a better lipid profile, and lower markers of inflammation and better health. The only advantage skimmed milk is the lower level of calories, but it seems more sensible to drink small amounts of healthier whole milk rather than larger amounts of unhealthy skimmed milk.

Yogurt and kefir: Fermentation with bacteria partially breaks down some of the lactose so this is a little better for the lactose intolerant. The lactobacillus bacteria is known to help maintain gut microbiota which has numerous benefits for the gut itself and the rest of the body. Studies have shown that triggering the fermentation by adding probiotic *Lactobacillus* to milk when drunk resulted in a four-fold lowering of IGF compared to drinking non-fermented milk.

Cheese: High fat content has meant that cheese has been vilified for years. but evidence of harm is lacking apart from contributing to weight gain if eaten in excess. It is rich in probiotic bacteria and in the blue veined varieties, healthy fungus and vitamin K2. These improve gut health, reduce chronic inflammation and improve immunity. A study from Texas reported regular consumption of cheese reduced the risk of liver cancer and was linked to a longer life expectancy.

Butter and cream: Apart from taste, converting milk into cream adds no additional health benefit and by removing the buttermilk it concentrates the saturated fats and cholesterol and makes it highly calorific. However, the process does also concentrate other healthy fats and fat-soluble vitamins, particularly A and K, so unlike margarines made from trans-fats there is some benefit. The recommendation to ditch butter for lower saturated fat margarine is certainly unfounded but excess can increase cholesterol levels.

Dietary phytosterols: Phytosterols are structurally related to cholesterol. Plants manufacture phytosterols, which can compete with cholesterol for reabsorption in the intestinal tract, thus potentially reducing cholesterol reabsorption. When intestinal lining cells absorb phytosterols, in place of cholesterol, they usually excrete the phytosterol molecules back into the gut. Sitosterol and campesterol are the most frequent plant sterols and respectively constitute about 60% and 35% of plant sterols in food. Plant stanols are the saturated form of plant sterols, meaning they have no double bond in the sterol ring. Saturated sitosterol is known as sitostanol, and saturated campesterol is campestanol.

Plant foods that are particularly rich in phytosterols (stanol or sterol esters) include avocados, flaxseed, peanuts, soybeans, chickpeas, pumpkin seeds, beans and buckwheat, but they are also found in whole grains, vegetables, fruits, nuts and other seeds. An Australian study found that eating a bowl of tomatoes every day lowered LDL by up to 10%. A recent meta-analysis of 41 similar trials reported that regular intake of phytosterol-rich foods was linked conclusively with lower serum cholesterol. From this data, it appeared that 2-3 g/day seemed to be the optimal amount to lower LDL by about 10%, with higher intake not seeming to reduce levels much further. The beneficial effects, however, were found to be additive with other lifestyle interventions.

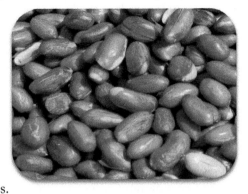

For example, eating foods low in saturated fat and cholesterol, and high in phytosterols, reduced LDL by up to 20%, while eating them with statin medication almost doubled their cholesterol-lowering capacity. In addition, a growing body of scientific evidence also suggests other positive health outcomes, including the reduced risk of certain types of cancer. Although further research is needed to determine whether this reduction in LDL will lead to a reduction in heart attacks, numerous organisations promote their intake, including the American Heart Association (AHA), Spanish Cardiology Society, the Association of Clinical and Public Health Nutritionists in Finland, and the National Heart Foundation in Australia.

Plant sterol and stanol supplements are as a convenient way to boost daily plant sterol intake, especially those who do not like eating these foods. Some yoghurts also have small quantities of sterols added, but many of these products also contain added sugar and flavours. The studies above show that, if combined with other lifestyle measures, the 10-20% drop in LDL may be enough to mitigate the need for statins. Sterol supplements would also be very useful for individuals who are already taking statins but are suffering side effects. Instead of stopping statins altogether, people with side effects may be better off lowering the statin dose and taking a concomitant plant sterol supplement at the same time. This compromise may be enough to stop side effects and maintain normal serum cholesterol levels. There are some safety issues related to very high intake of plant esters sterols (>3g / day). This high intake could increase serum plant sterol levels, which some argue may increase arterial fat deposits. This risk is largely hypothetical, and any increase due to the small increase in plasma plant sterols is more than offset by the decrease in plasma LDL. The reality is that, in a western diet, the consumption of plant sterols is usually much less than 0.5g / day, so individuals can safely be advised to eat considerably more of these foods and even take a sterol supplement.

Another potential concern with very high doses is that they could potentially affect the absorption of carotenoids and fat-soluble vitamins. This can, in theory, constitute a hazard to children and pregnant and breastfeeding women. Because of this theoretical risk, labelling advises these individuals to avoid consuming these products. Despite this theoretic risk, meta-analyses have not demonstrated any lowering of vitamin A, D, E and K levels after plant sterol intake. Nevertheless, general advice if taking a sterol supplement is to ensure adequate intake of carotenes rich foods such as carrots, pumpkins, squash, broccoli, apricot and mango.

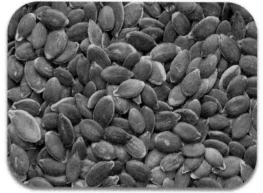

Stanol esters are less absorbable plants which not only reduce serum cholesterol on their own but also reduce plant sterol levels in the bloodstream. The safety and efficacy of plant stanol esters have been confirmed in more than 70 clinical studies which show that daily intake of 2 g plant stanol ester lowers LDL-cholesterol by about 10% on average. They are now recommended by a number of academic bodies, including the American Heart Association, to assist serum cholesterol control. For optimal cholesterol lowering, plant stanol ester should be used daily, in sufficient amounts, with a meal and in combination with other recommended dietary

Tips to help increase healthy fat and reduce cholesterol levels

Ensure a healthy energy balance
- Don't overeat and try to fast for 13 hours overnight
- Try not to snack between meals, put up with an empty stomach
- Be more physically active and on sedentary days eat less

Lower animal saturated fats and cholesterol intake by reducing:
- Processed palm oil ridden biscuits, cakes, muffins and pastries
- Deep-fried or fatty snacks – crisps, pakoras, bhajis, pies and sausages
- Fatty "thin" chips and hash browns, batter from fish and chip shops
- Curry dishes containing ghee and rich creamy dishes
- Meat intake in general. Should be <3 times/week

Remember to also reduce processed sugar and refined carbohydrate intake:
- Stop adding sugar to tea or coffee, avoid sugar cereals in the morning
- Although whole fruit is good – Avoid dried fruit or fruit preserves
- Avoid sweet foods on an empty stomach – restrict to after meals

Increase unsaturated fatty acid intake:
- Oily and white fish - cod, sea bass, mackerel, herring, swordfish, salmon, sardine
- Algae, krill and brown algae (kelp)
- Seeds - Linseeds (crushed), sunflower, sesame and pumpkin seeds
- Walnuts, almonds, Brazil nuts, hazelnuts, Macadamia nuts and cashews
- Dairy and eggs from free range animals, wild or fed on grass
- Use cold pressed olive oil, rapeseed (canola), soya and sunflower

Increase plant sterols and stanols:
- Avocados, flaxseed, peanuts, soya beans, chickpeas mushrooms, beans
- Grains, vegetables, buckwheat fruits, nuts and pumpkin seeds.

Eat more polyphenol-rich foods:
- Colourful fruits – avocado, pomegranates, tomatoes, strawberries
- Leafy and cruciferous vegetables – broccoli, Brussels sprouts, asparagus
- Herbs and spices – hemp, turmeric, chilli, parsley, sage and perilla
- Teas, mushrooms, sugar-free chocolate

Eat more healthy bacteria:
- Sauerkraut, kefir, miso soup, kimchi or a quality probiotic supplement

Blood pressure (hypertension)

Lowering excess blood pressure: Recent research suggests a role in cardiovascular health. A meta-analysis of nine studies published in the journal 'Hypertension', tracked 543 adults with both normal and high BP and found that those taking probiotics had lower average systolic and diastolic BP by about 3 mmHg. The greatest effects were seen in subjects with BP above 130/85. 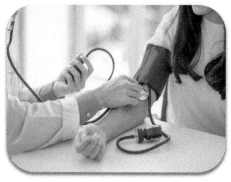 Those who took probiotics containing four or more strains were also more successful at lowering BP than those taking single-strain sources.

Some treatments, such as abiraterone and enzalutamide, can increase blood pressure (BP) soon after starting. Other biological and chemotherapy agents can affect long-term BP. A raised BP can add to the cardiac risks caused by chemotherapy. Over time, high BP can cause blood vessel damage, leading to heart failure, kidney disease and stroke among other problems. Many risk factors for high blood pressure such as age, family history, gender, and race, are beyond an individual's control, yet there also factors which people can control, including ensuring adequate relaxation, engaging in exercise and avoiding obesity. Nutritional influences on BP are highlighted by the DASH guidelines (Dietary Approaches to Stop Hypertension). A recent meta-analysis of 17 studies found that followers of the DASH guidance had significantly reduced systolic and diastolic blood pressure. These dietary measures include:

Avoiding sodium-rich foods or habits which increase sodium intake include:
- Adding salt when cooking or using canned vegetables and beans
- Processed ready meals, salted nuts, canned or cured meats
- Ham, frankfurters, sausages, frozen breaded meats

Consuming potassium-rich foods: Because leafy green vegetables are high in potassium, magnesium and fibre content, they help reduce BP by encouraging the excretion of sodium. Those with notably high levels include:
- Romaine lettuce, arugula and kale
- Turnip and collard greens
- Spinach, beet greens and Swiss chard

Fruits and berries tend to be rich polyphenol flavonoids, low in sodium and higher in potassium. One study found that drinking a cup of fresh pomegranate juice once a day for four weeks lowered blood pressure by an average of 5mmHg. Another study reported that two bananas a day reduced BP by 10% after only 6 weeks. Watermelon is a rich natural source of the amino acid L-citrulline, which has been shown to help regulate blood flow and blood pressure. The fruits and berries which can particularly help BP include:

- Berries – Blueberries, raspberries strawberries
- Bananas – Low in sodium and high in potassium
- Watermelon, avocados and dates

Plant nitrates provide a natural means of increasing blood nitric oxide (NO) levels. NO is absorbed by endothelial cells lining the arteries and then penetrates the underlying smooth muscles, acting as a potent vasodilator which relaxes the arteries. NO plays a critical role in controlling BP, improving overall circulation and oxygenating the heart, muscles and brain during 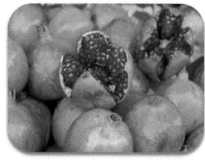 exercise. Studies in humans have demonstrated that the NO generating properties of nitrate-rich foods are likely to be responsible for improvements in cerebrovascular blood flow, improved erectile function and lower cognitive deficits. A study of older adults with high BP found that after just 18 weeks of eating a small amount of dark chocolate every day, BP was reduced by 20%. Foods containing nitrates include:

- Fruit – Apples, cherries, pomegranate, blackberries, strawberries
- Herbs - Turmeric, ginger, green tea, cocoa (Dark chocolate)
- Salad - Spinach, kale, watercress, rocket, arugula lettuce
- Vegetables – Beetroot, radish, celery, broccoli

Coffee, alcohol and tea: The DASH guidance suggests no more than one alcoholic drink per day for women and two drinks per day for men. Caffeine in coffee is reported to cause a transient increase in BP, but people who drink coffee regularly are not more at risk. In fact, a study which gave men with pre-existing high BP 3 cups of tea/day saw a decrease in BP.

Unsalted seeds, nuts and legumes that are high in potassium, magnesium and other minerals are known to reduce BP. Pistachios reduce peripheral vascular resistance (blood vessel tightening), as well as heart rate. One study found that because of these factors, one serving a day helped reduce blood pressure. In another study, adults eating ½ cup of walnuts - rich in healthy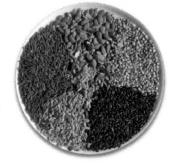

fats, magnesium and fibre - daily for four months, had lower BP. Encouragingly, participants did not gain weight even though they added over 350 calories to their daily intake. Eating three tablespoons of crushed flaxseeds daily for six months, lowers BP by an average of 10% according to one study published in the journal 'Hypertension'. Sunflower, pumpkin seeds, flaxseeds, pistachios and walnuts are particularly beneficial help with gut health and reduce inflammation

Allium vegetables (Onions, garlic and leeks) are particularly rich in the polyphenols quercetin, gallic acid, ferulic acid and kaempferol. Regular intake has been shown in cohort studies to be associated with lower blood pressure and a reduced need for anti-hypertensive drugs. A meta-analysis of 25 RCTs published in 2008 found garlic to have a sizable effect on lowering blood pressure when compared with a placebo. Another study, involving patients with poorly controlled BP, reported that 1g of garlic supplementation resulted in a significant

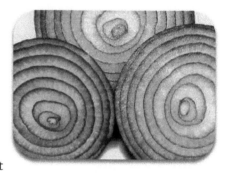

reduction in blood pressure levels. This effect is due to garlic's polysulfides, which have a vasodilatory action on blood vessels, widening them and lowering vessel wall tension.

Yoghurt is an excellent source of calcium and is low in fat, both of which are useful to help with BP control. According to the American Heart Association, women who ate five or more servings of yoghurt a week experienced a 20% reduction in their risk of developing high BP.

Egg whites contain a peptide which lowers blood pressure. A study presented by the American Chemical Society revealed egg whites lowered BP as much as a commonly prescribed drug.

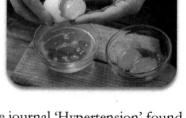

Gut bacteria: There is emerging evidence to suggest that probiotics may have a role in cardiovascular health. A meta-analysis of nine studies published in the journal 'Hypertension' found that, on average, taking probiotics lowered systolic BP by 3.5 mmHg and diastolic blood pressure by 2.4 mmHg. The greatest effects were seen in subjects with BP above 130/85. Multiple strain probiotic supplements were more effective than single-strain sources.

Blood clots – Thromboembolism

The increased risk of blood clotting in the deep veins (thrombosis) is especially high following a recent operation or if there is a disease of the lower abdomen or pelvis. The risk is also greater among individuals who don't exercise, are overweight, smoke, have a previous history of thrombosis, have varicose veins, are undergoing chemotherapy, receiving hormone therapies or have had long periods of immobility. Extended plane

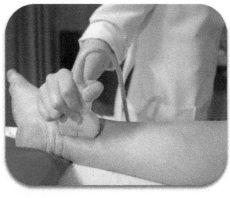

journeys are notorious for causing the blood clots, but being stuck on a motorway in a traffic jam for just a couple of hours can also significantly elevate risk. Individuals are more likely to form clots if their platelet count is high or they have a hereditary abnormality of the blood. Blood can clot in the deep or superficial veins:

Superficial vein damage and thrombosis: Patients may experience a darkening of the veins in the hands and arms after chemotherapy. This is normal, and the dark colour should fade once the course of treatment has been completed. Of more concern are veins that start to feel hard and 'cord-like'. This is caused by blood clotting in the superficial veins of the hands or arms. This can be associated with painful inflammation and may prevent the oncology nurse from finding a good vein. This thrombosis may take several months or sometimes years to resolve. Fortunately, although uncomfortable, this sort of thrombosis is localised and does not result in clots embolising to the lung or elsewhere. If painful, an anti-inflammatory cream. Squeezing a soft sponge repeatedly for 5 minutes, 3-4 times a day, will help pump blood through the veins and open up collateral vessels. A mini aspirin (75mg) taken three times a week can also help to dissolve the clots and speed up the healing.

Deep vein thrombosis (DVT): The most common veins affected are those in the deep veins of legs (particularly if there's a history varicose veins), yet thrombosis can also occur in the deeper veins in the arm, chest abdomen and even veins within the head. In the leg, DVT tends to cause swelling, redness and discomfort.

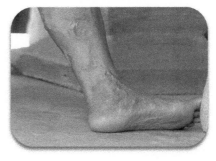

Pulmonary embolism (PE): Clots can potentially break off and travel to the lungs where they become trapped. This can cause considerable damage and even be fatal.

The classic presentation of a PE is sudden breathlessness, chest pain and coughing up blood. In reality, however, most people just start feeling increasingly breathless on exertion and start feeling generally unwell, sometimes with dizzy spells or faints. It's important to report this to a doctor who can arrange an urgent CT scan.

What can reduce the thrombosis risk?

Medical interventions such as warfarin, low molecular weight heparin and the newer oral anticoagulation agents such as apixaban are usually effective. If the risk of thrombosis is high, ask your doctor to consider an injection of heparin before travelling. Provided you do not have a history of aspirin allergy or stomach ulcers, taking 75mg of aspirin before you take a long car, coach or plane 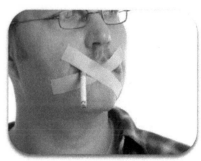 journey may also be wise. In terms of lifestyle, exercising and stopping smoking are the two most important factors involved in reducing the risk of thrombosis.

Summary – Tips to prevent blood clots

- Avoid long periods of inactivity
- If working a desk job, try and stand regularly
- Avoid confined spaces for long periods of time
- Walk briskly for >20 minutes at least twice a day
- Remember that any form of exercise reduces risk
- Compression stockings are recommended when travelling
- When in a car, keep the legs moving and avoid being cramped
- While travelling, if possible, take regular breaks to walk and stretch
- In airports, walk around for as long as possible before boarding
- Prolonged periods of immobility should be avoided
- Smoking – stop immediately

Tips for superficial thrombosis:

- Exercise arms – it gets blood pumping through your veins
- Exercise hands – use a specific hand grip device or a tennis ball
- Oil and moisturise – regularly rub pure olive oil into your arm
- Gently massage your skin and veins when applying the oil

Chapter 6

Skin care after cancer

The skin and chemotherapy

Chemotherapy attacks rapidly proliferating cells. This is why normal cells that have higher growth rates such as skin, bone marrow, the lining of the gut, the cornea, nails, hair and mucous membranes tend to be more susceptible to damage. Chemo can affect the skin in several ways and with varying degrees of severity. At the very least it can make skin dry and blotchy, and rashes are fairly common. Some chemotherapy and biological agents (e.g.

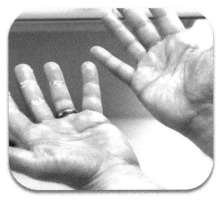

capecitabine, Caelyx, sunitinib and sorafenib), cause inflammation, reddening and splitting of the palms of the hands and soles of the feet (Palmer-Planter Syndrome). This is thought to be caused by the small blood vessels of the extremities being damaged, a process which causes chemotherapy agents to leak into the tissues. On the feet, because of friction from walking, the skin tends to peel off, creating raw painful blisters. Your doctor may reduce the dose of chemo for a while to allow your skin to recover.

Other drugs, such as Erbitux for bowel cancer, can cause acne. In this situation, topical anti-acne creams or antibiotic tablets may be prescribed. Most chemotherapy drugs will also make your skin more sensitive to the sun during their administration, and some drugs, such as bleomycin, capecitabine and fluorouracil, can increase sensitivity for several months afterwards.

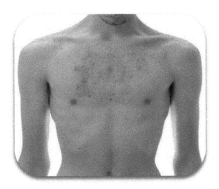

What can you do to help?

In order to improve dryness or blotchiness, five basic principles apply; stop smoking, eat well, exercise, nourish and moisturise the skin. As a rule, people who are healthy tend to look healthy. Smoking, for example, reduces oxygen to the skin and increases the appearance of ageing. The amount of haemoglobin carrying carbon monoxide instead of oxygen is increased, and this produces a grey/brown pallor particularly on the face and around the eyes. There has to be common sense when it comes to sunlight. While intense exposure can be dangerous, light regular sun on the skin is healthy as it increases vitamin D levels, helps bone density and may also have a direct anti-tumour effect.

For the acne associated with some drugs, topical probiotic creams are worth a try as either an alternative or to complement the antibiotics prescribed by the medical team. For the hand-foot syndrome, no cream has proven better than another in clinical studies, but due to its DNA protective properties, an olive oil cream is recommended.

Summary – Skincare advice during chemotherapy

- If you smoke, stop. It is the worst thing you can do for your skin
- Avoid excess alcohol, especially hangovers, as this can dry the skin
- Take extra care in the sun - many chemotherapy agents photosensitise skin
- Eat a well-balanced healthy diet with plenty of oily fish and polyphenols
- Gently wash skin in warm water with a mild, non-perfumed soap
- Avoid harsh shower gels and detergents
- Do not use a coarse washcloth, bath oil or bubble bath
- Dab the skin with a soft, clean towel
- Wear loose-fitting clothing, preferably made with a natural fibre e.g. cotton
- Clothes should not rub or cause friction
- Use a mild detergent to wash clothes that will be next to your skin
- Exercise and stretch regularly
- Rinse the skin after swimming in chlorinated pools
- After swimming, shower and apply oils
- Use chemical-free natural oils
- If healthy oils are not available, use extra virgin olive oil before a shower
- Massage your skin gently when applying oil
- Consider a probiotic skin cream

Chapped lips and cold sores

Chapped lips are a common condition where they become dry, cracked and sore. If marked, this can lead to bleeding and secondary infection. Lip soreness during chemotherapy is an understated symptom as it can cause considerable distress and an unfavourable appearance for the sufferer.

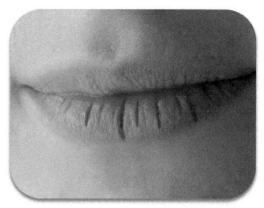

There may be many contributory causes for chapped lips, ranging from dehydration to the dry air in hospitals, but the most likely reason is that chemotherapy damages the rapidly dividing basal cells in the deep layers of the skin (vermillion border) of the lips. This means that it does not grow fast enough to replace skin which is shed or rubbed off through everyday activities such as eating, speaking and breathing. The lips consequently become thin and vulnerable. On top of this, between chemotherapy cycles the skin-producing cells recover but can then go into overdrive, producing too many skin cells which pile up and thus cause scaling and cracking, leading to secondary infection.

Despite being so common, sore lips are generally regarded by medical teams as a trivial condition and are rarely mentioned in patient information materials. Within oncology units, there is very little advice on how to prevent or alleviate lip soreness. During a study of 100 individuals at the Primrose Unit, 30% said they developed troublesome sore lips – more than double the incidence reported among the general population. Over 80% of these individuals used petroleum-based lip balms, and only 10% reported that they were helpful. The other 20% used natural oil-based creams and a far more encouraging 60% reported a benefit.

There appeared to be an association between sore lips and cold sores, as 82% of the patients who were prone to cold sores were 2.5 times more likely to have regular episodes of chapped lips, suggesting that preventing chapped lips may also prevent cold sore episodes. Patients who developed cold sores during chemotherapy said the episodes

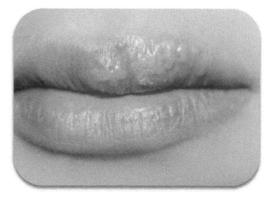

were worse than normal for them. Other strategies to prevent an attack of cold sores have so far been unsuccessful, but topical or systemic anti-viral agents such as acyclovir or valacyclovir have been shown to shorten the length of the attack if used early in an episode.

What can be done to help?

Basic preventative precautions listed below are encourgaed before the start of chemotherapy to prevent soreness from happening in the first place. It is always more difficult to treat chapped lips once they have started. The trial mentioned above suggested that a natural oil-based balm is likely to help, but ensure it is made from natural oil bases such as olive oil and shea butter, rather than petroleum, and has anti-inflammatory essential oils rather than perfumes and colours. It's also important that there are very low concentrations of botanicals, as in many natural balms levels are too high which can also cause irritation. An ideal cream can be found on the keep-healthy.com website.

There is an association between chapped lips brought on by chemotherapy and exacerbation of cold sores, so it may be worth applying topical anti-virals after each chemotherapy cycle if there is a history of cold sores. Also, ask for a prescription of oral and topical antivirals which can be dispensed from the chemist and used as soon as the tell-tail tingling starts.

Summary - Advice to help avoid chapped lips and cold sores

- Avoid dehydration – drink regularly and often (unsweetened drinks)
- Avoid licking and rubbing the lips
- Avoid wind, as well as excessive cold and sunlight
- Apply a sunblock when walking, cycling, skiing or running
- If you have a history of chapped lips, apply salves more often
- If you are prone to cold sores, apply salves more often
- If prone to cold sores, ask for an antiviral prescription
- Apply topical antivirals and start tablets as soon as the signs appear
- Natural oil-based salves are preferable to petroleum-based salves
- Avoid salves with colours, perfumes, hydrocarbons or preservatives

Nail damage and chemotherapy

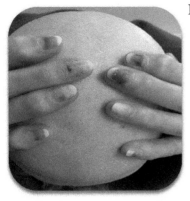

Distressing nail damage can occur in up to 44% of patients receiving chemo, especially during regimens which contain taxanes, commonly used for breast, lung and prostate cancer. Nail damage is often unsightly and affects body image. More serious consequences include pain, interference with activities of daily living and secondary infection, a particular concern if patients are also neutropenic as this could be a source of systemic infection.

Damage typically starts after the second and third cycles and gets worse as chemo progresses. It begins with a burning sensation under the nail beds and patients often initially describe their nails as being hot, uncomfortable and oversensitive. In most cases, the first visible signs of damage are ridges in the nails that correspond to the timings of chemotherapy episodes, known as Beau's lines. This can be associated with some brittleness and

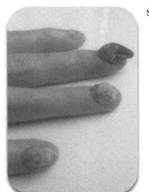

splitting of the nails but fortunately, once chemo has finished, the damage, although unsightly, grows out, leaving normal nails. More pronounced nail damage can lead to discolouration, painful subungual haemorrhages and distortion. Later, if the damage is marked, the nails can separate from the bed, causing considerable pain as well as secondary bacterial and fungal infections. If secondary infection sets in, the surrounding and underlying skin becomes red, inflamed and seeps pus.

Chemotherapy-induced nail damage (onycholysis) is caused by disorganised inhibition of the rapidly dividing cells in the nail bed. Further damage is thought to be caused by the blood vessel and nerve damaging properties of taxanes, which trigger an excess local inflammatory reaction. The secondary bacterial and fungal pathogens which enter the nail beds after disruption of the normal anatomy cause further damage.

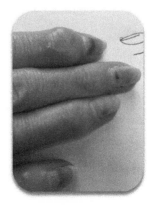

A variety of anecdotal strategies are recommended to patients during chemotherapy. The Primrose oncology unit published a report highlighting how cooling the nail bed with pots of iced water helps to reduce the severity of damage. Cooling gloves are commercially available but are not popular with nurses as they cover the veins of the hands and prevent assessment of the patient's extremities.

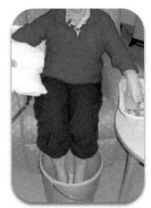

Many patient advocacy groups suggest wearing dark nail varnish, despite no evidence in support of this and the knowledge that nail polish removers dry the nails and cause further damage. Others recommend massaging moisturising balms into the nail bed, on the assumptions that it may prevent splitting and damage. Unfortunately, there are no studies to support this practice, and most patients use petroleum-based balm which may actually be irritating. Once nail damage has set in, soaking fingers and toes regularly in salt water, keeping them as clean as possible and avoiding trauma may help until the nails start to fall off.

The development of Polybalm

Given the lack of practical measures to prevent or relieve nail damage, a scientific committee was established to design a potential solution. The committee consisted of oncologists, nurses, a dermatologist and a herbalist. It collaborated closely with advisors from the Department of Biological science at Coventry University and liaised with the UK Government funded National Cancer Research Institute behavioral change committee. Over 18 months, the laboratory

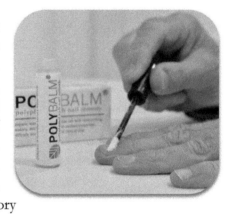

and clinical data from standard and traditional medical studies was critically reviewed before the choice of the blend of oils and waxes natural oils decided. The oils were

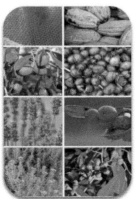

steam extracted from plants, before being gently blended to avoid overheating in order to maintain their rich phytochemical content. It was important that the balm contained no preservatives, parabens, petroleum or perfumes which could have potentially irritated the nail beds. It consisted of wax bases of unrefined shea butter (Butyrospermum parkii); organic beeswax (Cera alba); extra virgin, organic, cold-pressed olive oil; Organic cocoa seed butter (Theobroma cacao). The added essential oils included African sage (Tarchonanthus camphoratus); Wintergreen leaf (Gaultheria procumbens); Lavender flower (Lavandula spica); Eucalyptus leaf (Eucalyptus globulus).

These ingredients are particularly rich in phytochemicals, especially the phenolic 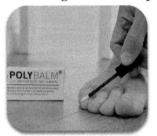 polyphenols group, which, in addition to their ability to moisturise the skin and prevent drying, splitting or cracking of the nail, also have anti-inflammatory, DNA repair and anti-oxidant properties. It was hypothesised that oils with these properties, applied locally to the nail bed, would be absorbed and act as a local antidote to the chemotherapy, preventing damage to the proliferating stem cells. Additionally, their anti-microbial properties would help prevent secondary infection. By including different plant extracts, each with a range of phytochemicals, it was felt that their different modes of action would have a synergistic effect.

The Polybalm trial: Sixty men and women receiving chemo for breast or prostate cancer were randomised to either Polybalm or a simple placebo moisturising balm to apply to their nail beds twice a day. The trial was a double-blind design, so none of the patients, doctors, research team or statistician knew which balm was assigned to which participant. Both groups were given general advice on

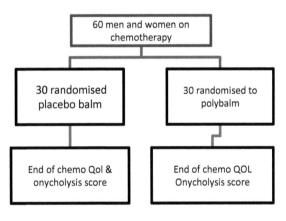

how to protect their nails during chemotherapy. An information video demonstrated how to apply the balm onto the nail beds of the hand and the feet (see polybalm.com). The balm was commissioned specifically for a study, was produced by a UK manufacturer. Its quality assurance, stability and microbial tests were performed by an additional laboratory in order to comply with EU standards.

Trial measurements and outcomes: The health of the nails were measured by four validated independent tools. Patients recorded their own nail health with a Dermatology questionnaire, plus a simple linear severity scale that emphasised how the nail damage affected their daily activities and quality of life. Physicians recorded the physical condition of the nails using the national Nail Psoriasis Index. Photographs of the nails were also sent to three doctors from other hospitals for further independent verification.

Trial results: In all but 2 of the 30 patients in the Polybalm group, there was no troublesome nail damage, and only 4 reported minor asymptomatic ridging. More than half in the placebo group suffered significant damage and distress. Nail quality was eighty times better in the Polybalm group, and formal, independent statistical analysis stated this difference had a 10,000 to one probability of happening by chance. One of the patients using Polybalm actually felt that the condition of their nails improved despite the chemo.

Conclusion: The polyphenol-rich essential oils and plant-based waxes in this balm were sufficiently absorbed into the nail beds, to enabling their bioactive properties to protect them from the harmful effects of chemo. This resulted in profoundly reduced chemo-related nail damage and improved nail-related quality of life compared to a plain petroleum-based balm. Although this was a scientific evaluation, the regulatory authority class these products as a biocosmetic, meaning it cannot be prescribed by doctors. The balm, however, is now distributed by an independent organisation via the website polybalm.com.

Other condition: Since this initial landmark trial, the balm is being investigated for other conditions which effect nails including psoriasis, distortion caused by chronic fungal infection after numerous anecdotal reports of benefit from individuals who have used it. In particular, one man from Germany who send in the adjacent 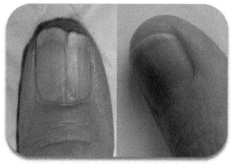 photograph. He had been to three dermatologist for a longitudinal split in his nail which was unsightly and caught on his clothes and was told nothing could be done. Within 4 months of using Polybalm the ridge resolved.

Summary - Tips for nail damage during chemotherapy

- Keep nails clean and cut short
- Avoid trauma, so protect them when washing dishes or gardening
- After chemotherapy, keep the nails cool for 2-4 hours
- Between cycles avoid excessive cold - wear gloves in the winter
- Moisturise the nails beds with Polybalm before and during treatment
- Stop smoking
- Avoid nail varnish remover
- There is no evidence for wearing dark nail varnish – so best avoid
- Eat a healthy diet

Chemotherapy nerve damage

Certain types of chemotherapy agents can damage the nerves. In most cases, symptoms tend to start away from the head (fingers and toes) but move closer over time, which is why the condition is referred to as chemotherapy-induced peripheral neuropathy (CIPN). When affecting both hands and both feet, it has a stocking-glove distribution. CIPN can begin at any time after treatment starts and often gets worse as treatments go on. Typical symptoms include:

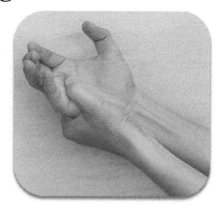

- Shooting or stabbing pain
- Distressing burning (hyperaesthesia)
- Pins and needles or an electric shock-like sensation
- A feeling of walking on cobblestones
- Numbness or a reduced ability to sense pressure and touch
- Increased sensitivity to heat or cold

CIPN can affect your ability to write, button up shirts, pick up coins, play a musical instrument and even walk. In advanced cases, it can increase the risk of falls because it impairs spatial awareness (especially in the dark or with the eyes closed). Many drugs can cause this distressing symptom, particularly:

- Paclitaxel, docetaxel and cabazitaxel, carboplatin, cisplatin and oxaliplatin,
- Eribulin vinblastine, vincristine, vinorelbine, and etoposide
- Bortezomib and carfilzomib

Factors that increase the risk of CIPN
- Increasing age
- Having other medical conditions such as; Diabetes, HIV infection, Vitamin B deficiency and excess alcohol intake and autoimmune conditions
- The cancer itself can cause nerve damage
- Ciprofloxacin antibiotics (often given with chemotherapy)

What can be done to help?

Talk to your doctor or nurse right away about any symptoms of CIPN that you might have. They will want to exclude and treat other causes of neuropathy which may be aggravating the CIPN. Otherwise, they may reduce the dose or stop chemotherapy altogether. Sometimes, extending the duration of the infusion, or giving it in small frequent doses rather than one big one every three weeks, can help - you could ask your oncologist about the practicalities of doing this. Calcium, magnesium, vitamin E and glutathione, have previously been reported to help symptoms, although any apparent benefit from these substances has since been discredited. If pain is a problem, your doctor may offer you anti-neuralgia drugs such as gabapentin, anticonvulsants such as carbamazepine or antidepressants such as venlafaxine. Unfortunately, the likely benefits from these are often small.

Diet: Ensure a adequate intake of vitamin B rich foods to avoid deficiency, and it is also best to stop drinking alcohol until symptoms are resolved.

Acupuncture: Two small trials have reported benefits and there have been no cases of harm. So if other measures have failed it may be worth signing up for a course. Most GP's will have a list of registered practitioners or more information can be found on the British Medical Acupuncture Society website (www.thwbmas.com).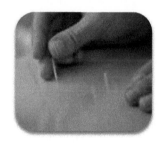

Exercise: A cohort study from Holland, examined the data of 1,648 colorectal cancer survivors and found that those who undertook at least 150 minutes of moderate to vigorous exercise per week experienced fewer of these symptoms. A controlled trial from Germany saw 355 patients, receiving either taxanes or platinum-based chemotherapy regimens, being randomised to receive either an exercise intervention or standard care. They found a significantly lower level of tingling and numbness in the exercise group. A trial from the USA involved 230 women receiving chemotherapy being randomised and given either a supervised high-intensity exercise regimen, a home-based self-initiated regimen or standard care. Despite the burden of chemotherapy, women in the intense exercise regimen had less fatigue, less nausea, greater muscle strength and reduced CIPN.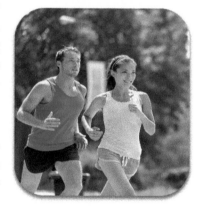

CBD oils: Two RCTs have been conducted looking at the impact of inhaled oils on patients with peripheral neuropathy or neuropathic pain. Both found that pain was reduced among those who used the oils, compared to placebo. Two additional trials of inhaled cannabis have also demonstrated a benefit in HIV-associated neuropathic pain. There has not been a study specifically involving participants with CIPN but, as CBD oils are often well tolerated, it would be worth a try.

Managing hair loss

Chemotherapy often causes hair loss (alopecia) because it damages the fast-growing cells in the hair follicles. Hair loss is usually not permanent and will grow back once your treatment has ended, although it may be slightly different from before in terms of colour (more grey) and texture (finer and curlier). With radiotherapy, hair loss occurs in the treated area only, and it may be permanent. Some people experience hair thinning with hormone drugs when it is not 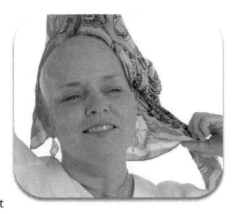 expected. Not all chemotherapy agents cause hair loss, some just cause thinning, while others cause dramatic hair loss, including body hair and eyebrows. People have different tolerances to the drugs but the ones more likely to cause alopecia should have been explained when consenting for treatments and include:

- Adriamycin, epirubicin, paclitaxel, docetaxel, cyclophosphamide, ifosfamide
- Etoposide, vinorelbine, topotecan

What can help?

Cold caps: The availability and types of cold cap vary between units. The cap is put on before chemotherapy and is kept on for up to 1-2 hours afterwards. Not everyone can tolerate wearing the cold cap and wearing it has no bearing on the outcome of treatment. In some situations (e.g. leukaemia), doctors may advise against it.

Wigs and head scarfs: There are a wide variety of wigs and headscarves available from most oncology centres. Wigs can be made from either synthetic hair, human hair or a combination of both. Wigs made from human hair often require a specialist shampoo and set, whereas synthetic ones can be shampooed at home and, when dry, fall naturally into place. They are also considerably cheaper than human hair wigs.

Hair loss can start at any time after chemo. It usually begins growing back within a few weeks of the last cycle of chemotherapy but can surprise many people when it starts growing back before that. Don't be concerned - this does not mean the chemo is not working. If the hair does not grow back after chemotherapy has finished, it may be worth asking for an appointment with a dermatologist as there may be other causes such as hereditary pre-disposition hormone imbalances such as an excess of testosterone, thyroid disorders or aberrant mineral fatty acid levels.

Summary - Advice for coping with hair loss

- Before undergoing treatment, your hair can be cut into a shorter style
- Thinning hair causes an itchy scalp – try cool showers, moisturising
- Avoid harsh chemicals and shampoos - they increase discomfort
- A perm should be avoided for at least six months after treatment
- Avoid irritating and scratching your scalp, use a soft hairbrush
- Cotton is a good alternative to nylon pillowcases which may irritate
- Hairdryers and rollers can damage brittle hair, avoid sleeping with rollers
- If some long stringy hairs remain on your scalp, cut them off
- As your hair starts growing, clip it short - it grows back the same length

Wearing a wig:
- A well-fitted wig should stay in place by itself. If not, consider replacing
- If a little loose, hypo-allergenic double-sided tape is available
- If the lining irritates your scalp, wear a thin cotton skullcap underneath
- Your wig may need to be adjusted as more hair is lost

If hair does not grow back after chemotherapy:
- Measure hormone, thyroid, mineral and vitamin levels
- Ask for a referral to a dermatologist
- Consider a referral to a private hair clinic

Dupuytren's contracture

This is slow growing chronic inflammatory thickening on the palm of the hand that eventually creates a deformity starting in the ring and little finger. The skin on the palm initially appears puckered or dimpled, before a painless firm lump of tissue forms. In later stages, cords of tissue form under the skin and extend up to the fingers. As these cords tighten, the fingers are pulled toward your palm, sometimes severely. Once this occurs, the fingers affected can't be 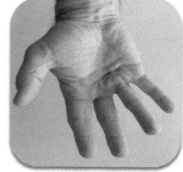 straightened completely, which can complicate everyday activities such as placing hands in your pockets, putting on gloves or shaking hands.

The exact reason why Dupuytren's occurs is unknown, but it's a local chronic inflammatory process and is more common in:

- Older age and mainly men of Scandinavian ancestry or other family history
- Long term hormone therapies such as aromatase inhibitors
- Other medication such as phenytoin for epilepsy
- Smoking and alcohol intake or other Pro-inflammatory habits

Medical treatment are detailed on the website keep-healthy.com and include:

- Needling to puncture the cord of tissue that's contracting a finger.
- Injections of an enzyme, collagenase clostridium histolyticum
- Local radiotherapy or surgery

Lifestyle and self-help strategies

As soon as signs of Dupuytren's appear, lifestyle strategies will prevent it progressing to a troublesome form. In fact, my contracture, which started 15 years ago, has actually improved which regular attention, despite close relatives, over the same time period, progressing to needing painful surgery. Here is what helps:

Stretching: This should be performed 2- 3 a day but do not overstretch and cause pain. Gently bend your fingers backward from your palm. With your fingers on the edge of a table, palm down, lift the palm upward gradually, keeping your fingers flat. Rotate the wrist from side to side. Put your hand in a prayer position pushing the palms and fingers together (see video on keep-healthy.com).

Massage with natural oils: Before stretching, warm up your hands in water or with a heat pack. Use a balm without scents, hydrocarbons and preservatives which may have an irritative effect. A specifically designed plant-based balm is available on keep-health.com.

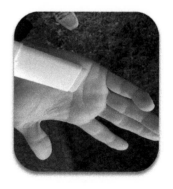

Protect your hands: Avoid a tight grip on tools by building up the handles with pipe foam or cushion tape. Use gloves when gardening.

Reduce inflammation in the body: The earlier chapter explains the importance of avoiding pro-inflammatory activities like smoking, eating chargrilled meat and excess alcohol and sugar. Exercise, eating omega fats and polyphenols, and ensuring intake of healthy bacteria, all help to enhance anti-inflammatory activities.

Carpal tunnel syndrome

This condition is due to compression of the main nerve as it travels through the wrist into the hand via the narrow carpal tunnel. The main symptoms are pain, numbness and tingling in the thumb, index finger, middle finger and the thumb side of the ring fingers. Symptoms typically start gradually and during the night. Pain often extends back up the arm. Eventually, the muscle supplying the thumb wastes and grip strength deteriorates.

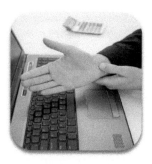

The cause is largely unknown, but chronic inflammation plays a major part and is more common with hormone therapies such as aromatase inhibitors, obesity, underactive thyroid, diabetes, arthritis, and previous trauma to the wrist

Medical treatments include physiotherapy, splinting, steroid injections but eventually surgery can be required

Self-help strategies: As soon as symptoms of carpal tunnel appear, measures should be taken as this will prevent it progressing to the state which causes muscle wasting and permanent pain. The following strategies help.

Stretching: This should be performed 2- 3 times a day and particularly before an activity which normally aggravates symptoms. Do not overstretch and cause pain as this may be counter-productive. Gently bend your hand backwards and forewords, then side to side, then rotate the wrist to the right then the left. Hold each turn for two seconds, adding a stretch in each direction. Try to do these with the arm elevated (the hand above

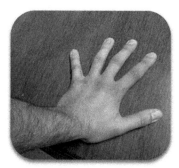

the level of the head). Another useful stretch is to put the hand flat on a desk and lean forward until a stretch is felt – repeat 10 times (see video on keep-healthy.com).

Massage wrist with natural oils: As with Dupuytren's, use a balm without scents, hydrocarbons and preservatives, all of which may have an irritative effect. The same natural plant-based balms mentioned above would be ideal.

Reduce inflammation in the body: Avoid smoking, eating chargrilled meat and excess alcohol and sugar. Take more exercise, eat omega fats and polyphenol-rich foods, and ensure high levels of healthy bacteria.

Chapter 7

Breast care after cancer

With Gillian Horton

Advancements in breast surgery and radiotherapy have reduced complications. Better preoperative imagery, such as MRI, has helped improve decision making over which type of surgery is needed. Chemo, hormones, Herceptin, pertuzumab for HER +ve, and PARP inhibitors such as olaparib for triple –ve, are now more frequently given before surgery (neoadjuvant), enabling more women to have a lumpectomy and avoiding mastectomy. For the armpit, testing one or two sentinel nodes has lessened the number of women requiring more extensive surgery (axillary clearance). Technical improvements in radiotherapy have evened out the dose across the breast, reducing skin reactions and avoiding hot spots which can lead to tissue damage. Despite these technical improvements, some issues, which will be covered in this chapter, include breast tenderness, lymphoedema and issues with bras

Breast tenderness

Some women have persistent breast pain or tenderness after treatment. There are a number of different underlying causes which produce a variety of different types of pain. The tumour itself, along with surgery, would have disrupted the normal architecture of the breast, disturbing the flow of fluid around it. This causes a throbbing, aching discomfort, but it also makes the breast heavier and hotter, straining the underlying muscles. Surgery also cuts the minor

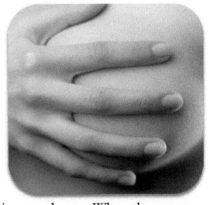

nerves in the breast and under the arm, often causing numbness. When these nerves attempt to repair themselves, the numbness usually gives way to a burning-type pain (hyperaesthesia) which can last for several years. As well as all this, the disrupted nerves often send sharp, jabbing pains into the breast. Some of these pains can be fluctuate at different times of the month even if the periods have finished. These neuralgic pains may only last seconds, but they are enough to make your toes curl! If these neuralgic pains get severe, medication, such as gabapentin, can be prescribed. During radiotherapy, the skin can become red and itchy and, in the long-term, treatment can contribute to the underlying thickening and fibrosis of the tissues, especially in smokers.

What can you do to help?

Whatever the cause of the breast pains, it's important to diminish the scars and fibrosis between the breast tissue and the surrounding tissues. Avoiding trauma, stopping smoking and wearing a comfortable, well-fitted bra are sensible measures. More specific strategies involve:

- Local exercises and stretches
- Local massage
- Lifestyle measures to reduce inflammation

Exercise and stretching, if performed regularly, will improve the blood supply, aid lymphatic drainage, and improve the mobility, flexibility and compliance of the breast tissue, skin and the underlying muscle, nerves and ribs. It is important to realise that this is a slow process. Most people give up stretching and exercising after 6 weeks if they cannot feel a benefit, but clinical trials show us that improvements are usually only noticed several months later. After surgery, moving your arm or upper chest is often associated with an aggravation of pain because the tissues do not glide smoothly across each other. However, over time this discomfort will ease especially if the exercises described below are continued long term.

Local massage: Gently massaging the breast and armpit will help break down fibrosis tissue and improve mobility between the breast tissue and muscles of the chest wall. When doing this, it's important not to use creams or oils with oestrogenic properties and there is evidence that these can be absorbed. The chemicals of concern, include aluminium (a metaloestrogen) which is responsible for the anti-sweating effect of antidepressants, and parabens which are included as preservatives. Both aluminum and parabens have been shown to increase chronic inflammation, alter gene expression, stimulate angiogenesis and cancer invasion in lab rats. More relevant to breast cancer, they have been shown to have xeno-oestrogenic effects which stimulate normal breast cells to grow faster. chemicals commonly found in cosmetics, topical creams, gels and shampoos, which may have weak oestrogenic and negative effects, include:

- phthalate esters in moisturisers and plasticisers
- polycyclic musks, nitromusks and benzyl benzoate in fragrances
- triclosan - a preservative used in fragrances, toothpastes and cosmetics
- UV light filter chemicals - benzophenones, octyl-methoxycinnamate
- camphor, octamethylcyclotetrasilazane as conditioning agents

General measures to reduce inflammation: It would be useful to reduce the amount of chronic inflammation in your body by reducing exposure to harmful chemicals and adopting the anti-inflammatory lifestyle tips summaries below.

Summary – Tips to help breast tenderness

Local measures:

- Regularly perform local breast shoulder and neck exercises
- Consider physiotherapy if self-help measures fail
- Consider medication for neuralgic (shooting) pains
- Improve your fitness, but wear a good fitting bra when exercising
- Gently massage your breast and armpit with olive-based natural oils

Breast and skin care with radiotherapy

Radiotherapy will only affect your skin in the treated area. Most regimens cause no obvious skin damage as advances in techniques have significantly reduced the dose of radiotherapy to the skin. The area's most likely to be affected are the head and neck, skin creases such as under the breast, the groin and between the buttocks.

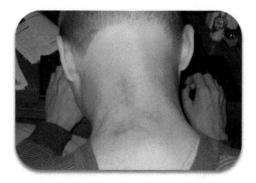

Radiotherapy side effects can occur during treatment (acute), or come later and be life-long (late). Acute skin reactions may make your skin red, itchy and dry. If severe, however, the skin may break down and form superficial ulcers, known as moist desquamation. In this situation, the skin can sometimes develop a secondary fungal or bacterial infection and treatment should be considered if the reaction is inappropriately severe or the redness spreads outside the actual treated area. In the vast majority of cases, the skin heals completely and returns to normal, albeit with some reduced hair and sweat formation. Long-term damage may occur, and the skin may become thin, developing small, abnormal blood vessels (telangiectasia).

What can you do to help?

All patients should be given the skin care guidance, summarised in the table below. During radiotherapy, moisturising may improve the condition of the skin. It is particularly important not to rub or scratch the area even though you will be very tempted. If the itching becomes unbearable, you should report this to your medical team who can prescribe a mild steroid ointment. If the skin worsens before the end of the radiotherapy, the dose or technique can be modified. Otherwise, anti-fungal cream can be prescribed or, if there are signs of a bacterial infection, antibiotics can be taken. The skin care guidelines listed in the box below will help limit damage to the skin as the treatment progresses.

Smoking during radiotherapy will significantly increase the chance of an acute skin reaction. If patients cannot give up completely, they should, at the very least, avoid smoking four hours before the radiotherapy and four hours after. This will reduce levels of harmful smoke chemicals at the time of radiotherapy.

Moisturising the skin helps during radiotherapy and gives patients a focus, especially if creams are kept in the fridge as the cooling effect provides some relief. Many radiotherapy centres advocate aqueous cream or products similar to E45. These are non-perfumed and regarded as 'simple'. No trial has shown they are harmful but, on the other hand, no trial has shown they are any better than using nothing at all.

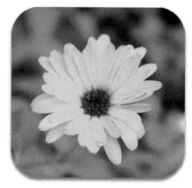

Botanical creams: In general, be cautious of using creams with high concentrations of additives (even if labelled natural) unless they have been tested as they could make the skin worse. There have been a number of trials comparing Aloe Vera-containing creams with aqueous cream, most of which demonstrated little difference between the two, while one study showed it actually made the skin reaction worse. As a consequence, Aloe Vera creams or gels are not recommended despite their anti-inflammatory properties. A calendula (marigold) cream called Trolamine, commonly used in France, has been shown to be effective at reducing moderate-to-severe dermatitis when compared to a standard moisturising cream. Creams containing calendula are not generally supplied in UK oncology units but can be bought online. Another randomised trial involving 50 patients with head and neck cancer found a cream containing turmeric and sandalwood oil both reduced dermatitis and significantly improved the time it took for the skin to improve after radiotherapy.

Emollient creams: such as Xonrid gel have been shown in scientific studies to relieve the burning and itching experienced with radiation dermatitis. It has been granted FDA approval and helps to maintain a moist wound and skin environment beneficial to the healing process.

In the long-term, certain lifestyle measures can improve the quality of the skin and underlying tissues. A healthy diet of fruit and vegetables, rich in vitamins and polyphenols, is important in order to protect your skin from both further damage and increased skin cancer risk. Smoking, in particular, increases the thickness of the skin (fibrosis) and contributes to on-going pain and lymphoedema in the areas affected. General exercise improves whole body well-being and will have a beneficial impact on the skin. Specific daily exercises and stretches relevant to the area of the body irradiated will help prevent fibrosis and damage to the blood vessels in the underlying muscles, tendons and joints. Olive oil applied directly to the skin can offer 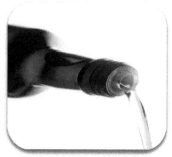 protection after radiotherapy. It has strong antioxidant and skin-protecting properties and is capable of reducing the risk of skin cancers, skin wrinkling and ageing. A good tip is to buy a high quality natural oil-based moisturising cream and then add some extra virgin olive oil yourself. Mixing these together into a paste, applying to the skin and massaging for 5-10 minutes before a shower or bath will leave the skin soft and smooth.

Summary – Advice to help the skin during radiotherapy

During radiotherapy

- Gently wash skin in warm water with a mild, non-perfumed soap
- Do not use a washcloth bubble bath; use a mild detergents only
- Air dry or dab the skin with a soft, clean towel
- Wear loose-fitting natural clothing such as cotton
- Avoid friction in the treated area e.g. rubbing, scratching
- Avoid the use of adhesive tape (e.g. Elastoplast) in the treated area
- Avoid extremes of heat in the area e.g. ice packs, hot water bottles
- Moisturising creams (aqueous cream or E45) may help
- Applying olive oil before a shower or bath is sensible
- Consider a calendula or turmeric and sandalwood oil-based cream
- Avoid using aftershave, perfume, deodorant and makeup in the area
- Avoid swimming in a chlorinated pool during radiotherapy treatment
- Eat a healthy diet, do not smoke

To reduce the risk of long-term damage after radiotherapy

- Stop smoking, eat a healthy balanced diet, avoiding excessive alcohol
- Exercise frequently and regularly stretch the tissues in the treated area
- Avoid sunburn in the treated area
- Massage olive oil-based creams into the treated area before a shower

Exercise after breast surgery and radiotherapy

The types of exercises depend on how recent surgery was and whether complications have developed. Done properly, they can speed up recovery, reduce pain and fibrous tissue in the armpit, help prevent lymphoedema and reduce the risk of breast pain. The following may be helpful:

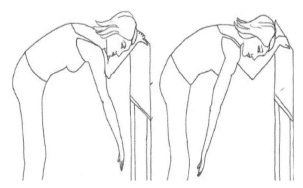

The monkey swing: This exercise is for the first few days after surgery. Stand squarely and bend forward at the waist leaning on a chair/table. Circle entire arm clockwise, then anti-clockwise. Swing forwards and backwards. Swing arm sideways, away from the body, and back again.

Walk the wall: Stand straight facing a wall. Stretch upright as far as comfortable. Place your hands on the wall, ensuring a comfortable stance. Walk your hands up then down the wall. Repeat ten times.

The fan: Put your hands out horizontally in front of your body. Take them up above your head as far as possible. Drop them down to the waist.

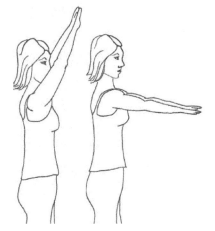

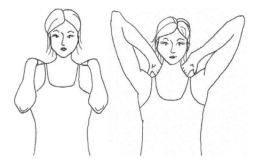

Small bird: Place your hands on your shoulders (or at the level of your shoulders). Move the elbows forwards and upwards, then down and inwards. This should look like a small bird flapping its wings slowly. Repeat each movement ten times.

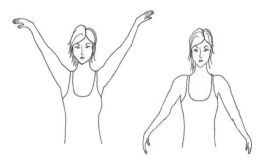

Big bird: Place arms by the side of your body, standing upright. Raise and lower your straight arms as high as possible. This should look like a big bird flapping its wings slowly. Repeat ten times.

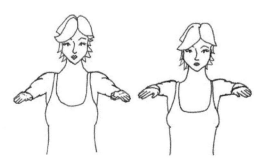

Show me the money (front): Raise the arms straight out to the front of your body, from the shoulders. Rotate the palms of your hands to face upwards then down. Repeat ten times This should look like asking for money to be put in the hand.

Finger walking (neck): Stand straight, with your head slightly bent forward. Take each hand to the back of your neck alternately. Walk fingers down your spine as far as comfortable. Walk them back up to your head. Repeat ten times.

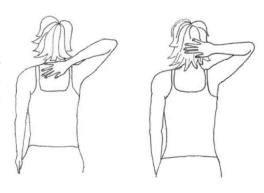

Finger walking (back): Stand straight, with your head slightly bent forward. Take each hand to the lower back alternately. Walk fingers down your spine as far as comfortable. Walk them back up to your head. Repeat ten times.

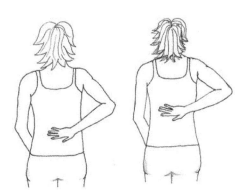

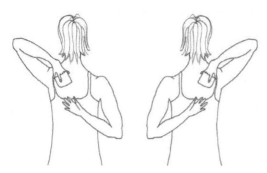

The hand over: Put your right hand behind your back. Pass a small, light object across your back, over your left shoulder to the other hand. Repeat and swap hands. The ability to do this may depend on previous flexibility.

In addition to these exercises and stretches, which concentrate on the chest and shoulders, it is worth considering the neck exercises described in the joint pains section below. Furthermore, generally exercising the whole body will help recovery from the surgery, reduce the risk of blood clots, improve overall well-being and reduce the risk of cancer returning.

Neck and shoulder exercises

Neck stiffness is fairly common following cancer therapies. Steroids may have impaired core strength and posture, chemotherapy, while some hormonal therapies can generally cause joint discomfort, particularly with aromatase inhibitors. During radiotherapy,

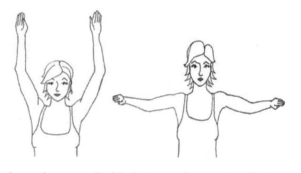

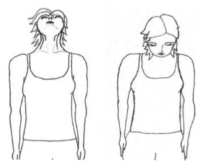

patients have to hold their neck straight during treatments which can cause some stiffness. Finally, as we all get older, our necks become very prone to stiffness and pain. The neck consists of complex series of joints which, if weakened or inflamed, can lead to muscle spasm, pains down the arms and discomfort radiating up the back of the head – a not infrequent cause of headaches.

Exercise 1: Stand straight and as upright as possible, stretching your arms towards the ceiling as high as possible. Hold for 3-4 seconds, then bring your arms to the horizontal position and push your elbows back. At the same time, keep your chin towards your chest – this should arch the upper thoracic spine and straighten your neck. Repeat three times.

Exercise 2: Facing straight ahead, look up as high as possible. Hold for 3-5 seconds and then look down as low as possible. Repeat three times.

122

Exercise 3: Facing straight ahead, turn your head to the right as far as possible (hold for 3-5 seconds), then move it slowly up and down for ten nods. Then turn your head to the left and repeat three times.

Exercise 4: Facing straight ahead, tilt your head to the right, as if trying to put your ear on your shoulder. Hold for three to four seconds, and then repeat on the left. Repeat on both sides three times. It is very important to get into a routine and perform them every day – even if only for 10 minutes.

These neck stretches can be combined with the breast exercises above, or other good shoulder exercises, such as shrugging. To do this, sit or stand squarely. Bring your shoulders up towards your ear. Relax and repeat. Sink your shoulders downwards.

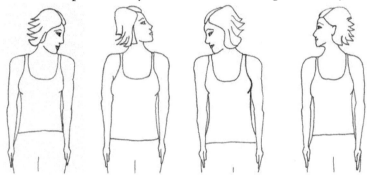

Relax and repeat. Ease shoulders forwards. Relax and repeat. Pull shoulders back. Relax and repeat each movement five-ten times. It is also a good idea to perform neck exercises in front of the mirror in order to achieve the optimal posture.

The effect of head posture: The weight of the average adult's head is between four and five kilograms, but when it is tilted forward its effective weight increases, placing greater pressure on the neck. A 30-degree tilt of the head, commonly done when writing a text message on a phone or working on a laptop, is the equivalent

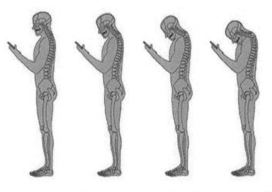

of holding 18 kilograms of weight. This exaggerated yet common head position will increase chronic musculoskeletal pain, especially after cancer, so it's important to be aware of the neck position and try to spend less time on electronic devices.

Massage: Gentle manipulation of the breast and surrounding skin can help to stimulate blood supply and break down adhesions. Although this should be avoided during radiotherapy when the skin may sensitive, there is no evidence at all that massage is harmful or should be avoided after cancer. Use a natural oil, such as extra virgin olive oil, rather than commercial oils containing perfumes and additives. Apply the oil with the fingers gently, trying to roll the skin over the ribs – you should be as firm as possible but without causing any pain or bruising as this would be counter-productive. At first, there will not be any noticeable improvement, but with daily persistence the pain and mobility will improve.

Lymphoedema

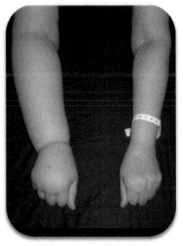

To understand how lymphoedema occurs, it is helpful to know a bit about the lymphatic system. Your body's tissues are bathed in lymph, a slightly yellowish, watery fluid. Lymph travels along tiny channels called lymph vessels or lymphatics which, like blood vessels, join together to form larger channels. Eventually, lymph is filtered through a number of lymph nodes before draining into the bloodstream. The job of the lymphatic system and the nodes is to collect and filter out unhealthy matter such as bacteria, other micro-organisms and cancer cells. These are carried in lymph through the nodes, where the lymphocytes will try to attack and break them down before they are carried away by the bloodstream and filtered out along with other body waste. If lymph nodes trap an infection or cancer, they will usually swell. With infection, the swollen nodes are usually hot, painful and tender to touch. With cancer, however, the nodes are often painless and do not cause any discomfort when touched.

The presence of cancer in the lymph nodes of the armpit is the most important prognostic factor in breast cancer, and thus the removal and evaluation of these lymph nodes are integral components of breast cancer management. However, removal of the lymph nodes can result in a number of side-effects, including lymphoedema. The more lymph nodes that are removed, the higher the risk of developing the condition. Fortunately, the risk of lymphoedema is significantly less with the development of better surgical techniques such as sentinel node biopsy.

Lymphoedema usually manifests as a swelling to the affected arm, but can also occur in the hand, trunk and breast. It can develop immediately or many years after treatment. Whenever it develops, lymphoedema is a chronic, debilitating condition that can cause severe physical and psychological morbidity as well as a reduction in quality of life. If you have lymphoedema, you should be referred to a specialist unit for evaluation and therapy, which will include the fitting of compression garments and sleeves. Massage is an important part of the treatment of lymphoedema, but it is essential to use the correct technique. Deep, firm massage, for example, is harmful as it stimulates blood flow and increases the amount of fluid produced. The aim of massage is to stimulate or move the excess fluid away from the swollen area so that it can drain away normally. This type of massage is called manual lymphatic drainage, and because it is a specialised form of massage, it should be given by a trained therapist who should be trained in the Vodder, Foldi, Leduc or Casley-Smith method.

What can you do to help?

Various self-help strategies can help prevent and treat lymphoedema. The main interventions include protecting the arm, weight reduction, aerobic exercise, weight lifting, stretching and massage.

Protect the arm: Breaks in the skin can allow bacteria to enter your tissues, leading to infection which can cause lymphoedema to either start or continue to deteriorate if already present. Reduce your risk of scratches and cuts by being aware of this extra risk. For example, if you are washing dishes with a pan scourer, gardening or playing with the cat, always wear gloves. If you shave your 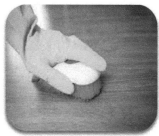 armpits, use an electric razor as there is less chance of nicking or cutting your skin. If you need to have an injection, ask to have the needle inserted in your other arm.

Weight reduction: A study from Royal Marsden Hospital compared women with lymphoedema who had weight loss counselling against a group who continued their normal diet. After the 24-weeks of dietary intervention, there were notable differences in body weight, skinfold thickness and percentage body fat between the control group and both the weight-reduction and low-fat groups. There was a significant reduction in excess arm volume in women who had lost weight. Several other studies have also been published which show that maintaining a healthy weight and avoiding obesity is one way to help avoid and treat lymphoedema.

Stretching: A study published in 2006 compared a group of women who had no intervention with a group who were taught stretching exercises to increase range of motion. Stretching did not make the lymphoedema worse, and the range of movement and comfort improved.

Aerobic exercise: One study found that 2 hours of steady exercise increased lymph clearance rate 2-5-fold. This was supported by a further study which demonstrated increased lymphatic clearance in the hands of healthy women who performed arm crank ergometry for five minutes each day. Vigorous aerobic exercise such as running, group fitness and dance have all been shown to be safe and effective.

Exercise combined with compression garments: Two studies in 2004 reported that anaerobic and resistance exercises while wearing a compression garment demonstrated a reduction in arm volume and no harmful effects were reported.

Weight lifting: A review of the published evidence concerning the safety of weight lifting among ladies with lymphoedema concluded that a wide variety of strenuous exercise can be safely undertaken by those either suffering from or at risk of lymphoedema. The most convincing evidence for the benefits of weight lifting was published in the prestigious New England Journal of Medicine. 141 women were randomised to either 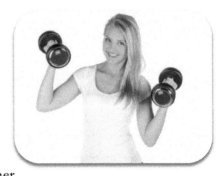 join a control group or take part in a supervised weight lifting programme. They had all received an axillary node clearance or radiotherapy. Both groups received standard lymphoedema advice. The intervention group received twice weekly supervised exercise sessions for six months. Weight lifting started with a warm up and warm down which included particular stretching exercises. The initial weight and escalation was determined at each session by a certified exercise professional. At six months there was a significant difference in the number of lymphoedema flares which required acute intervention (either infection or sudden deterioration in symptoms).

A combination of aerobic and weight lifting exercises are ideal, but there are many other exercises that may help you, depending on your fitness and preferences. What is right for you depends on your agility and general condition. Ideally, seek help from a qualified professional before starting exercise.

Massage: In addition to massage by a lymphoedema specialist, self-massage can be helpful and convenient. The skin should be moved by gentle, circular movements of your fingers (if the skin becomes reddened the movement is too hard). Using your fingers in a relaxed scooping movement, push gently towards the head or the direction of the unaffected side. Start on the non-swollen tissue as close as possible to the swollen area, often in the armpit, then move down the limb. Move the skin across and then release the pressure to allow the skin to come back. Repeat this technique with a slow and gentle rhythm. Start the massage at position one and repeat five times being careful with rings or sharp nails as these could damage the skin. Hand-held massagers, although not as effective as using your hands, are particularly useful for people who have restricted movement of their hands. Aim to use it for at least 15 minutes a day, don't use harsh oils or creams, don't use the heat setting and use a gentle circular movement covering the areas of the body described for self-massage, all the while taking care to avoid abnormal or broken skin.

Summary – Tips to prevent and improve lymphoedema

- Reduce your risk of scratches and cuts that could cause infection
- If you are washing dishes with a brush, always wear rubber gloves
- Be careful with pets and gardening
- If you shave your armpits, an electric razor will avoid nicking the skin
- If you need an injection or blood sample, avoid the at risk arm
- Ensure you are referred to a specialist lymphoedema expert
- Lose weight if overweight, stop smoking if you smoke
- Don't take diuretics (water tablets) for this purpose as they do not help
- Take regular aerobic exercise
- Regularly and gently stretch the shoulder, elbow and wrist of the limb
- Embark on a regular, supervised weight-training programme
- Wear a well-fitting bra (see below)

Finding the right bra

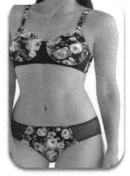

The thought of shopping for bras after breast cancer can fill women with dread. Bra shopping can become a daunting and very emotional task. I (Gillian Horton) remember my first bra and breast form fitting after my mastectomy in 2008. I was filled with trepidation of not knowing what to expect and disappointment at the lack of bra choice. Despite the lack of choice, I felt like me again, something which greatly helped my confidence and self-esteem. Because of this, I established a company dedicated to supplying and fitting bras and swimwear for ladies post breast cancer surgery. I now offer advice based on my experience with hundreds of women who have had various types of breast surgery. Fortunately, the choice of lingerie after surgery has greatly improved, and there are now many styles and colours available.

Prior to surgery, the best place to start is to ask your breast care nurse, surgeon or breast cancer support group for advice on where to buy a post-surgical bra. There are lingerie shops which specialise in after breast surgery bras, swimwear and clothing but these may not be accessible to you depending on where you live. If you cannot visit a store in person, look for online retailers which sell post-surgical bras. Contact them to discuss your needs. Experienced and professional bra fitters should be able to advise on the most suitable bra for your type of surgery. Don't forget to check their returns policy as you may need to order bras in different cup sizes if you are having a reconstruction. The types of bra vary depending on the type of surgery and time after surgery. One which may fit initially may not several months later.

Specific post-surgery bras will not give you the support of your usual bra but will be comfortable following surgery and can also be worn through radiation. They are front fastening with soft cups (wire-free) and no seams. As well as being comfortable, seamless, soft cup bras will stretch over surgical dressings and be less likely to cause irritation at the wound site. The front fastening also allows easier access to the wound dressing. Additionally, bras without back fasteners are more comfortable to sleep in, while not 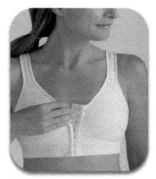 having to reach behind your back for hooks is also an advantage as your arm movements may be restricted after surgery. If you are having a mastectomy, a post-surgical bra which has a pocket either side will allow you to wear a very lightweight breast form (prosthesis) if you wish. This will provide shape until you are ready to be fitted with a silicone breast form.

Breast reconstruction bras provide compression to help the swelling and healing process. A compression bra is front fastening and gives a firmer pressure and more coverage of the breast, back and underarm tissue than a post-surgical bra. Compression over the breast and incision site can help prevent swelling from fluid building up as you recover from your surgery. A good compression bra will hold your skin in place as you heal and prevent it from stretching around the stitches. The front fastening allows access to the wound dressing and makes it easier to put on and take off. Compression bras can also help all types of surgery if there is swelling, a build-up of fluid or lymphoedema.

Bras from six weeks after surgery will be different from those used immediately post-op, although the ideal time for a change depends on the wound site, residual infection and resolution of surgical swelling. Once the swelling has resolved, if your breast size or shape hasn't changed too much it is worth trying the bras you previously wore as these might still be comfortable. However, underwire bras are not recommended for twelve months or longer depending on the initial swelling. In some cases, you may never be able to wear an underwire bra again depending on the location of your surgical scar, effects of radiation or general discomfort.

Bras for the longer term depend on the shape of the breast, type of surgery, any lymphoedema or ongoing discomfort. Bras designed for after breast surgery have a pocket to fit a breast form. The pocket offers greater thickness to the bra cup and prevents nipples showing, something which many women prefer, especially if they only have one nipple. After breast surgery bras should be comfortable, offer support and have the following features:

- Soft, wire-free, cups to prevent irritation of scar tissue
- Wider side bands under arms to help hide surgery scars
- Wider, thicker or padded straps for greater comfort.
- Better designed side seams, helping to prevent lymphoedema
- Cups which offer greater coverage of the breast

Sports bras: Exercise is highly recommended not only after treatment but also during treatment, and finding a good sports bra can make all the difference. Sports bras following surgery should preferably be wire free and offer support which prevents bounce. There are some great front zipping sports bras which will give you good support and prove easy to take on and off.

In conclusion, there are many lingerie options which will allow you to continue to dress the same way as before. The key to comfort is to wear a well-fitting bra.

Summary - Tips for choosing the right bra post-surgery

- One step at a time – there is no rush to be fitted
- Let the swelling after surgery or radiotherapy settle first
- Trust yourself to know when you are emotionally and physically ready
- Take your old bras to your first bra fitting to see if they still fit
- Ask advice from women who have been diagnosed with breast cancer
- Find a lingerie retailer which offers as much choice as possible
- Look for experienced fitters who know and can find what is best for you
- If you don't have a lingerie shop near you, find one online
- Don't be afraid to call them to discuss your needs
- If you feel that you're not being understood, try another retailer
- If you have a dress for a special occasion, take it with you to your fitting
- Once you have the right size, buy a range of bras for:
  - Day to day; during exercise or for special occasions

Soya & phytoestrogenic foods after breast cancer

The two food groups **lignans and isoflavones** which have multiple healthy attributes of their own, but they share a common ability to weakly bind to oestrogen receptors. Because of this, for years, women with breast cancer have missed out on the wonderful benefits offered by these foods, as doctors were concerned that their oestrogenic properties could stimulate breast cancer cells. Research has shown the opposite 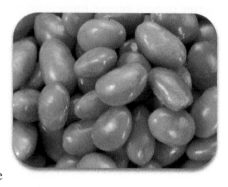 effect. In moderation, they actually reduce the risk of breast and prostate cancer as well as decreasing the risk of relapse after radical treatments.

Lignan polyphenols are found in many healthy foods, particularly in the outer layers of grains and seeds. People who only eat refined grains and seeds with the outer husks removed are likely to have an inadequate intake. Lignin-rich foods include:

- Flaxseeds and sesame seeds, pulses such as beans, lentils and peas
- Pumpkin, sunflower, poppy seeds, quinoa and buckwheat
- Unrefined whole grains such as rye, oats, barley

Isoflavone polyphenols such as genistein and daidzein are found in:

- Fermented soya produce - miso, natto, tempeh
- Unfermented soya produce - tofu, soy milk, soybeans (edamame)
- Peanuts, chickpeas, fava beans, alfalfa, kudzu tea

Several observational studies have reported an association between a regular intake of plant lignans and isoflavones, and a lower risk of developing lifestyle-related diseases such as cardiovascular disease, osteoporosis and cancer, as well as lower menopausal symptoms such as hot flushes. After cancer, soya products, particularly the more easily digested such as fermented 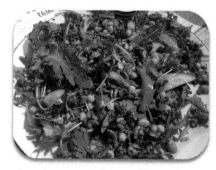 varieties reduce the risk of relapse rate and improve the chances of overall survival. In sensible amounts, phytoestrogens in these foods attach to the oestrogen receptor (ER) but only have weak activity. They consequently dilute the effect of the body's own oestrogen by blocking the receptor. Genistein (from soya) attaches to the ER in the same way as tamoxifen – inhibiting the oestrogen effect on tumours.

Women with breast cancer who had the highest serum lignan levels, reflecting good intake of legumes, cereals, cruciferous vegetables, and soya, were reported to have better overall survival after established cancer than those with the lowest levels. I particular, a major study conducted by the Roswell Park Cancer Institute found that as well as a lower overall breast cancer amoung in regular lignan food consumers, there was a particularly low incidence of the worst types of breast cancers, all of which require more intensive treatments and carry a poorer prognosis. Regular intake was found to decrease the risk of other cancers such as oesophagus and bowel.

Lignan polyphenols may also protect patients from the adverse effects of radiotherapy. A lab study found they reduced radiation, decreasing inflammation, lung injury and eventual fibrosis in mice with cancers. Patients receiving radiotherapy to the rectum have a lower than expected toxicity if they ate lignan-rich foods. However, it's better to avoid foods which produce gas during prostate cancer radiotherapy, as this could change the shape of the rectum and reduce accuracy. Instead, consider foods such as quinoa and flaxseeds rather than pulses and grains.

In terms of what soya products to eat, a large cohort study in 2009 linked a lower risk of prostate cancer with higher consumption of both soya products and non-fermented products such as tofu, soy milk and whole soybeans (edamame), but not fermented products such as miso, natto, and tempeh. Since then, another large meta-analysis concluded that soya and total isoflavone intake was associated with a lower prostate cancer risk among Asians but not men from Western populations. As mentioned above, two large cohort studies, from China and the USA, demonstrated that women with the highest intake of phytoestrogenic polyphenols, isoflavones and flavanones, found in soya and other beans, had a significantly reduced risk of breast cancer recurrence and death from any cause, compared to those with the lowest intake at a median follow-up of 4 years. Similar findings have been observed following a high intake of green tea (containing small amounts of isoflavone) after breast cancer and colorectal cancer.

One analysis of a dataset from California linked a higher total isoflavone intake with a higher prostate cancer risk, yet this data is likely to be influenced by the use of cheap soya products, phytoestrogenic supplements and highly sugared ice tea, which the authors included in the questionnaire as a recognised isoflavone source.

Concerns with phytoestrogenic food supplements
Although phytoestrogenic-rich foods are generally healthy, their benefits are not replicated by phytoestrogenic foods supplements. These supplements were previously promoted by some enthusiasts to help hot flushes and improve prostate health. Well-conducted placebo-controlled studies involving patients with breast

cancer have shown no reduction in hot flushes with phytoestrogenic-rich food supplements. More worryingly, the oestrogenic effect can become overpowered, leading the oestrogen receptor to become stimulated rather than weakly blocked. This was highlighted in an experiment with monkeys which, after being given a high dose of phytoestrogen extract, began to experience a thickening of the uterus after several months, indicating a negative oestrogenic effect. Likewise, a RCT from the Memorial Sloan-Kettering Cancer Centre in New York gave a group of women with early-stage breast cancer either a supplement containing high-dose genistein (the main isoflavone in soya) or a placebo for a period of 30 days prior to surgery. The supplementation was found to induce changes in the expression of 21 genes, potentially leading to increased signals for elevated growth rate. Furthermore, blood serum obtained from women in the supplementation group, added to laboratory tumour cells, caused the tumour cells to proliferate faster.

In men, the data for phytoestrogenic supplements is conflicting. One small crossover RCT found that a dietary supplement containing isoflavone-rich foods, including 60 mg of soya and 15 mg of lycopene among other phytochemicals and antioxidants, administered 4 times a day for treatment periods lasting 10 weeks, significantly delayed PSA progression among men whose PSA relapsed after radical therapies. A subsequent larger study of men with prostate cancer on active surveillance, using mixed isoflavones and other nutraceuticals, reported no effect on PSA. Of some concern, a study involving men with rising PSA after prostate radiotherapy reported no slowing after taking a supplement with high dose genistein, while IGF levels actually went up (a chemical often associated with cancer development).

Saw palmetto: Supplements containing the liposterolic extract from Saw Palmetto are widely rumoured to help prostate health, based on the hypothesis that it has anti-androgenic properties via inhibition of 5α-reductase. However, there are no clinical studies that show any decrease in serum testosterone or prostate-specific antigen after taking saw palmetto extracts. Its efficacy in the treatment of lower urinary tract symptoms has also not been conclusively proven. While several small commercially sponsored studies suggest that Saw Palmetto may help symptoms relating to benign prostatic hypertrophy, larger trials found little or no evidence that it affects prostate enlargement or symptoms. This includes a robust study sponsored by the prestigious National Cancer Institute. This is why this organisation and many others do not recommend supplements containing phytoestrogenic foods and was one of the principal reasons why they were not included in the Pomi-T trial.

Chapter 8

Bone and joint health after cancer

With increasing age, the daily wear and tear on our skeleton leads to bone loss, joint pain and arthritis. After cancer and its treatments, the rate and magnitude of bone and joint problems significantly accelerates. Medical interventions for bone issues are often necessary so monitoring of bone density is important. Lfestyle factors can significantly influence the rate of development, reduce the severity of symptoms, improve physical functioning and prevent fractures

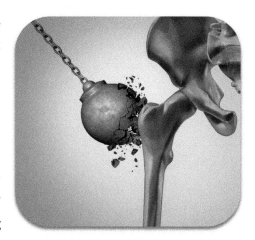

Loss of bone density

Bone is a dynamic organ, continually remodelling itself in response to trauma, weight bearing, exercise and metabolic and environmental processes. A person in space, for example, without the influence of gravity, will develop osteoporosis within 6 weeks. The bony matrix comprises of protein (collagen) and mainly calcium phosphate, with less than 1% consisting of other minerals such as magnesium and zinc. Loss of bone density is a

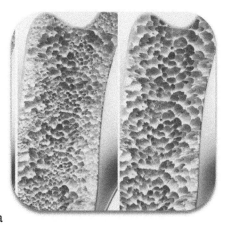

silent disease until the bones start crumbling or breaking, by which point it can be devastating. The three most common osteoporotic fractures occur in the wrist, hip and spine. A crush fracture of the spine can occur suddenly, be very painful and even

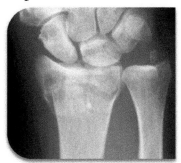
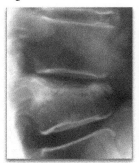
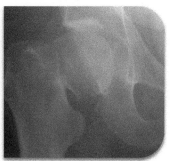

cause nerve damage, while it can also crumble over time, causing deformity and loss of height. Fractures of the hip can lead to hospitalisation and secondary complications which carry a high death risk among the elderly.

Diagnosing bone loss: There are no blood tests available which detect bone loss. It can be seen on a plain x-ray, but the most reliable test is a bone density scan (Dexa). This does not require an injection, is painless and safe as the amount of radiation used is much less than a normal x-ray. Patients lie on a bed for a few minutes, and the machine provides a scale called a T-score:

- 0 to -1 normal
- -1 to -2 osteopenia (mild loss)
- < -2 osteoporosis (significant loss)

What factors affect bone health?
Bone health depends on our age, gender (women are more at risk after menopause), a family history of weak bones, medical conditions, medications and lifestyle factors.

Medical illnesses linked to lower bone density:
- Chronic illnesses that cause disability and make a person less mobile
- Premature menopause or testosterone deficiency
- Diabetes, asthma and rheumatoid arthritis
- Inflammatory bowel diseases, Crohn's disease and ulcerative colitis
- Chronic liver or kidney disease, overactive thyroid disease
- Eating disorders such as anorexia nervosa

Medical interventions which increase the risk of bone loss:
- Surgery or radiotherapy to the ovaries or testis
- Hormones which stop sex hormone production (e.g. Zoladex)
- Aromatase inhibitors for breast cancer (e.g. anastrozole)
- Chemotherapy which damages ovaries
- Chemotherapy directly damaging bones (e.g. methotrexate)
- Biological therapies directly damaging bones (e.g. imatinib, nilotinib)
- Drugs such as phenytoin, warfarin, omeprazole and lansoprazole

Lifestyle factors which increase the risk of bone loss:
- Lack of weight-bearing physical activity
- Too much non-weight-bearing exercise (e.g. cycling)
- Low body weight (BMI<20kg/m^2)
- Drinking more than 3.5 units of alcohol / day
- Smoking, poor gut health, lack of sun exposure
- Calcium and protein poor diets

Interventions for bone loss

Excluding and treating contributory medical conditions is an important first step. The bone health of post-menopausal women can be helped by Hormone Replacement Therapy (HRT) for a limited period, although prolonged use can increase breast cancer risk. It particularly helps women who have been made prematurely post-menopausal by surgery or chemotherapy. If a man has a low testosterone level, he can be given testosterone replacement treatment. Testosterone replacement is usually regarded as unsuitable for men with prostate cancer as it can encourage prostate cancer cells to grow. However, evidence is emerging that correcting a low level in men with low-risk prostate cancer may be appropriate and improve quality of life as well as bone density.

Calcium supplements can help, but there is conflicting information regarding their benefit. One study involving women taking aromatase inhibitors found that high dose vitamin D with calcium helped reduce joint pains. Conversely, a recent comprehensive summary of 59 RCTs concluded that calcium supplements had very little clinical benefit for either improving bone density measurement or decreasing risk of fractures. Of more concern, another comprehensive summary, published in the BMJ, reported calcium supplements were associated with an increase in cardiovascular issues such as angina and heart attacks. Evidence suggests that they should only be taken if someone lacks calcium in their diet or to support bisphosphonates therapies.

Dietary calcium of around 700mg is recommended every day for adults. If you have osteoporosis, it's important to ensure adequate daily calcium by eating one or more portions of these calcium-rich foods:

- Dairy products (milk, cheese, yoghurt)
- Shellfish (oysters, mussels, clams), tinned oily fish with edible bones
- Leafy green vegetables (broccoli and curly kale)
- Nuts, legumes, soya beans, tofu, kidney beans and baked beans
- Dried fruit (apricots and raisins)

If you have a dairy-free diet, make sure you eat non-dairy foods that contain added calcium including some types of fortified non-dairy milk. Always shake the carton well before use to ensure calcium is mixed throughout the drink. Conversely, its best to avoid foods and drinks which can reduce calcium including caffeine, red meat, salt and fizzy drinks that contain phosphates.

Bisphosphonates are drugs that interfere with the cells which break down bone (osteoclasts), thus increasing bone density and reducing the risk of fractures. They have been shown to help age-related osteoporosis and prevent bone loss caused by hormonal therapy and other cancer treatments. They are also used to prevent or treat cancer that has spread to the bone. A rare side effect of bisphosphonate treatment is osteonecrosis of the jaw which is when the jaw bone begins to starve from a lack of blood. This rarely happens with oral tablets or bi-annual administration used after breast cancer – which incidentally also has a small but significant benefit in reducing relapse. It frequently occurs with 3-4 weekly IV administration, especially if there is another disease of the jaw including cancer itself or dental caries. It's usually necessary to take calcium and vitamin D supplements whilst on these drugs otherwise the calcium will drop in the blood stream.

Denosumab is a targeted antibody treatment which also impairs osteoclastic activity. They only require a subcutaneous (under the skin) injection once every six months. Although they have the same benefits for bone, they do not have the same anti-cancer properties as bisphosphonates.

Exercise interventions for bone loss

A number of intervention studies have highlighted how exercise protects bone density. In one RCT involving 66 women with breast cancer, a third walked briskly or jogged for 15-30 minutes for four days a week and also used resistance bands. A third just used resistance bands, and a third were given no exercise instruction at all. Bone Mineral Density (BMD) stopped declining in the aerobic exercise and resistance group, dropped 4% in the resistance training only group and dropped 6% in those who didn't exercise. Another study involved 223 post-menopausal women who had completed initial breast cancer treatment found that those randomised to an exercise class had a 20% better BMD in the femoral neck than non-exercisers.

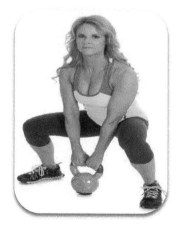

Try to find an exercise you enjoy so you will be more likely to commit to it long-term and not get bored. Exercise needs to be done regularly to have the most benefit. When exercising, try to challenge yourself and add some weights and resistance but do not push yourself too hard at first. With practice, you'll soon find you're able to do more. Weight-bearing and resistance exercise is best to send signals to the cells in the bone to lay down more calcium and harden them. Some examples of good exercise to prevent bone loss are now outlined.

High-intensity resistance and impact training (HiRIT) has been shown in a well-designed RCT from Australia to improve bone density (and physical strength) in both the hips and back with no increased risk of fractures, despite participants having established osteoporosis. The HiRIT program consisted of resistance exercises such as the deadlift, overhead press, and back squat, performed in five sets of five repetitions. The impact loading exercise was a jumping chin-up with a drop landing. This is something to work up to, preferably with supervision.

Balance and stretching: These can also help the joints, reduce fibrosis in the tissues, stimulate the mind and help people maintain their mobility and independence in later life. It also prevents falls – a big advantage if you have brittle bones. Yoga, tai chi, Pilates, body balance and qi gong are good examples.

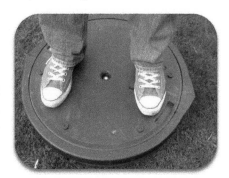

Aerobic exercises that raise the heart rate and get you breathless are excellent for general fitness. This type of aerobic activity strengthens and protects the heart, lungs and metabolism, helps maintain a healthy weight and should be undertaken for at least 30 minutes, five times a week. Weight-bearing aerobic exercises are the most effective at increasing bone density, and these include walking, jogging, skipping, climbing stairs, dancing and hiking.

Resistance exercises involve making your muscles work harder than usual against some form of resistance. They strengthen muscles, bones and joints. They may also improve your balance. The exercises can be done with hand weights, machines or elastic bands.

Anaerobic exercises: These are exercises which use up more oxygen than you can replace by making you breathe faster. When you stop anaerobic exercises, you have to breathe heavily until you have paid back the oxygen debt in your body. Examples would be fast running, cycling, rowing or swimming. It is good to introduce an element of this in every session but only after reaching a suitable level of fitness and warming up and stretching beforehand.

Safety issues while exercising with bone loss: Exercise is very safe, especially if you join a supervised exercise programme. If you get chest pain or extreme shortness of breath after starting you need to consult your GP. Remember to warm up and warm down with aerobic exercises and stretching. If you have severe osteoporosis already, it may be better to avoid high impact exercises such as jogging, skipping, racquet sports like tennis, and certain types of dancing until your bones start healing. Instead, start with low impact exercises such as walking (either outside or on a treadmill machine), climbing stairs and using a cross trainer. A Pilates instructor who has specific extra training dealing with osteoporosis would be a real advantage.

Vitamin D for bone health

Vitamin D helps your body to absorb calcium, so it's vital in helping maintain healthy bones and muscles. Over 80% of the body's vitamin D actually comes from the skin following exposure to sunlight. Chronically low levels of vitamin D increase the risk of bone loss (osteoporosis) in adults. In addition, low levels have been linked to infertility, dementia, heart disease, cancer and arthritis.

Natural sunlight to product vitamin D: As we mainly get vitamin D from the effects of sunlight on our skin, many studies have reported a high incidence of vitamin D deficiency in the UK, particularly by the end of the winter and especially if individuals:

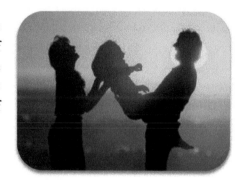

- Cover their skin when outside
- Are dark or black skinned
- Stay in-doors (housebound or those in care homes)

The most significant way to increase vitamin D levels is to get gentle regular sun exposure. Vitamin D has a half-life of 6 weeks, so by mid-winter, unless other precautions are made, most people in Northern climates will have suboptimal levels. Investing in a winter holiday in the sun, budget allowing, is one sensible approach. Only 10-15 minutes of exposure to outdoor sun is necessary to start the production of vitamin D, but precautions need to be taken to avoid burning as this will this create thin, sun-damaged skin, premature ageing and an increased risk of skin cancers. Also try to expose areas of the skin that get the least sun such as the tummy, while avoiding the face, hands and upper chest which generally get too much exposure. Take particular care to put total barrier sunblock on areas which have received radiotherapy. Some chemo agents can sensitise the skin and make burning more likely so take particular care. Here are some other factors to consider when sunbathing.

Smoking whilst sunbathing: If you want to look ten years older, smoke. If you want to look 20 years older, smoke while sunbathing. The ageing and carcinogenic chemicals in cigarette smoke enhance the harmful aspects of the sun. Obviously it is best to stop smoking altogether, however, if you can't, at least don't smoke while in the sun. For the opposite reason, it is worth increasing polyphenol and olive intake if sun exposure is anticipated, such as during a summer holiday or skiing.

Sun exposure and chemotherapy: During and shortly after chemotherapy the skin can be more sensitive to the sun. The chemotherapy drug most likely to photosensitise the skin is fluorouracil, used to treat bowel and breast cancer. Sensitivity to chemotherapy agents usually wears off after three months.

Sun exposure and radiotherapy: Be very careful with skin specifically treated with radiotherapy. Although better with modern techniques, the skin is still at increased risk of sun damage. For example, with breast cancer, the upper cleavage area is treated, so take care when wearing a V-shaped top. The sensitivity to radiotherapy will be life-long. Wear a high factor sunscreen or preferably barrier cream on irradiated tissue.

After sun lotions: While massaging lotion into the skin after sun exposure is a viable way to avoid peeling and make the skin feel better, there is also evidence that some products may reduce the risk of skin cancer. Natural plant products have been shown to reduce the risk of sun damage via two separate mechanisms. In one experiment, olive oil was massaged into the skin of hairless mice for 5 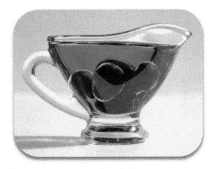 minutes every evening, after exposure to UV light. Another group had the same UV exposure but no olive oil. There was a major difference in the number of subsequent skin cancers between the two groups. They discovered that the oleic acid reduced the formation of 8-hydroxy-deoxyguanosine (8OhdG), a marker of DNA damage. In other words, the olive oil helped repair the damage the sun had inflicted on the DNA, preventing the mutations which would have gone on to cause cancer. In another experiment involving sunbathing mice, scientists applied the antioxidant resveratrol after the UVB exposure and also found this inhibited skin damage and decreased skin cancer incidence.

It would make sense to regularly use an olive oil-based lotion after sun exposure or, failing that, olive oil itself. It also makes sense to avoid lotions packed with hydrocarbons and potentially carcinogen chemicals just when the skin is most vulnerable to DNA attack.

Tanning beds to boost vitamin D: The benefits of tanning beds are unlikely to counterbalance the risks. However, a recent study in The Lancet Oncology commented that sunbeds pose as big a risk as tobacco and asbestos. It reported a new analysis of about 20 studies, which concluded the risk of skin cancer jumps by 75% when people start using tanning beds before the age of 30. Researchers from the WHO found that all types of ultraviolet radiation (UVA, UVB, and UVC) caused worrying mutations and have classed them as Group 1 carcinogens, issuing a warning that people younger than 18 years should avoid tanning beds and older people should use them with caution.

Dietary sources of vitamin D: Small amount of vitamin D can be found naturally in foods, while others such as breakfast cereals, breads and soy products often have fortified vitamin D. Some supermarkets have introduced a mushroom which has had its vitamin D levels enhanced by sun exposure, while sun-dried mushrooms (Porcini) are available in select delicatessens. Other natural food sources include:

- Oily fish such as mackerel, sardines and anchovies
- Grass-fed meat and liver
- Free range chicken or game egg yolks

The recommended daily amount (RDA) of vitamin D for adults is 600-800 iu /day, but more is necessary if there is a history of deficiency or bowel malabsorption. It's advisable to take an over the counter vitamin D supplement, unless you are able to get a sunny holiday, during autumn and winter. People who have a higher risk of vitamin D deficiency are advised to take a supplement all year round and at a higher dose of 1000 iu, which is safe as toxicity has only been associated with megadoses of vitamin D e.g. over 50,000 iu a day for several months. To be on the safe side, however, it's best not exceed 3000iu / day. Unless you have a known vitamin E deficiency, ensure the supplement you take does not contain added vitamin E.

Milk and bone health

Bones are constantly remodelling and repairing, so it's essential to have adequate levels of calcium. Diets chronically low in calcium are linked to osteoporosis. On the other hand, higher than needed calcium does not further improve bone health. A summary of several large meta-analyses published in the BMJ highlighted how >600mg per day (which is easily achieved without dairy products or calcium supplements) did not improve bone integrity. Other clinical

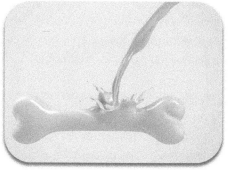

research, tracking the diets and physical activity of young girls for seven years, also concluded that high dairy intake or extra calcium supplements did not prevent stress fractures. Similarly, the Harvard NHS, which followed more than 72,000 women for 18 years, showed no protective effect of high milk intake on fracture risk. Of more concern, another large review also published in the BMJ showed that long-term calcium supplements were associated with an increased risk of heart disease.

Milk products are a good source of dietary calcium. Although the health concerns have been over emphasised in the past, there are some issues to consider. One of the main problems with milk intake is the reduced ability to digest lactose - commonly known as lactose intolerance. This results in abdominal symptoms such as intermittent diarrhoea and constipation, excessive intestinal gas, cramps, and bloating after drinking milk. If chronic and unrecognised, this leads to symptoms such as fatigue, low mood and even depression. A small amount of milk in a cup of tea is usually not a problem, but a large latte coffee often is. Live yoghurts and many cheeses (especially hard varieties) have already had the lactose partially broken down by the fermentation process, so are better tolerated. In view of the high saturated animal fat content, it does seem sensible to avoid excessive milk and milk products if you are overweight or have high cholesterol. In terms of cancer, like many foods, milk has ingredients which could be both potentially harmful or beneficial. Cohort studies have suggested a link between eating high animal fat and increased risk of breast cancer, but these studies have not determined a more specific association with milk as opposed to meat fats. Other studies report a link between very high milk intake and breast and ovarian cancer relapse, but no association with moderate intake. High milk and calcium intake are risk factors for prostate cancer, but it is protective for bowel cancer. Drinking cow's milk in the first few months of life may increase the risk of type 1 diabetes, but later in life, milk, and especially fermented milk products, seems to reduce the risk of type 2 diabetes.

Other dietary influences on bone density

Plant proteins: Protein is formed by the combination of building blocks called amino acids. The body needs 20 different amino acids to grow muscle, bones and function properly. Although all of these are important for your health, nine are classified as essential i.e. the body cannot make them. Meat, fish, milk and eggs contain all the essential amino acids, yet intake of protein from protein rich plants, can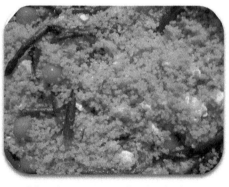
more than adequately supply them all if eaten in combination. Examples include:
- Quinoa (contains all the essential amino acids)
- Soybeans and soy products,
- Hemp, chia seeds, buckwheat, lentils, chickpeas, peanuts
- Butter beans, pinto beans, red kidney beans, black-eyed beans
- Peas, broad beans, corn, artichokes
- Seaweed, chlorella, spirulina, algae
- Whole grains and nuts, mushrooms, kale, spinach, broccoli

Osteoporosis is less common among Asian women and vegetarian populations, a trend thought to be a consequence of higher plant and lower meat consumption. The European Prospective Investigation into Cancer and Nutrition (EPIC) study has been following the dietary habits of 48,830 people over several years. It concluded that high consumption of animal protein harms bones, whereas a higher intake of vegetable protein is beneficial to bone health. The benefits of plant proteins, and particularly soy intake, were further confirmed in a number of other studies. Genistein, found in soya products, was specifically investigated in a double-blind placebo RCT involving 389 post-menopausal women. After 3 years, bone mineral density increases for both femoral neck and lumbar spine were greater within the soy extract group compared to the placebo group. From a safety perspective, genistein in soya foods did not change mammographic breast density or endometrial thickness, and BRCA1 and BRCA2 expression were preserved despite their potentially phytoestrogenic effects.

In reality, most men and women eat about 55% more protein than they need each day. There is certainly no benefit on bone health to having very high protein intakes, and individuals who require high energy intakes should consider how to increase energy without increasing protein consumption excessively. That said, eating enough protein can help with weight loss and increase muscle mass, so it is important to eat an amount which is adequate given an individual's age and exercise aims.

It must also be remembered that a low protein intake can also be a problem. If protein levels in the body drop, this can be a sign of advanced disease, especially if cancer has affected the liver. On a blood test, this is often referred to as serum albumin. If this drops below 30, fluid can seep out from the blood into the tissues, particularly the ankles, causing ankle or even leg swelling. Within the abdomen, fluid can seep into the cavity causing or contributing to ascites (free fluid in the abdominal cavity). A number of studies have shown that a low albumin level in someone with advanced disease is a worrying development. A study in 2016 also reported that women with early breast cancer who have a low protein intake have a higher risk of relapse and progression, so adequate intake is important at all stages

Polyphenol-rich foods: There are several ways these foods influence bone density. One laboratory study found that bone reabsorption activity was increased when animals were exposed to increased oxidative stress. However, when animals were pre-fed with berries rich in polyphenols, markers of oxidative stress reduced, glutathione activity increased and bone

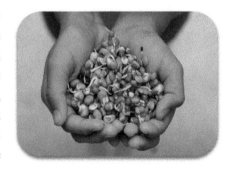

reabsorption reduced. In support of this, a separate study found that polyphenols decreased RANKL activation of osteoclasts, cells responsible for reabsorbing bone. In the longer term, polyphenols in green tea reduced chronic inflammation and insulin-like growth factor-1, both of which are associated with bone loss. The other polyphenol-rich foods which have the best benefit are the isoflavones and flavonoids. These have the advantage of additional plant proteins such as soya products and legumes. Turmeric appears to be particularly potent in protecting bone density in animals.

Probiotic bacteria have been shown to reduce gut inflammatory markers, making them particularly useful effective at improving bone density as there is a known link between chronic gut inflammation and bone health. In a number of lab studies, just 4-6 weeks of probiotic supplements significantly increased biochemical markers of bone and calcium metabolism, leading to either improved bone density in animals with established osteoporosis. Many authors are suggesting a possible benefit in humans, and randomised trials are eagerly awaited.

Vitamin K. Vitamin K1 (Phylloquinone) is essential for the formation of clotting factors. More recently, vitamin K has been found to be important for bone health, especially the vitamin K_2 (menaquinones) variant which is formed by bacterial fermentation foods. Although more confirmatory research is needed, it appears that vitamin K_2 helps harden the bones as it is required for the gamma-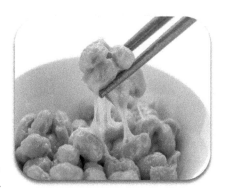
carboxylation of osteocalcin, a bone matrix protein which is made in osteoblasts to form bone. Numerous studies have reported that elderly people with hip fractures

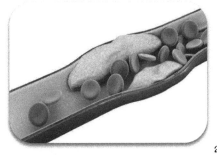 have a lower level of vitamin K_2 than the general age-related population. An animal study showed that a vitamin K_2 rich diet prevented bone loss caused by removal of the ovaries. Quite remarkably, vitamin K_2 has the opposite effect on arterial calcification. It inhibits the formation of calcified plaques in coronary and systemic arteries, likely explaining the cardioprotective links reported in population-based studies.

Dietary sources of vitamin K: Leafy dark green vegetables are one of the richest dietary sources. Cooking does not significantly damage vitamin K, while condensing foods can increase levels per gram. Vitamin K2 is found in fermented products including cheese. It is also made by healthy gut bacteria, another reason to optimise and improve gut flora. Common foods containing vitamin K and K2 include:

Dietary Vitamin K:
- Kale, mustard beetroot greens
- Spinach, chard, rocket, broccoli
- Cabbage, sprouts and green beans
- Chicken legs and wings
- Prunes, blueberries or blackberries
- Avocados, eggs and peas
- Kiwis, grapes, pomegranates,
- Olive, soy and safflower oils
- Peanut, cereals and sesame oils

Dietary vitamin K2:
- Fermented soya, natto
- Liver paste (grass-fed animals)
- Fermented cheeses, stilton, gouda
- Egg yolk, Natural yoghurts
- Soya beans, Curd, Sauerkraut
- Serrano ham
- Tempura, Kombucha, Kimchi
- Meat from grass-fed animals
- Butter from grass-fed animals

Toxicity: Excessive intake of vitamin K has not been reported to cause toxicity syndromes as the body is limited in the amount it can store. This lack of accumulation contributes to the safety of natural vitamin K. Even taking supplements of K and K2 in sensible amounts have no reported toxicity. Vitamin K-containing foods are safe for people taking warfarin, but vitamin K supplements are best avoided.

Other trace minerals and bone health: It is not just calcium and proteins which make up healthy bones. Other minerals have a role too, albeit to a lesser extent. Low magnesium intake has a detrimental effect on bones as it has direct action on crystal formation, stimulating activity of parathyroid hormones. Zinc, manganese and copper help maintain bone quality through their role in the synthesis of collagen and other proteins that form the structure of bone. Animal experiments inducing deficiencies in these trace minerals cause bone loss, but fortunately, we know from micronutrient tests in humans that these deficiencies are rare. Nevertheless, it's important to pay attention to foods containing essential minerals.

Smoking & alcohol: The list of health risks for smoking just gets longer and longer. Several cohort studies have linked lower bone density with smoking. On the other hand greater bone density was found in men consuming 7 alcoholic beverages weekly, suggesting a potential benefit of low to moderate alcohol consumption. Men with very high alcohol intake had worse BMD.

Avoid being underweight: A US study, reported that heavier people had better bone density. The same authors also reported that underweight breast cancer survivors (BMI less than 19) who smoked had a high risk of osteoporosis. If you are underweight, it would be worth bulking up with a combination of carbohydrates, proteins and weight-bearing exercises.

Summary – Advice to help bone density

- Avoid excess alcohol and try to stop smoking
- Reduce meat intake to < 3 times a week
- Avoid being underweight

- Exercise and stretch your joints every day; More weight baring exercise
- Consider a High-intensity resistance and impact training programme

- Increase plant proteins:
- Soy, legumes, beans, seaweed, quinoa, beans, mushrooms

- Ensure adequate vitamin D levels
- Regular sensible sunbathing take a vitamin D pills during Winter
- Oily fish, sun dried mushrooms

- Avoid calcium deficiency ensuring adequate intake of:
- Fermented dairy products such as cheese, yoghurt and kefir
- Shellfish such as oysters, mussels, clams, plus oily fish with edible bones
- Spinach, and curly kale, nuts, legumes, apricots and raisins

- Ensure adequate vitamin K2 levels:
- Soy, hard cheeses, blue veined cheeses
- Fermented soy (Natto), Yogurts, Tempura, Kombucha, Kimchi

- Increase other foods which also promote a healthy gut
- Miso, sauerkraut, kefir; Consider a good quality probiotic supplements
- More prebiotic foods such as artichokes, mushrooms, beans
- Increase polyphenol-rich foods Broccoli, tea, pomegranate, turmeric, other herbs and spices; consider a whole food supplement such as Pomi-T

Joint pains - Arthritis

Arthritis is a common condition that causes pain, stiffness and inflammation within a joint. In the UK, around 10 million people have arthritis at any one time. Existing medical treatments help the pain but not the underlying damage to cartilage, ligaments, tendons and synovial fluid which make up the complex joint structures. These medications also tend to have long-term 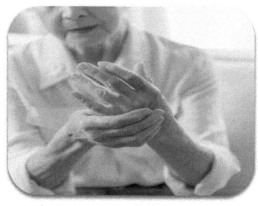 adverse effects on the heart, kidneys and stomach. In contrast, the lifestyle, exercise and nutritional advice emphasised in this book target the disease processes which cause deterioration of joint health.

Lifestyle factors which affect the development and progression of the most common type of systemic osteoarthritis are also the same ones which affect the development of arthritis after cancer treatments and include:

- Family history
- Pro-inflammatory foods
- High meat intake
- Low polyphenol food intake
- Poor gut health
- Smoking
- Processed sugar
- Excess alcohol
- Being overweight
- Stretching and exercise
- High vegetable intake
- Local trauma

After cancer, osteoarthritis remains the most common form of arthritis, reflecting its high incidence among the general public. The arthritis which develops in patients with no previous history of joint pains within months of cancer treatments has features of both osteo and rheumatoid arthritis. After the onset of arthritis, it is still worth talking to the doctor to exclude other rarer forms of arthritis such as infective arthritis, gout, polymyalgia rheumatica and arthritis associated with psoriatic arthritis and urinary tract infections.

Why is arthritis more common after cancer?

The Bedford Real World study found that over 50% of patients report joint pains as one of the most troublesome symptoms after cancer. The reasons for this are multifactorial. Chemo drugs such as Taxotere can cause generalised arthralgia, triggering longer-term painful joints, especially if women have been made prematurely postmenopausal or given additional Herceptin. Women treated for breast cancer can experience shoulder stiffness related to axillary surgery and radiotherapy. A third of women taking tamoxifen and 55% of those taking an aromatase inhibitor have arthralgia Men with prostate cancer on androgen deprivation therapy (ADT) report a 20% incidence of arthralgia.

Arthralgia affects compliance, potentially compromising the effectiveness of adjuvant therapies as highlighted by one of our research studies. Other institutes have also reported that arthralgia leads to poor adherence and drug discontinuation, with one USA trial showing that 20% of women discontinued treatment and 40% did not take the medications as prescribed because of the condition.

The damage of arthritis

Not only are the joint swellings, pain and stiffness troublesome, but it can also lead to an exacerbation of other symptoms by restricting an individual's ability to exercise. In fact, a study from Cambridge University found that arthritis was the main barrier to exercise after cancer treatment in up to 40% of patients.

Men on Androgen Deprivation Therapy (ADT) are prone to weight gain, hot flushes, impaired cognition and osteoporosis, all of which are helped by physical activity. Exercise after breast cancer has a range of benefits including reducing unwelcome weight gain, risk of thromboembolism and cancer-related fatigue, while also improving sleep patterns, quality of life and psychological wellbeing. Exercise has also been shown to relieve arthralgia itself. The HOPE trial, from New York, reported significant and specific reduction in arthralgia among 121 women given an exercise intervention. If arthralgia restricts physical activity, it may increase relapse rates and impair survival.

Medical treatments for arthritis

Analgesia: Simple analgesia include paracetamol, non-steroidal anti-inflammatory agents and if severe, stronger painkillers such as opioids. Although helpful, they have significant long-term cardiovascular and gastrointestinal risks and unwelcome effects.

Invasive procedures: Surgical interventions such as joint fusion and replacement prosthesis remain effective but intrusive. Steroid injections can help initially but cannot be repeated too often.

What can you do to avoid arthritis?

Exercise which involves stretching is the most effective way to slow the disease progress and help the swelling and pain. The problem is that at the start of exercise the pain often gets worse, giving the impression that it should be avoided. However, with persistence this wears off and the benefits are realised.

Stretching, yoga and Pilates significantly help to relieve joint pain and improve mobility. Participants don't have to be contortionists, and a good class should cater to all levels. Stretching the joints, tendons, ligaments and muscles, although sometimes uncomfortable, will improve the health of the joints, increase flexibility and reduce long term swelling and pain. Although classes are cheaper, a personal trainer can provide extra motivation and offer individualised stretching guidance.

In addition to formal instruction, it is worth putting aside ten minutes every day for stretching as part of a regimented programme aimed at ensuring all your joints are stretched. Start from the neck down, extending and flexing your joints to the fullest range possible without causing pain. Video clips of sensible stretches for individual joints are featured on the keep-healthy.com website.

Physical complementary interventions such as acupuncture, reflexology, chiropractic, osteopathy and massage offer emotional support, and there are some reports of improved pain and stiffness.

Topical chilli pepper extract (Capsaicin) has been investigated in three randomised trials, involving over 400 participants. Capsaicin gel (0.025 – 0.075%) was applied topically four times a day for between 4 and 12 weeks. In all three trials, capsaicin was found to be about four times more effective at improving pain, stiffness, joint tenderness and joint function compared to placebo gel.

Weight reduction: If overweight, diets which assist with weight reduction do have reported benefits by reducing the load on the weight-bearing joints.

Fasting: A notable recent clinical evaluation found that participants who fasted, reduced their salt intake and increased consumption of vegetables had a significant reduction in arthritis-related pain and stiffness. Another study confirmed fasting, followed by a diet of green and cruciferous-rich vegetables, helped reduce the number and severity of tender swollen joints, duration of morning stiffness and blood markers of chronic inflammation.

Avoiding ingested toxins: Once absorbed into the blood, a variety of chemicals can circulate and become caught in the microvessels of the joints. These toxins not only cause direct irritation themselves but can also trigger an immune attack from the body, causing collateral damage to delicate joint tissues. For these reasons, a diet avoiding man-made chemicals is certainly well worth a try if you have joint pains.

Carefully wash fruit and vegetables and eat more organic and less processed food if possible. Avoiding high temperature prepared snacks, burnt meats, sugary drinks and foods containing preservatives, colourings or flavourings.

Polyphenol-rich foods: Laboratory studies have demonstrated that polyphenols and other phytochemicals help prevent the progression of underlying joint damage via a number of biochemical pathways:

- Anti-inflammatory - reduces discomfort and stiffness
- Antioxidant - protecting the joint from oxidative damage
- Anti-apoptotic - stopping chondrocytes destroying themselves
- Metalloproteinase stimulation – makes extracellular matrix (cartilage)

A major study from the Mount Sinai School of Medicine demonstrated that polyphenol-rich plants. reduce chronic inflammation and improve joint pains especially if combined with other lifestyle measures such as maintaining a healthy gut, avoiding pro-inflammatory carcinogens. In addition, large population studies from the Far East which have linked fruit, vegetables, teas, herbs, spices, and pulses with a lower risk of osteoarthritis.   Foods which have shown particular promise include:

Turmeric (Curcuma longa) is a perennial plant native to southern Asia and originating from the ginger family. In one laboratory experiment, turmeric was administered on a random basis to rats prior to the administration of a toxin (streptococcal cell wall) which induces arthritis. The turmeric profoundly inhibited joint inflammation and peri-articular joint destruction in a dose-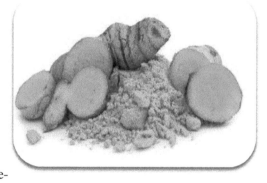
dependent manner. It also altered expression of NF-kappa which regulates genes which mediate joint inflammation and destruction. In humans, a double-blind RCT gave either a placebo or 50mg of turmeric in combination with other botanicals to 42 patients with established osteoarthritis. Those taking the turmeric combination demonstrated significant improvements in pain severity and disability scores. Another trial involved 100 men and women with a history of joint pain being randomised and given either a placebo or a supplement containing turmeric root, white willow bark, ginger root, boswellia serrate, cayenne extracts, methylsulfonylmethane (MSM), glucosamine sulfate and hyaluronic acid. They reported improvements in joint pain severity, the ability to perform daily activities, stiffness scores and knee pain after 8 weeks. A further trial, involving 107 participants with arthritic pains of the knee, randomly compared taking 2g of turmeric versus

800mg of ibuprofen per day for 6 weeks. Although both groups' pain levels improved when walking and climbing stairs, improvement was more significant in the turmeric group. These and other studies have prompted the European Food Safety Association [EFSA] to state that turmeric, "Helps to protect joints, maintain joint flexibility and improve joint health".

Green tea (Camellia sinensis) is a rich source of the catechin epigallocatechin 3-gallate (EGCG). Laboratory studies, using cartilage cells (chondrocytes) derived from joints affected by OA, have demonstrated that incubation with tea extract reduced pro-inflammatory cytokines when these cells were subsequently exposed to oxidative stress. Under normal circumstances, chondrocytes in the cartilage make extracellular matrix 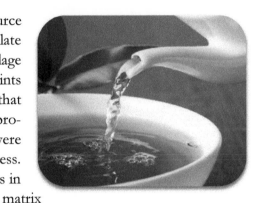 components such as aggrecan and collagen in response to mechanical pressure. Under conditions of high oxidative stress, an influx of pro-inflammatory cytokines activate an enzyme called matrix metalloproteinases (MMP) which promotes cartilage degradation. Tea catechins block activation of MMPs, protecting the joint. Several laboratory experiments have reported the modifying effect of EGCG on arthritis. Additionally, total immunoglobulins (IgG) and type II collagen-specific IgG levels were found to be lower in serum and arthritic joints of green tea-fed mice – this is particularly important for aromatase inhibitor-induced arthritis which is associated with raised collagen-specific IgG.

Broccoli and other cruciferous vegetables rich in isothiocyanate and its metabolite sulforaphane (SFN) have a number of health benefits. Firstly, they are known to be potent inductors of antioxidant enzymes, particularly glutathione, which binds free radicals formed by dietary or environmental carcinogens before they damage our DNA, including those within the tissues of our joints. Secondly, SFN is a potent inducer of the transcription factor 2 (Nrf2), reducing chronic 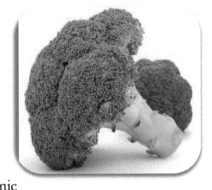 inflammation. More relevant for joint health, SFN has been shown to modulate MMP expression in chondrocytes. In animal models, mice fed an SFN-rich diet had significantly reduced cartilage destruction at 12 weeks compared with those fed a control diet.

Cordyceps militaris, a parasitic caterpillar fungus found in humid tropical countries, is rich in cordycepin. Various studies have focused on the pharmacological activities of cordycepin and revealed that it has anti-inflammatory, anti-angiogenesis, anti-ageing and anti-proliferation properties. Moreover, lab trials have found that it inhibits expression of MMP and also decreases glycosaminoglycan (GAG) release, preventing aggrecan and proteoglycan loss (important components of cartilage).

Boswellia serrate (Indian Frankincense) is a branching tree of the family Burseraceae, found growing in dry mountainous regions of India, Africa and the Middle East, which has disease-modifying effects on arthritis and other chronic conditions. In human chondrocytes, it has demonstrated an ability to suppress a protein known as RANKL which prevents cartilage and bone reabsorption. Boswellia has also been shown to suppress the release of MMP. A unique property of boswellic acid is its ability to reduce inflammation via the pro-inflammatory enzyme lipoxygenase (LOX) without affecting arachidonic acid. Boswellia serrata also inhibits NF-kB activation triggered by pro-inflammatory toxins. For example, in two laboratory experiments, animals fed with Boswellia had a 50% reduction in arthritis induced by the toxins formaldehyde and bovine serum albumin. In humans, in one RCT involving participants with established osteoarthritis, it improved pain and functional ability scores while also leading to a significant reduction in synovial fluid MMP. In another study, 300mg per day improved pain, knee flexion, analgesia use and walking distance compared to placebo.

Other nutritional supplements for arthritis

Concentrating healthy whole foods in a capsule, if made with sufficient quality control, is a convenient way to boost intake of certain foods to a higher level than can be realistically achieved with dietary measures alone. The Bedford Real World study reported that 50% of people with cancer took nutritional supplements, but this went up to 70% if they also suffered from arthralgia. There is a varying degree of evidence for their benefits, and the charity *Arthritis Research* published a comprehensive review of nutritional supplements, highlighting their potential benefits but emphasising the significant gaps in research.

CBD oil: Numerous laboratory studies have found that CBD reduces the production of inflammatory cytokines, some of which can trigger arthralgia and joint damage. There are widespread anecdotal reports of improved pain in humans, and it is often prescribed to dogs with arthritis. One study involving 58 patients with arthritis reported a significant reduction in pain compared to placebo. These findings have been encouraging, but more research is required to confirm that CBD oil is an effective treatment for arthritis.

Glucosamine is a monosaccharide amino sugar which as a major component of the exoskeletons of crustaceans, fungi and higher organisms. It is produced commercially by crushing crustacean exoskeletons. Glucosamine has been found in animal studies to delay breakdown and improve repair of damaged cartilage. It has also been evaluated in an early RCT involving 400 women with breast cancer, which demonstrated an improvement in pain and knee joint space. However, in 13 subsequent RCTs, the results were mixed, and two large summaries of the studies concluded that there were no meaningful symptomatic benefits or changes in radiological measures of arthritis.

Chondroitin is made from extracts of cartilaginous cow and pig tissues, particularly trachea, ear and nose, although alternative sources include bird and shark cartilage. Laboratory studies have found that chondroitin supplements reduced the activity of enzymes that break down collagen in joints. In humans, although some of the 22 RCT studies showed a benefit, two meta-analyses concluded that there were no clinically meaningful effects.

Fish oils have been reported to improve the pain of rheumatoid arthritis, but the evidence of a benefit for osteoarthritis lacks sufficient data. One study sought to evaluate the efficacy of fish oils, with women with arthralgia who were taking an aromatase inhibitor being randomised to receive either omega 3-rich fish oils or a placebo (soybean/corn oil) daily for 24 weeks. Although arthralgia scores in both groups improved, there was no difference between them.

Further studies

Phytochemical-rich whole food supplements have been evaluated for their anti-arthralgia properties, with emerging results somewhat encouraging. They are certainly popular among elite athletes, as there is evidence that they reduce reactive oxygenated species produced by vigorous exercise, aid muscle recovery and help protect joints. They are very likely to have a role in helping arthritis in non-athletes, but studies have tended to be small, underpowered and involved patients with advanced disease already. The evidence for turmeric, green tea and broccoli described above are three of four ingredients in the Pomi-T supplement described earlier in the book, so it was little surprise that men reported reduced joint discomfort during the original trial involving men with prostate cancer and afterwards. Countless people have also emailed or written to the research unit commenting on improvements in joint pain, especially women taking Aromatase inhibitor drugs for breast cancer. This was one notable email:

"I have taken Pomi-T for 3 months - I thought it may be a sensible option as I'm now in the risk age group for cancer. I have noticed such a great improvement in an arthritic knee condition that I will now avoid a total knee replacement for the foreseeable future. Along with this, my tendons have lengthened, enabling better knee flexion. I can touch my toes easily for the first time in years".

Considering their mode of action, it likely that their main benefits lay in arthritis prevention, so trials would have to take place over many years and involve many thousands of participants in order to be statistically robust. There have been no RCTs specifically addressing people after cancer, a group for whom arthralgia is commonplace and particularly burdensome. Because arthritis after cancer tends to develop within four months of starting hormone therapies, individuals at this stage represent a perfect group to investigate a nutritional intervention in humans. This was the rationale for a trial, described below, which is currently underway.

The arthritis and exercise study

This study hypothesised that a nutritional strategy, beginning at the same time as hormone therapies, may prevent the onset or deterioration of arthralgia enough to

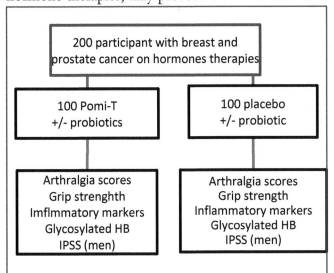

ensure a maintenance or even increase of exercise levels. With increased exercise levels a whole host of benefits could ensue. With this in mind, a clinical trial committee was set up, bringing together a panel of sports scientists, oncologists rheumatologists and nutritionists. A double-blind placebo-controlled RCT was then designed and is now underway. By the time it has fully recruited, it will involve 200 patients with cancer who have recently completed primary treatments. All participants are encouraged to undertake an exercise programme via written and verbal advice, behavioural change interviewing and referral to their local gym or another exercise group of their choice. They are being randomised and given either the polyphenol-rich capsule (Pomi-T) or placebo. In view of the limited evidence for probiotics, a sub-randomisation will allocate a probiotic supplement or further placebo. At six months, the change in arthralgia score will be compared between the two randomised groups of patients. In addition exercise levels between the two groups will be scored by an analysis of grip strength, a wearable exercise monitor and a two-minute walking test . Other late toxicities such as mood, urinary function and hot flushes will be recorded. Other tests will measure blood levels of inflammation and oxidative stress, as well as glycosylated Hb (a marker of sugar control), cholesterol and body fat. The final results of this innovative study will be available in 2020.

Summary – Advice to help joint pains

- Eat plenty of polyphenol-rich fruit and vegetables
- Identify food intolerances
- Reduce meat intake to less than three times a week
- Eat more oily fish
- Keep a diary of what foods can make your joints worse
- Reduce calorie intake if you are overweight
- Use fresh ginger and turmeric as much as possible
- Avoid food additives, pesticides and particularly sulphites
- Avoid excess alcohol and try to stop smoking
- Exercise and stretch your joints every day
- Improve your posture and consider joining yoga or Pilates classes
- Review medications with your doctor
- If these measures fail, nutritional supplements to consider include:
  - A polyphenol-rich whole food supplement such as Pomi-T
  - A good quality probiotic supplement

Chapter 9

Sugar intake and diabetes after cancer

With Dr Karl Neff

Diabetes after can cause several problems after a diagnosis of cancer; it adds to the complexities of care, it risks further toxicities such heart damage, dementia and stroke and actually increased the risk of relapse. The reasons why the type 2 version of diabetes (T2D) is more common after cancer include weight gain, co-administration of steroids during chemotherapy, surgery or radiotherapy to the pancreas. Several lifestyle factors contribute to the development of T2D, including exercise, body weight but one of the most significant is processed sugar intake:

Dangers of processed sugar:

Processed sugar and to lesser extent processed carbohydrates, in diabetics or prediabetics they lead to high blood sugars. In non-diabetics, the blood sugar rises rapidly but the rapid release of insulin ensures sugar levels do not significantly exceed normal levels. Over time, however, these high levels of insulin required to deal with these rapid rises in sugar lead to insulin resistance and type two diabetes (T2D). Foods with a high Glycaemic Index (GI), cause marked fluctuation in blood sugar levels because they are rapidly digested and absorbed which trigger a rapid insulin response. On the other hand, low 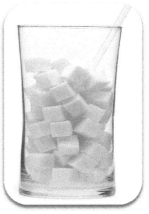 GI foods, by virtue of their slow digestion and absorption, produce gradual rises in blood sugar and insulin levels. In addition, food manufacturers are well aware that sugary foods are craved by many people, to a level some regard as addictive. As a result sugary foods and drinks tend to be eaten in excess – certainly more than is required. This increases the glycaemic load (GL) of meals, a term, which takes into account the amount as well as the type of food eaten.

It is particularly important to stop sugary fizzy drinks, boiled and chewy sweets, mints adding sugar to tea, coffee or cereals as well as cakes or muffin containing the sugars. Most sugary foods can be easily identified, as advertisers usually label them as "Luxury" or "Treats" or use terms such as "spoil yourself". Maybe it's time for governments to step in legislate advertisers to use the truth, although "Treating yourself to fatigue, dental caries, obesity, heart disease, diabetes and cancer" doesn't have the same ring to it. The sugar tax is a step in the right direction but the money raised should subsidise healthy drinks and foods. It's a senseless that on a hot summer's day, a thirsty customer is offered a sugary drink half the price as water and often almost quarter of the price of more tasty sugar free drinks.

Sometimes it's not so obvious were sugar has been added especially as some of these foods may be advertised as healthy – reduced fat ready meals, salad dressings, pasta sources, yogurt, breakfast cereals or muesli for instance. It is worth reading the label of processed foods such as "ready meals" or even crisps where sugar is often added to supposedly enhance the favour. Some restaurants add sugar to their curries and stews – you can instruct the waiter to ask the chef to omit the sugar.

The cancernetUK blog has a series of practical recipes, which maintain a high taste but have no sugar. They also emphasise phytochemical rich foods, which as mentioned above, also reduce the GI or carbohydrates. A number of natural nutritionist update the blog monthly with fresh ideas supported by a short video clip explaining how the dishes are made (blog.cancernet.co.uk).

Honey is a good example of a food which has both good and bad elements. It's high fructose levels, especially if consumed on an empty stomach, such as first thing in the morning causes rapid rises in glucose and subsequent insulin levels which could led to insulin resistance. It is also calorific so increases the glycaemic load and the risk of weight gain. On the 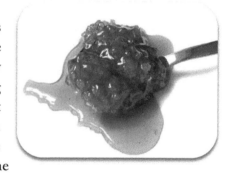 other hand, it contains oligosaccharides which act as prebiotics that encourage growth of healthy bacteria. So unlike sugar which increases growth of bad bacteria, increasing inflammation, it tends to improve gut health. Some brands such as New Zealand manuka honey have antimicrobial properties which explains why, despite its sugar content has a lower than expected risk of dental plaque and small studies even suggest it could even help reduce gingivitis. It has been used as an adjunct for wound cleaning and healing for centuries. Certain varieties have been shown to reduce of *H. pylori* related gastritis, thought to be due to its high polyphenols content which have been shown to stimulate antioxidant enzyme production particularly glutathione. The timing of honey consumption is important. A small quantity after a meal has a lower influence on GI yet still provides healthy prebiotics and polyphenols which could help with digestion. The composition of honey varies enormously reflecting its floral source. In general the darker, more aromatic honeys have a greater phytochemical composition. Many commercial honey bees have been fed processed table sugar which reduces its quality and these are best avoided.

Fructose in whole fruits: It must be emphasized that although fructose is present in whole fruit, no study has shown that eating a lot of fruit is harmful. In fact, quite the opposite, fruit is rich in vitamins, minerals and healthy phytochemicals. Compared to adding processes sugar to foods, the levels of sugar in whole fruit is still relatively low, even with as grapes, mango and pomegranate. At these concentrates it would near impossible to get to harmful levels of fructose by eating whole fruit. The fibre and pulp makes fruit satiating deterring the individual from eating other foods because they feel full. The pulp and fibre slow down gastric emptying and reducing the GI. There are a number of ways humans have managed to make fruit potentially unhealthy:

Dried fruit: The process of drying fruit removes water and damages some of the nutrients but more importantly concentrates the fructose. Some manufacturers also add more sugar and sulphites as for taste and preservation. The table below show the 5 fold increase in sugar by this process (e.g. fresh figs 7% to dried figs 55%). On the positive side however, despite this high in sugar content, they still have their fibre, polyphenols and pulp.

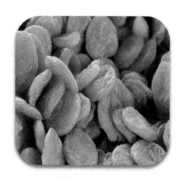

Fruit juices: Many of the fruit juices on the market aren't even "real" fruit juices. They consist of mixed concentrates with extra sugar liberally added. Even 100% real fruit juice, has a high levels of fructose because so many more fruits are used. A 300ml orange juice may contain 4-5 oranges, the same sugar content as a fizzy cola drink. There is also little chewing resistance to slow down consumption, making it very easy to consume a large amount of sugar quickly. This lack of pulp significantly speeds up its GI. There is certainly some truth in the commonly used Californian expression "Eat your fruit – Juice your vegetables"

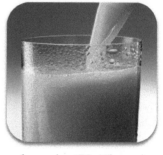

Smoothies; Those where the whole fruit has been put in the blender are better as they maintain the pulp and fibre. They still have a high fructose content especially if sugary fruits such as grapes, pears, apples and mangos are used. To overcome this, the smoothie aficionados often add less sweet fruits such as avocado, vegetables such as kale and spices such as ginger, which lowers the sugar content and enhances the polyphenols content.

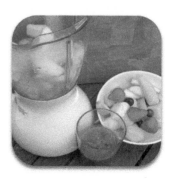

Why processed sugar is harmful

Obesity, metabolic syndrome and inflammation; Several well-conducted cohort studies have linked consumption of high sugar foods and drinks with obesity. Sugary drinks pack on the pounds because this high energy source is less satiating (signaling to body to stop eating when you have had enough calories) resulting in higher consumption. Sugary drinks or meals also trigger a damaging yo-yoing effect on blood glucose and insulin levels. The body responds to an initial sugar rush by rapidly increasing insulin levels that triggers metabolism of the excess sugar, into energy storage such as glycogen in the liver. As sugar has only been around in the human diet for the last 150 years, our body thinks that this level of sugar hitting the blood stream must be associated with a very large meal so it over produces insulin which then causes sugar levels to drop which then stimulates hunger and fatigue. The natural reaction to this is to reach for another high calorific snack or drink, which gives instant relief but starts the process all over again as highlighted in the adjacent graph. Weight gain caused by high calorific and glycaemic index foods increases the

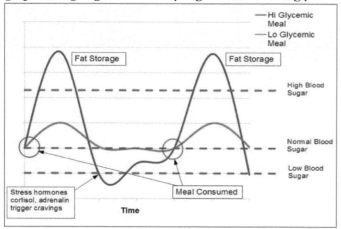

risk of weight gain and metabolic syndrome which is defined by the Adult Treatment Panel III criteria as a combination of abdominal obesity, high triglyceride and hyperglycaemia. This combination leads to a higher risk of insulin resistance, diabetes, heart disease, cancer, dementia and stroke. People living with this syndrome have a significantly higher inflammatory markers. The cause of this is thought to be that cells too full of fat are more fragile to physical trauma, and cell rupture evokes the accumulation of macrophages in fat stores. Organs such as the liver and pancreas, when heavily infiltrated with fat, suffer from reduced functioning which contributes to impaired insulin regulation. Increased metabolism to deal with greater amounts of food increases free radical production and oxidative stress, particularly when poor dietary choices lead to deficiencies in essential micronutrients and anti-inflammatory polyphenol-rich foods. Moreover, overweight individuals tend to have a suboptimal microbiota; have an increased risk of chronic infections, such as those of the urinary tract or candida in the skin folds; and are at greater risk of psychological disturbances, all of which affect inflammatory regulation. The role of inflammation after sugar intake was highlighted by an experiment where half a group of mice were fed sucrose with their usual meal at comparable levels to Western diets, and the other half a normal (mouse) diet. The Western diet led to increased ex pression of inflammatory markers, including 12-lipoxygenase (12-LOX) and its metabolites (arachidonic acids). Reassuringly, fruit containing fructose did not promote inflammation in similar experiments. This is because the bulk of the fruit slows inflammatory progression through the gut, while the polyphenol content slows the transfer of sugar across the gut wall – both reducing the GI. It is particularly harmful to eat sugar, sugary drinks, processed white bread and white rice on an empty stomach, so it's important to have a completely sugar-free, non-processed breakfast.

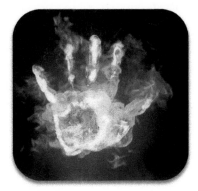

Insulin like growth factor (IGF) The section above explained how sugar increases the risk of obesity, which is associated with higher levels of several hormones, which can trigger cancer. Many of these biological changes can also be generated directly, not necessarily with associated obesity. High sugar and insulin levels also lead to direct overproduction of IGF. After binding to its receptor tyrosine kinase, IGF activates several signalling pathways, leading to the inhibition of apoptosis, the promotion of cell growth and angiogenesis. Higher levels of IGF-1 in humans has been linked with a greater cancer risk. Furthermore, two very large international studies involving people with treated bowel cancer both reported those who eat higher GL diets had higher IGF levels and an increased relapse rate.

Genetic damage Studies have found suggested that high sugar levels can result in the formation of oxidative metabolites which increase intracellular free radicals. Certainly markers of single strand DNA breaks have been reported in the presence of hyperglycaemia. Other lab experiments using Vitamin B6 deficient flies (more susceptible to genetic damage) found that feeding them with sugar triggered direct DNA damage.

Diabetes and glucose intolerance: Independent from obesity, high sugar intake directly increases the risk of diabetes by overloading the insulin pathways. Individuals with T2D have higher serum insulin levels (hyperinsulinemia) as the pancreas produces more to try and overcome cellular insulin resistance, considered to be independent risk factors for cancer development, probably related to insulin receptor stimulation on cancer cells. In addition, hyperglycemia-related oxidative stress promote malignant transformation. It is not a surprise, therefore, a study involving 872,706 Australians cross referenced the National Diabetes Service Scheme with the National Death Index and found a significant link between T2D and fatal cancer. Likewise, in the UK, a total of 62,809 patients with diabetes were found to have a higher risk of colon and pancreatic cancer compared to a similar population without diabetes especially if also obese. Because of these, and many other data, the American Diabetes Association and the American Cancer Society have issued a consensus report stating that 2TD infers a two fold higher risk for cancers of the liver, pancreas, and endometrium, and a 1.5 fold increased risk for cancers of the colon and rectum, breast, bladder and leukaemia. Even without a formal diagnosis of diabetes, research, funded by the WCRF, found that amoung half a million people from Norway, Austria, and Sweden, those with glucose intolerance or pre-diabetes, particularly if overweight were significantly more likely to develop a range of fatal cancers.

Factors which lower GI:

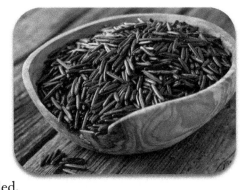

As well as the type of carbs, the timing and total content of the entire meal can influence GI. Carbs eaten alone will be absorbed quicker but eaten with fat, protein, and fibre slows gastric emptying, which has less of an impact on blood sugar. Wholemeal bread has a slower absorption, as well as more vitamins and fibre, than typical thin white bread which to add to the insult, often has table sugar added.

Whole meal or fava bean enriched pasta as well as *al dente* pasta have a slower GI than overcooked white pasta. Processed sugar, especially sugary drinks on an empty stomach, such as first thing in the morning, is particularly harmful as they are absorbed rapidly. Conversely, a small sweet dish after a healthy meal will have less of an impact as the stomach has a plenty of other food to minimise the effect. Likewise, as mentioned above, eating the whole fruit will reduce the impact of the sugar as the pulp and fibre slow gastric emptying.

Polyphenols lower impact of sugar:
Higher intake of natural polyphenol rich foods such as turmeric, cinnamon; broccoli, tea, coffee, chocolate, pomegranate, red wine and berries are linked to a lower risk of type two diabetes T2D. This data is collected from cohort studies which, although can be subject to bias, nevertheless provide interesting insights into the benefits and

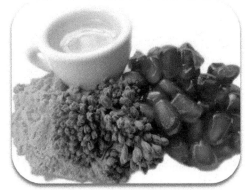

risks of foods certain food which are difficult to evaluate in formal RCT's. The most notable studies included The Nurses' Health Study, which investigated urinary excretion of eight polyphenol metabolites and found that anthocyanins, flavanones and flavonols (broccoli, grapes, tea, berries, pomegranate) as well as the phenolic acid, caffeic acid (cinnamon, coffee, vanilla), were associated with a significantly lower T2D risk. This was in accordance with the HPFS, which found that higher polyphenol intake such as curcuminoids (turmeric) was significantly associated with a lower risk of T2D. Both the Women's Health Study and a large Finnish cohort study reported that ≥1 apple/day (rich in kaempferol) had a lower risk compared with no apple consumption. In addition to these large cohort studies, a laboratory study demonstrated that glucose transport in gut cells was inhibited by flavonoid glycosides and non-glycosylated polyphenols such as ECCG, in green tea. A further study amoung human volunteers both with and without diabetes reported that polyphenols, especially condensed tannins significantly reduced the GI of simultaneously consumed carbohydrates.

The benefits of polyphenols are not just restricted to lowering blood sugar. One of the pathogenic mechanisms that explain the development and progression of micro and macro vascular complications in diabetes is oxidative stress; caused by increased generation of free radicals coupled with an impaired antioxidant defense system. Inhibition of these oxidative processes by polyphenols with antioxidant properties is known to help prevent the onset and development of long-term diabetic complications. The underlying mechanisms of how polyphenols have sugar lowering properties include inhibition of α-amylase and α-glucosidase, inhibition of glucose absorption in the intestine by sodium-dependent glucose transporter 1, stimulate insulin secretion and reduce hepatic glucose output. Polyphenols may also enhance insulin-dependent glucose uptake, activate 5' adenosine monophosphate-activated protein kinase.

Diabetic treatments and cancer

Numerous epidemiologic studies and subsequent meta-analyses have repeatedly indicated that T2DM patients receiving metformin, compared to those taking other anti-diabetic medications, have a decreased risk of the occurrence of various types of cancers by 30-50%. Most notably, in the UK, a total of 62,809 patients with diabetes were found to have a higher risk of pancreatic cancer, particularly if also obese, but a lower risk if they were taking metformin monotherapy as opposed to gliclazide or insulin. This finding was substantiated by a pooled analysis of 108,161 patients with T2DM, which reported that metformin treatment was associated with a significantly lower risk of colorectal cancer. Data from 3,837 men obtained from several databases from Canada noted that a longer duration of metformin after prostate cancer was associated with a lower in all-cause mortality. Women with diabetes participating in Women's Health Initiative had, a lower risk of breast cancer if taking metformin opposed to other diabetic drugs.

One proposed indirect mechanism for metformin's benefit lies in the fact that it improves cellular sensitivity to insulin and hence reduces IGF in those developing insulin resistance. Other studies have demonstrated a direct anticancer via inhibition of the (mTORC1) which plays a pivotal role in metabolism, proliferation and antiestrogen hormone resistance in breast cancer cells. Although RCT confirming the protective benefits of metformin have not been completed, these data are very convincing, especially as they involved such large numbers and are from independent prestigious organisations. It would be common sense, if diabetic, to ask your doctor to take metformin as opposed to glyclazide, if otherwise medical feasible.

Summary – reducing processed sugar after cancer

- Wean yourself off adding sugar to tea or coffee
- Eliminate all processed sugar for breakfast
- Never add sugar to savoury foods or veg during cooking
- Avoid pre-packed ready meals if they add sugar
- Avoid food labelled as "low fat" as they may contain sugar
- Throw out boiled and chewy sweets, from the house
- Restrict cakes, sponges and muffins biscuits to after lunch
- If you do eat cakes cut off the icing and sugary toppings
- Refrain from sweet fizzy drinks
- Stop eating in restaurants which add sugar to their meals
- Try not to drink fruit juices with the pulp removed
- Don't eat white toast and jam for breakfast
- Eat salad and vegetables with white pasta to slow its GI
- For treat consider 100% chocolate melted on fruit
- Make cakes without sugar - use fruits, dates or banana instead.
- For snacks, consider sticks of crunchy vegetables or nuts
- If you are craving something sweet – restrict to post meal times
- For a snack easy-to-eat nuts and wholes fruits
- When making smoothies have more veg than fruit.
- Eat plenty of polyphenol-rich fruit and vegetables
- Don't overeat I- f very active eat more if sedentary eat less
- Avoid white rich and white pasta
- Eat foods with a low glycaemic index
- Quinoa, wholemeal bread
- Wild rice, wholemeal pasta, buckwheat

<table>
<tr><td>

</td><td>

Sexual and hormone issues

</td></tr>
</table>

With Dr Catherine Zollman

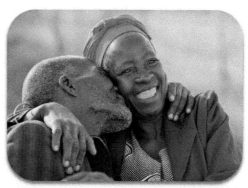

Sexual intimacy is a key element of quality of life for most people, yet they often find it difficult and embarrassing to discuss in a medical setting. Cancer and its treatments cause sexual dysfunction in a greater proportion of patients than most health professionals appreciate. Both patients and partners often miss out on the physical, psychological and bonding benefits of a sexual relationship, and this may lead to other relationship difficulties, emotional problems, depression and demotivation to comply with medical treatments or embark on lifestyle strategies. Maintaining sexual activity can be a sign of overall wellbeing.

Research suggests that although sexual issues may not be a patient's main concern during treatment, they are still an important issue and can persist long after treatment is completed. Despite this, sexual issues are rarely discussed in routine oncology appointments. Healthcare professionals often perceive discussion of sexual issues as disrespectful or inappropriate due to the patient's age, gender, religion, culture or socioeconomic status. Time constraints are also a concern. Sexual issues are not given priority in the clinical setting, meaning healthcare professionals struggle to make time and often do not feel they have the skills to discuss these issues. Finally, a lack of available resources to manage identified sexual problems is another possible barrier to discussion. There have, however, been recent moves to ensure that sexual function is covered during a patient's Holistic Needs Assessment, a process people should be offered routinely after completion of treatment which explains several interventions that can help. The most common types of sexual dysfunction caused by cancer and cancer treatments, alongside some of the most relevant lifestyle approaches, are highlighted in this section.

Types of sexual dysfunction

Erectile dysfunction (ED): There are several physical reasons why men can have difficulties with erections following cancer treatments. Surgery to the pelvic region, prostate, bladder or rectum can damage veins and nerves needed for sexual function. Drugs given for prostate cancer can reduce male hormone levels, the most common culprit being LHRH modulators (e.g. Zoladex), but other drugs for depression and high BP can also compromise sexual function. Radiotherapy to the pelvis or pressure on the spinal cord caused by a tumour in the spine can both have an adverse effect on the nerves to the penis. Erectile dysfunction has also been reported after taking drugs to improve bladder function (e.g. tamsulosin).

Performance-related anxiety: Psychological well-being is very important for a healthy sex life. Depression, lack of self-esteem, low mood, guilt and anxiety all contribute to loss of libido and erectile dysfunction. If a man experiences loss of erection or a woman experiences pain or soreness, he or she may worry that it will happen again. This is called performance-related anxiety and may lead to chronic problems during sexual intercourse.

Retrograde ejaculation: Surgery and sometimes radiotherapy to the prostate can cause semen to enter the bladder instead of exiting through the penis during orgasm. Men can still climax, but they may ejaculate very little or sometimes no semen. This is sometimes called a dry orgasm. It is not harmful but may cause male infertility and can upset some men.

Vaginal dryness and fibrosis: A drop in oestrogen caused by cancer treatments such as aromatase inhibitors (Arimidex, Aromasin and Femara), often results in dryness and thinning of the lining of the vagina. Drugs such as tamoxifen can cause vaginal discharge. Radiotherapy can damage the mucous glands in the vagina, leading to dryness and soreness. As well as causing dryness and soreness, radiotherapy to the pelvis can sometimes cause inflammation, shrinkage and fibrosis of the vagina, leading to pain and sometimes bleeding which make sexual intercourse painful or impossible. If you have received radiotherapy to the pelvis, or are taking drugs which cause dryness, consider regular vaginal dilators with plenty of lubricants or, if possible, have sexual intercourse regularly. Regular gentle stretching of the vagina has been shown to improve function and lubrication.

Body image: Although any cancer diagnosis can cause sexual problems, breast cancer is a unique case in that the breast, although not directly a sex organ, is seen as a symbol of femininity and plays a role in pleasure and stimulation. Most treatments for breast cancer involve surgery to remove all or part of the breast. Surgery can impact on a patients' body image which in turn may affect sexual functioning. Women receiving breast conserving surgery or reconstruction report greater satisfaction with sex life compared to women who receive mastectomy. Other changes in body image including hair loss, weight gain, scars and stoma bags can all have varying impacts on an individual's confidence and sex life.

Loss of libido: Cancer and its treatments can often have a profound effect on libido, even if the *machinery* still works. The desire for sex can be impaired, sometimes as a direct result of reduced hormone levels, or sometimes because of other consequences of cancer treatments such as fatigue or depression.

Vaginosis: The vagina is an ecological niche where several aerobe and anaerobe microorganisms co-exist. It's composition being influenced by age, menarche, menstrual cycle, pregnancy, infections, methods of birth control, sexual activity, use of medication and hygiene. In fertile, premenopausal, healthy women, the vaginal flora is dominated by lactobacillus salivarius, and other lactobacillus strains. On the pathogenic side, common undesirable organisms include yeasts (Candida), anaerobic bacteria responsible for vaginosis (Gardnerella vaginalis, Mycoplasma hominis, and others), uropathogens (Escherichia coli, Proteus and Klebsiella) and sexually transmitted pathogens (syphilis, gonorrhoea, chlamydia, HIV).

By preventing the overgrowth of pathogenic organisms, lactobacilli play an instrumental role in maintaining the normal vaginal microflora. Principally by:

- Stimulation of the immune system
- Competing with pathogens for nutrients
- Competing with pathogens for adherence to the vaginal epithelium
- Reduction of the vaginal pH (make lactic and other organic acids)
- Producing natural antimicrobial chemicals and hydrogen peroxide

Bacterial vaginosis (BV) can afflicting all women but particularly those who are premenopausal, are taking hormonal therapies such as tamoxifen or have recently concluded chemotherapy. It is caused by an overgrowth of vaginal anaerobes which increase production of amines and become more damaging at an alkaline pH (the opposite to the mouth which likes an alkaline PH). Women who have discomfort and notice a strong malodour with a green discharge should go to the GP for a swab and, if an infection is found, receive antibiotics. Therapy with oral or local antibiotics, however, is often associated with failure and high rates of recurrence. Hydrogen peroxide (H_2O_2), produced by commensal lactobacilli bacteria, lowers PH and protects against pathogens. Once vaginosis sets in, H_2O_2 levels drop by up to 85%.

The dominance of lactobacilli in healthy vaginal microbiota, and its depletion in cases of BV, has given rise to the idea that probiotic lactobacillus strains could be utilised in the treatment and prevention of BV, especially following antibiotics, steroids and chemotherapy. Lactobacilli probiotics can be used over a long time without adverse effects, making them an attractive alternative to antibiotics, particularly in addressing the problem of high recurrence rates. The majority of clinical trials using probiotic preparations containing lactobacilli, administered either vaginally, orally or both, have generally yielded positive results. Notably, in two RCTs, women who took an oral probiotics pill demonstrated better vaginal colonisation of lactobacilli, displacement of pathogenic bacteria and reduced vaginal inflammation.

Another single-blind study compared intravaginal probiotics with metronidazole gel. A BV cure rate of 65% was achieved after probiotic treatment, compared to 33% following metronidazole therapy. In three out of five further studies, when oral and intravaginal probiotics were used following antibiotic treatment, the BV cure rate was increased and recurrence rates were reduced. The authors of these trials tend to agree that a combination of oral and intravaginal probiotics would provide the best results.

What else can be done to help sexual health?

Exercise: Being unfit can be a physical barrier to sexual activity. Regular exercise also improves psychological wellbeing which is a major factor in sexual health. The penis is very sensitive to changes in oxygen and blood supply. In fact, ED is often the first sign of hardened arteries and can precede angina by two years unless intervention has taken place. It is known that, in general, men who maintain a higher level of physical activity and who don't smoke are less likely to have erectile dysfunction (ED). A study from Cambridge University Hospital reported that men who were physically active during and after their radiotherapy had much lower ED rates as well as less urinary and bowel symptoms. More specifically, pelvic floor exercises are useful as these directly stimulate the muscles around your penis or vagina. If performed correctly these can be a great help. The problem is that most people give them up after a few days or are very sporadic with them. They need to be performed correctly for at least 10 minutes a day on a long-term, ongoing basis. Even then, an improvement only usually starts appearing after six to eight weeks – it is important to keep going.

Avoid excessive vaginal douching: An estimated 30% of women between the ages of 15 and 44 in Europe, UK and the USA use a vaginal douche. Higher rates are seen particularly among teens, African-American and Hispanic women. Despite its popularity, health experts, including those at the American College of Gynecologists, advise against regular douching. Having some vaginal odour is normal. The acidity of the vagina will, in most cases, naturally control bacteria, and hygiene can be maintained simply by washing the vagina with warm, salted water or mild soap. Douching with antiseptic liquids upsets the natural balance of bacteria in the vagina and washes away healthy bacteria, merely encouraging the growth of bacteria which cause infection. Studies have found that women who stopped douching were less likely to have bacterial vaginosis.

Dietary interventions: Although a small amount of alcohol can increase libido in some people by reducing inhibition, excessive alcohol intake can compromise erectile function and reduce libido. There may be some indirect truth regarding the supposed aphrodisiacal properties of oysters, with the high zinc and selenium content important for a number of enzymatic functions, including those in the fertility pathways. Some people choose to get their selenium and essential mineral blood levels checked so they can adjust their diet accordingly. Foods rich in plants nitrates can improve blood flow, and there are some reports they can help with erections. Some women find that omega 7 sea buckthorn oil capsules taken by mouth can help reduce vaginal soreness and dryness.

Drugs interventions: In men, medication such as PDE5 inhibitors, Viagra and Cialis can help achieve a satisfactory erection. They also aid performance-anxiety related ED because once a man has the reassurance that he can get an erection with medication, just the thought of this backup option is often enough to help. Partial erections or erections which are not sustained are usually restored to normal after these tablets, but for those unable to get an erection at all, tablets are often less effective. Some surgeons recommend taking them every day (whether you are having sex or not) for a month, as this seems to help in the longer term. If these drugs do not work or aren't appropriate, it is worth asking for a referral to a specialist urologist or nurse who may be able to offer a number of other interventions ranging from penile pumps to intra-penile injections. In women, using prescribed or over-the-counter lubricants can be very helpful. It is worth trying a few different varieties to see which works best for you.

Hormone replacement therapy (HRT): As noted above, many cancer treatments interfere with ovarian and testicular function. In people whose cancers are not hormone-sensitive, replacing deficient sex hormones, either by mouth, by skin patches or applied directly to the vagina using creams or pessaries, can usually be a safe and very successful way to improve hot flashes, reduce vaginal dryness and improve libido and overall satisfaction with sexual function. Despite this, HRT remains an under utilised option among this group of cancer survivors. However, many types of cancer, including most prostate and womb cancers, as well as many breast cancers, are hormone sensitive, and in these cases, the pros and cons of any hormone replacement strategies should be carefully discussed with your doctor.

Counselling: Several RCTs have evaluated the benefits of the two main types of counselling. *Supportive counselling*, typically delivered to individual patients, aims to help

167

patients deal with diagnosis and treatment and improve self-confidence and body image. *Sexual counselling* can be delivered to couples and involve encouraging them to discuss their ideas for a mutually satisfying sex life. Both these techniques have demonstrated some improvement of sexual function, especially if combined with other lifestyle manoeuvres.

Summary – Advice to help preserve sexual function

- Discuss medications with your doctor (including BP tablets)
- For men, consider extra medications such as Viagra, Cialis etc.
- For men, if ED continues, ask to be referred to a specialist urologist
- In women, simple lubrication may help
- Consider HRT if regarded as safe by your oncologist
- Look after your general health;
  - Stop smoking, eat well, lose weight and exercise regularly
- Perform pelvic floor exercises regularly, correctly and indefinitely
- Avoid excessive alcohol or other recreational drugs
- Reduce general anxiety – see the 'anxiety' section
- Women should discuss medications such as aromatase inhibitors
- Consider seeing a sexuality counsellor

Hot flushes

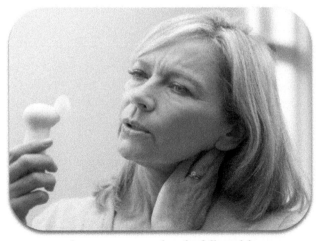

One troublesome consequence of falling natural levels of oestrogen and testosterone is an imbalance in the body's cooling system, causing hot flushes (flashes) and night sweats. These are described as a sudden and unpleasant sensation of heat spreading across the face, neck and chest. Hot flushes are common among women during natural menopause when oestrogen levels fall and hormones from the pituitary gland in the head rise. Cancer treatments may also cause premature and more dramatic menopausal symptoms. Hot flushes can range from a mild heat intolerance to prolific sweating throughout the day and night, disrupting sleep, causing embarrassment and sometimes even leading to fainting and exhaustion.

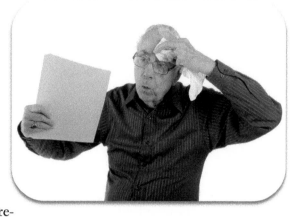

In women and men, the cancer treatments that can damage the ovaries or testes include surgery, chemotherapy, radiotherapy and hormone therapy. Hormone therapy is given to reduce cancer growth in people whose cancers are "hormone sensitive", which means that their cancer cells grow when exposed to hormones circulating in the blood. In pre-menopausal women, cancer treatments can cause an early menopause. In post-menopausal women who are given aromatase inhibitors, oestrogen levels can drop even further. Tamoxifen commonly causes hot flushes via its ability to bind to the oestrogen receptors. Hormone injections with LHRH modulators (like Zoladex) stop the pituitary gland in the brain from telling the ovaries and testes to produce hormones. Bone hardening drugs (bisphosphonates) can cause or aggravate hot flushes by a completely independent mechanism.

Medical treatments: If the hormones you are taking are causing unbearable hot flushes, and the lifestyle measures described below do not help, it would be worth discussing again the benefits they are providing. In some cases, they are only reducing the risk of relapse by 1-2% and balancing this against quality of life may not be worth it. Obviously, this is a discussion best had with your oncologist. If the lifestyle strategies highlighted below have not helped, it is also worth discussing with your doctor a trial of different versions of the initially prescribed hormone drugs, or the addition of other drugs such as progesterone, clonidine or antidepressants (Venlaflexine). Some of these certainly help but can have side effects of their own.

What can you do to help?

It is useful to keep a diary of your hot flushes, in order to prepare for or, better still, avoid the common trigger factors. If you know entering a warm room, drinking hot drinks or eating spicy foods can spark a flush, loosen the collar, take off a jumper or open a window first. Exercise to a level which makes you sweat, while a sauna (with sufficient cooling afterwards) can also help and gives the sweat glands a good flush.

Hypnosis, yoga and relaxation: Using self-hypnosis techniques such as imagining being in cool air or water has been shown to be helpful for some people. One single-arm pilot study explored the use of hypnosis in the treatment of hot flashes. Participants received four weekly 45-minute hypnosis sessions. They found that regular hypnosis reduced the frequency of 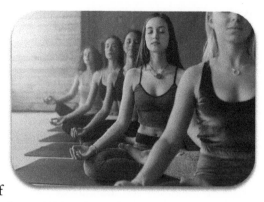 hot flashes and the impact they had on daily activities, including sexual functioning. Yoga and relaxation classes have had limited success.

Other complementary therapies: Acupuncture may be worth considering, as one study suggests that it is at least as effective as antidepressants. Homeopathy involves the use of preparations which are given at very low doses, which means that they are very safe as they do not interact with conventional medications and do not cause stimulatory effects on cancer cells. While there is considerable controversy about the mechanism by which homeopathy may work, and whether its effects are simply attributable to placebo, there are a number of published research papers which show beneficial effects in some people.

Nutrition and herbal interventions: Several studies have suggested that women who have diets high in phyto-oestrogens generally have fewer hot flushes or other menopausal symptoms. Despite this, a well-conducted scientific trial examining the effects of phyto-oestrogen supplements (which contain high levels of phyto-oestrogens difficult to obtain using food 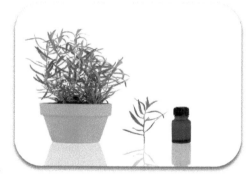 alone) in breast cancer patients with hot flushes showed no benefit. In a less robust trial, Sage (a natural anhidrotic which reduces sweating) has been reported to reduce hot flushes and other menopausal symptoms in some women. Black cohosh is also widely used for menopausal symptoms, and some trials report a benefit. One study of Dong Quai, a traditional Chinese medicine, report no benefit but another which combined it with chamomile did find it to be significantly more effective than placebo. It is uncertain how evening primrose oil, which is often recommended for hot flushes, could affect menopausal symptoms, with one placebo-controlled RCT trial finding that it did not reduce the frequency of hot flushes any more than placebo.

Two RCTs comparing ginseng with placebo found that it did not alleviate mood, or improve cognition in post-menopausal women, although it did help fatigue.

Many oncologists are not comfortable with recommending phyto-oestrogen supplements, as in theory they could stimulate residual cancer cells. There is no evidence for this in humans, but some animal studies have shown that phytoestrogen supplements can stimulate the lining of the uterus. There are numerous ongoing studies to help decide whether phytoestrogens can be used to help hot flushes or whether prolonged use could be harmful. In the meantime, it is probably best to avoid phyto-oestrogen supplements in tablet or powder form (sometimes these are marketed as soy isoflavone supplements) and stick to whole, healthy foods which contain phyto-oestrogens in their natural state and concentrations instead. Examples of these include soya-based foods, other pulses and ground flaxseed.

On the other hand, non-oestrogenic phytochemical supplements are safe and can help menopausal symptoms by reducing excess inflammation and elevating mood. The original Pomi-T trial did not measure hot flushes as the men involved were not taking hormones, but this testimonial was sent to the research unit:

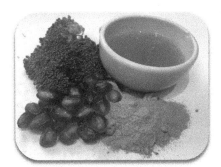

"After watching a TV program featuring Pomi-T, I thought I would give it a go, simply to help get rid of free radicals. After taking it for a short while, I noticed that I no longer had ANY hot flushes. I hadn't taken any prescribed medication for this. The only change I had made was taking Pomi-T twice daily. I was amazed but thought I would stop them and see what happened. Within a day or two, the flushes came back! I started the Pomi-T immediately, and within two days they had completely stopped again. I have taken them now for six months and have not had a single flush. I would never at the outset thought this would have happened. I cannot thank you enough, flushes are debilitating and this truly has transformed my life".

Other women have contacted the trials unit reporting a similar benefit which although very interesting, is not proof of effectiveness. Nevertheless, it has prompted a forthcoming study by the Institute of Sports Science at Bedford which will evaluate men and women taking hormone therapies.

CBD oils are extracted from the cannabis plant but do not have the psychotropic (THC) component. Current research suggests there are biologically active networks of endocannabinoids and cannabinoid receptors in the central and peripheral nervous systems. These influence a number of physiological and cognitive processes including heat regulation. CBD is thought to help reduce hot flushes by increasing an enzyme called fatty acid amide hydrolase (FAAH) which falls as oestrogen falls. While CBD increases levels of this enzyme, it does not increase oestrogen itself and is consequently regarded as safe. Formal trials in women are lacking, but there are numerous anecdotal reports of benefit. It may be worth a try, but remember to get an organic brand from a reputable supplier (such as that found on keep-healthy.com).

Summary – Advice for hot flushes

Clothes and environment
- Wear cotton clothing rather than polyester or other man-made fibres
- Wear layers of clothes that can be taken off or put on quickly
- Use layers of bedclothes (natural fabrics) that can be removed
- An electric fan placed on a desk or table helps
- Adopt sleep hygiene tactics if you are not sleeping
- Avoid warm or stuffy rooms as they can make flushes worse
- Take plenty of cool baths, showers and saunas (cooling afterwards)
- Use sprays or wipes to help lower skin temperature
- Remove a coat or jumper before entering a warm room

Diet and liquids
- Keep a note of what foods trigger a flush e.g. Chilli, hot drinks
- Avoid large meals excess sugar, especially at night
- If you are overweight, it is more difficult to regulate your temperature
- Alcohol and caffeine in coffee or strong tea can trigger a flush
- If sweating a lot, drink plenty of healthy fluids e.g. water and tea
- Evening primrose oil, Vitamin E and B6 supplements may help

Exercise and complementary therapies
- Regular exercise helps to reduce the severity of hot flushes
- Massage, reflexology and aromatherapy are safe and de-stress
- Acceptance – hot flushes are normal and most people don't notice them
- Acupuncture has been shown to help but needs to be done regularly
- If the above measures fail, some supplements are worth a trial:
  - Sage supplement can help, but there are oestrogenic concerns
  - Polyphenol products such as Pomi-T are saver
  - Organic CBD oils

Chapter 11

Exercise after cancer

With Daniel Bailey

The benefits of exercise do not stop after a cancer diagnosis. A number of studies have shown that patients who exercise regularly have a lower risk of relapse and have longer overall survival. The Melbourne Collaborative Cohort Study analysed the exercise habits of 526 patients with bowel carcinoma and found that while 57% of patients were alive at five years in the non-exerciser group, 71% were still alive in the exerciser group. This 14% difference was

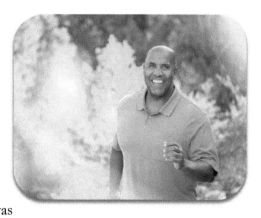

statistically significant. As regards to death, one of the largest US trials evaluated exercise habits in people with bowel cancer who had received chemotherapy. They found a 12% lower risk of dying (61 v 73%) in those who took part in recreational activities one or more times per week that made them sweat or feel out of breath. This benefit was seen across all stages of cancer and took into account other risk factors such as weight, smoking, tumour grade and stage of cancer.

A similar finding was demonstrated in another American study involving 816 patients with higher risk, resected local colon cancer. Those who took part in the most physical activity were 35% less likely to relapse and were more likely to have improved overall survival compared to those who took part in the lowest amount of physical activity. This study also evaluated blood samples and revealed major differences in inflammatory markers and oxidative stress between exercisers and non-exercisers, both of which are important for improving cancer outcomes. Other studiesAs regards the amount of exercise, an analysis of activity among 2,686 men with prostate cancer showed that those who jogged, played tennis, or enjoyed other comparable exercise for an average of three or more hours per week, had a 35% lower death rate than those who exercised less or not at all. As for walking, those who did so for four or more hours per week had 23% lower overall death rates than those who walked for fewer than 20 minutes per week. This suggests that people with cancer can take part in a wide range of different types of exercise to lower their risk of death.

Exercise and side effects of treatment

Exercise is also one of the main self-help factors which can reduce many of the risks and side effects associated with cancer treatments. A large analysis, summarising the findings from 34 RCTs, found that cancer patients who took part in exercise programmes had significantly improved levels of fatigue, mood, muscle power, hand grip strength, fitness and quality of life. A similar analysis, conducted by the American College of Sports Medicine, reviewed 85 studies and concluded that physical activity could safely be performed during and after cancer treatment and that it led to significant improvements in aerobic fitness, quality of life, body image, flexibility and strength, and reduced anxiety, depression and fatigue. Other important studies have also reported that exercise during and after cancer treatments, especially if supported by a supervised exercise programme, reduced the risks of:

- Blood clots - thrombosis
- Weight gain
- Reduced muscle power
- Cancer-related fatigue
- Heart problems
- Joint pains and arthritis
- Hot flushes
- Other menopausal symptoms
- Osteoporosis
- Urinary urgency
- Erectile dysfunction
- Heartburn and indigestion
- Peripheral neuropathy
- Diminished hand grip strength, fitness
- Reduced Cognition (chemo brain)
- Mood, anxiety and depression

A well-designed exercise programme can increase the degree of empowerment for patients and carers. It creates an overall sense of well-being and improves social integration and self-esteem. Physically active people are more likely to recover sooner, putting less strain on family dynamics and enabling them to return to normal activities after treatment. What's more, the benefits of physical activity span across several common cancer types involving a range of treatments including surgery, radiotherapy, chemotherapy and hormonal and biological therapies.

How does exercise fight cancer?

Over 180 biochemical changes occur after exercise. Most of these are beneficial against cancer and other chronic diseases such as heart disease and diabetes. A summary of these will now be highlighted and divided into those which directly influence cancer, and those which have an indirect pathway.

Indirect anti-cancer pathways

A number of studies have shown that supervised exercise programmes help individuals lose weight (about 6-10% per year). Vitamin D and sunlight exposure are both higher among those who exercise regularly outdoors. The chapter addressing vitamin D has already summarised the health benefits of maintaining adequate levels.

Regular exercise, especially if in groups and combined with relaxation, mindfulness and healthy eating programmes, has been shown to help improve mood and reduce anxiety and fear of relapse. As well as being distressing, cohort studies from California involving men with prostate cancer, and from Korea involving men with head and neck cancer, reported higher relapse rates and lower survival in those with anxiety or depression. The mechanism by which exercise helps fight depression has not yet been firmly established, but theories include increased endorphin and monoamine release, mental distraction and rises in core temperatures. In addition, light exposure, which increases with outdoor exercise, has been linked to a reduction in non-seasonal depressive disorders. Less depressed patients are also more likely to comply with medical interventions, which explains the improvement achieved with supervised exercise programmes.

Direct anti-cancer pathways

An array of direct biological, epigenetic, metabolic and inflammatory changes occur in the body after exercise, both acutely and over time. It's not been established which one, or combination of these, has the most influence on cancer pathways. The most notable pathways involve:

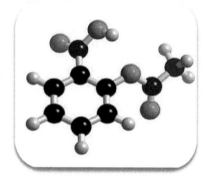

Insulin-like growth factor: The biological risks of raised IGF levels and cancer have been highlighted already in several sections of this book. Exercise has been linked with lower IGF in the HPFS, and this, in turn, was linked with a 48% reduction of cancer-specific deaths. Decreased levels of IGF in physically active patients after bowel cancer have also been linked to improved survival.

Epigenetic effects on gene expression and DNA repair: Exercise has been shown to have a significant impact on how genes are expressed (activated or not) in both cancer and normal cells. The GEMINAL study, a pilot trial involving men with low-risk prostate cancer, found a set of *RAS* family oncogenes to be down-regulated after an exercise and lifestyle programme. In the prostate, a *RAS*-related nuclear protein (RAN) appears to function as an androgen receptor activator, and its expression is increased in tumour tissues. Another study, involving men on active surveillance, demonstrated that 184 genes were differentially expressed between individuals who engaged in vigorous activity and those who did not engage in any physical activity. Genes particularly sensitive to exercise included those involved in signalling cell cycling and those supporting DNA repair including BRCA1 and BRCA2. The same up-regulation of BRCA expression following exercise has been demonstrated in women who were even BRCA 1 or 2 mutation carriers, making exercise even more important in this group. Markers of an improved cellular repair

175

process were also reported in a study which showed that exercise up-regulated the key regulator gene p53 and, by doing so, encourages damaged cells to repair or, if not possible, self-destruct. Telomere length has been shown to be a prognostic marker among men with prostate cancer on active surveillance. Moderate exercise and a healthy eating programme increased telomere length in blood and this correlated with reduced PSA progression.

Vasoactive Intestinal Peptide (VIP) is a neuropeptide that stimulates growth in cancer cells. Patients with breast and prostate cancer have been found to have higher VIP titres compared with matched pairs in the general population without cancer. Serum VIP has been shown to increase transiently after exercise. This transient rise leads to the production of natural anti-VIP antibodies, explaining the observation that individuals who regularly exercise in the long-term have lower VIP titres.

Oxidative stress and antioxidant pathways: Exercise can initially increase production of reactive oxidative species (ROS) and, therefore, can initially increase oxidative stress in the cell. In response to this transient increase, provided individuals have adequate levels of polyphenols, minerals and vitamins, an adaptive up-regulation of antioxidant enzymes occurs. These increased levels of superoxide dismutase and catalase not only restore oxidative stress but help maintain lower stress levels in the longer term. In a pilot study at the University of California, men who participated in at least three hours per week of vigorous physical activity had reduced markers for oxidative stress in their prostate tissue. Other studies confirm that trained individuals, and those embarking on a sensible graduated programme, have lower cellular stress.

Immunity: During exercise, increased levels of catecholamines stimulate the recruitment of white blood cells (leucocytes) into the peripheral blood. One study reported that individuals who regularly perform >2 hrs of moderate exercise per day had a 29% reduction in risk of upper respiratory tract infection compared with a sedentary lifestyle. On the other hand, if exercise is too strenuous for that individual, it is followed by decreased concentrations of lymphocytes and temporary impaired cellular-mediated immunity. One particular study highlighted how there was an increased risk of infection among subjects in the weeks following a competitive ultra-endurance running event. Overall, most long-term studies suggest that the effect of moderate exercise has little influence on immune function in healthy populations. However, its benefits are certainly felt among the obese or elderly whose immune function is often less efficient. This suggests exercise has an important role to play in boosting the immunity of individuals after cancer treatments.

Chronic inflammation and prostaglandins: There is a general consensus that the reason for a lower immunity in the elderly stems from overcompensation by an ailing immune system trying to maintain immunosenescence. Exercise is known to enhance natural killer cell activity and increase T-cell production, reducing the need for the immune system to increase circulating inflammatory biomarkers – it is therefore anti-inflammatory. Chronic inflammation can also be caused by excess prostaglandin levels which are biologically active lipids generated from arachidonic acid via the enzyme cyclo-oxidase (COX). Moderate, regular, non-traumatic exercise reduces serum prostaglandins. Most notably, a study in patients who, for various reasons needed a rectal biopsy, showed that leisure-time physical activity was linked with lower tissue prostaglandin concentration. This study also showed that overweight individuals, in particular, had increased mucosal prostaglandins, but increases in activity levels led to a 28% decrease in mucosal levels. Another reported anti-inflammatory mechanism concerns a mediator with the unlikely name of "apoptosis-associated speck-like protein containing a caspase recruitment domain", or ASC for short. ASC, via a number of biochemical steps, activates the release of ILs and other inflammatory cytokines, including TNF. The activation status of the ASC gene is influenced by epigenetic factors, particularly methylation, and exercise upregulates the methylation of ASC, resulting in its decreased activity in white cells and hence a lower inflammatory response.

Heat shock proteins (HSP) are produced in tissues in response to a wide variety of physiological and environmental trauma including infection, hypoxia, hyperthermia, dexamethasone and chemotherapy. They have protective functions including blocking apoptosis and allowing the cell to survive potentially lethal events. Consequently, they are substantially overexpressed following a myocardial infarction. They are also increased acutely following a bout of exercise. This acute rise in HPS is significantly lower in trained athletes and is most pronounced after severe anaerobic exercise, especially if the participant is previously unfit. An increase in HSP is the likely mechanism by which exercise protects the hearts of patients receiving chemotherapy. An increase in HPS is also the suggested mechanism behind exercise reducing cognitive impairment during chemotherapy, by protecting the astrocytes and supportive cells within the brain.

There is a potential albeit unlikely downside to this pathway, as some doctors suggest that HPS could protect cancer cells as well. This was based on one laboratory experiment which suggested that the addition of high levels of HPS to cell lines increased resistance to chemo. However, this experiment does not reflect a real life situation, because cancer cells produce their own HPS in much higher quantities than can ever be produced by exercise, so it is unlikely that the changes in serum HPS levels after exercise have any influence on levels inside cancer cells. Furthermore, increased serum levels are highly likely to help normal cells much more than cancer cells, helping facilitate higher chemo doses. This is supported by a recent experiment in mice that reports a better cancer response to adriamycin chemotherapy with concomitant exercise. Researchers in Phoenix, USA are now investigating whether administering chemo while patients are exercising on a stationary bicycle could allow higher doses of chemo to be used without greater normal tissue damage. Some cancer cells have also learned to harness the protective properties of HSP and even become HSP-dependent for their survival, which makes them an interesting potential therapeutic target. Until further research is published, however, it is probably wise to advise patients to avoid unaccustomed anaerobic or rigorous exercise just before or immediately after chemotherapy. Instead, build up exercise gradually.

Testosterone and oestrogen: Excess levels of androgens are associated with a higher incidence of prostate cancer, but what happens to testosterone after exercise is complex and depends on the underlying level of fitness, exercise intensity and even mood at the time of training. It is widely stated that serum testosterone increases immediately after vigorous exercise, but this has not been confirmed in all studies. This effect also appears to be very short-lived, with testosterone returning to pre-exercise levels by two hours. It is also often quoted that resistance training increases testosterone more than endurance exercises, yet there is very little to substantiate this in scientific experiments. In fact, both endurance exercise and resistance training have been reported to cause a transient increase in testosterone levels in men and women in a number of studies. It is important to note that these studies report that testosterone binding protein also rises with exercise but the free, biologically active testosterone proportion changes very little. Furthermore, this transient testosterone rise has not been reported in men over 55 years, when men are at a higher risk of prostate cancer. More importantly, over time, regular moderate or intense exercise actually lowers testosterone due to a negative feedback mechanism. This may be a bonus for men with prostate cancer but is a problem for many endurance athletes.

Some studies have reported that exercise and a healthy lifestyle delays the natural, age-related decline in testosterone. However, these studies involved subjects with conditions such as obesity, metabolic syndrome, diabetes and dyslipidaemia which had dropped testosterone levels below normal. In this case, exercise simply helped restore normal levels. There is evidence that, even before weight reduction occurs, exercise directly lowers serum oestrogen and leptin levels. In one clinical study, this was quantified as every 100 minutes of exercise causing a 3.6 % lowering of serum oestrogen.

Irisin is a messenger protein produced in muscle cells in response to exercise. One study reported that higher levels were linked to more favourable breast cancer prognostic risk at diagnosis. In laboratory studies, irisin significantly reduced cancer cell proliferation, migration and viability in malignant cancer cell lines, without affecting non-malignant cells. In another study, irisin enhanced the cytotoxic effect of doxorubicin when added to malignant breast cells, which again was not observed in non-malignant cells. Recent experiments, using highly sensitive and specific mass spectrometry, found far lower levels of irisin among inactive participants than in individuals who had followed programmes of aerobic interval training.

Energy metabolism and insulin resistance: A number of RCTs have shown that exercise improves insulin sensitivity and glucose metabolism even in patients taking androgen deprivation therapy (ADT) for prostate cancer. Androgen deprivation treatments for men with prostate cancer may cause a rise in circulating insulin, triglycerides and abdominal obesity, features of metabolic syndrome which carries a poor prognosis. Men randomised to an exercise programme after starting ADT can counterbalance these biochemical changes, lowering their risk of weight gain and metabolic syndrome. It has long been known that exercise, combined with dietary modification, not only reduces triglycerides but also total cholesterol and improves the ratio of high-density lipoprotein (the good cholesterol) to low-density lipoprotein. Large population studies have suggested that high levels of cholesterol in the blood are associated with an increased risk of cancer.

Designing your exercise programme

Whichever exercise you decide on, the essential point is that it should become a part of your regular routine. The choice depends on numerous practical factors such as local availability, ability, previous experience, preferences, cost, time pressures and what friends and family like to do as well. If an activity is to be sustained it should be enjoyable and convenient. There is little point putting yourself through torture, as even the most motivated person will give this up fairly quickly. After overcoming the initial barriers, exercise will be the norm and not exercising will feel unusual.

Depending on your condition and ability, try to build up to 2-3 hours of moderately intense exercise per week. Not everyone can achieve this, especially shortly after intense cancer treatments, but set yourself a realistic target and try and stick to it. You can start off with a small amount then gradually build this up. Any exercise is better than none. If you get pain when starting to exercise or have a specific disability which hinders exercise, don't be afraid to ask for help from a physiotherapist or exercise professional.

The type of exercise programme you choose depends on your preferences, goal and abilities, as well as available time and facilities. Whether exercising at a gym or at home, alone or supervised, within each session the emphasis should be on whole body conditioning. A typical session should ideally last about an hour at an intensity which gets you a little breathless, hot and sweaty. Ideally, each session should include:

- A warm-up
- Aerobic exercises such as walking, jogging, cycling or swimming
- Lifting weight using the large muscle groups in your body
- Balance
- Flexibility
- A cool down with general and specific stretching

Many people like to alternate between a longer run, swim or row on one day, and more resistance weight the next. In terms of order, resistance training should generally be performed after the aerobic exercise or, at the very least, after a good warm up. Balance training may be integrated into the resistance training portion of the session. Within the cool down session, as well as general stretches, those relevant to previous treatments can be emphasised.

Exercise goals: Specific exercises are a vital part of rehabilitation after surgery or radiotherapy to the breast, abdomen or pelvis and these are described in detail in the next chapter. If your goal is to lose weight, emphasis should be on regular and prolonged aerobic exercise combined with calorie restriction. If your aim is to prevent or correct osteoporosis, it is essential to consider squatting with weights as part of your regimen. A large

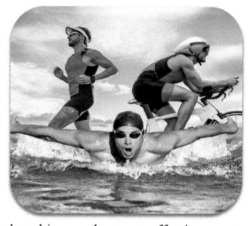

intervention study from Australia showed that this was the most effective way to harden bones and was safe even in people with established osteoporosis. Also, try to exercise outdoors to help improve Vitamin D levels. If arthritis or joint pains are an issue, spend more time stretching and consider yoga and Pilates. To improve coordination, make social contact and stimulate mental agility by considering a team game such as walking football and a competitive sport such as table tennis, bowls or even tennis. If aiming to combat the side effects of hormones such as androgen deprivation in men, consider more resistance and core exercises to maintain strength.

Aerobic exercises: Aerobic conditioning should be taken at a moderate level in both intensity and duration. In a gym, treadmills, cross trainers, arm cycling, and rowing machines are all suitable, as is outside jogging or strides in the local park. Aerobic exercise can improve heart and lung fitness, reduce fatigue and improve psychological distress. The duration of a bout of specific aerobic exercise depends on the emphasis of the session for that particular day and how much aerobic exercise has been performed by the individual during their activities of daily living. On training days that include resistance training, 20–30 minutes of aerobic exercise is ideal. On non-resistance training days, 30–60 minutes of aerobic exercise is appropriate, as recommended by the American Cancer Society. Aerobic exercise duration may also be limited by the presence of fatigue. In this case, it may be necessary to recommend shorter bouts of exercise throughout the day such as three 10 minute sessions jogging or walking briskly in the morning, afternoon and evening. This has been shown to obtain similar improvements to one longer gym session without the associated fatigue.

Resistance training: Light regular resistance (weight) training is an ideal way to increase strength, reduce fatigue and can be combined with core and balance exercises. Although many factors lead to the development of cancer-related fatigue, skeletal muscle wasting resulting from cancer is a major contributing factor. An exercise intervention that focuses on 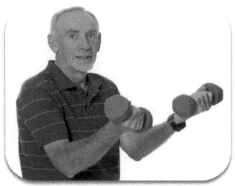 resistance training to stimulate protein synthesis is especially valuable for individuals experiencing cancer muscle wasting. Resistance training also slows down the common age-related decrease in muscle formation.

Balance training: Cancer treatments can impair balance by:
- Weakening the core strength muscles
- Damaging the nerves sensing the position of the limbs (proprioception)
- Damaging the sensory nerves to the limbs (peripheral neuropathy).

Loss of balance can be exacerbated by a general lack of confidence in physical ability. Balance training requires the use of both the core muscles and large muscles of the lower body. There are a wide variety of balance and core devices available in most gyms, yet simply standing on one leg and combining this with light bicep curls can be just as effective. The use of walking poles 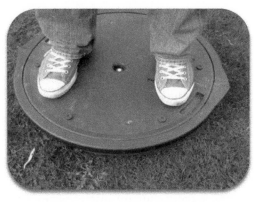 (nordic-walking.co.uk) can provide confidence and prevent falls at the start of balance training. As people get more advanced, a half ball balance trainer is very helpful. It can be used in two ways. Stand on two feet with the flat surface uppermost then squat slowly up and down. This can be made harder by carrying some dumbbells. Alternatively, put the flat surface on the ground and stand with one leg in the centre, then step on and off repeatedly. Another advanced exercise consists of throwing and catching a light medicine ball while seated or standing on a stability ball. Moving farther apart will make this exercise more difficult. To integrate balance training into resistance training, try bicep curls while standing on the balance trainer.

Flexibility stretches: Training sessions should aim to try and stretch the entire body. Try to introduce an order to ensure areas are not missed. For example, start with the right hand, wrist, arm, elbow, shoulder, then repeat on the left side. Move to the neck, thoracic spine, then feet and knees, hips and lower back. In addition to generally 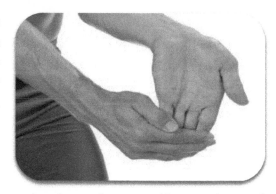 increasing your flexibility, there are some situations where specific exercises and stretches will aid recovery, improve local symptoms and help prevent long term complications such as neck or shoulder stiffness. It is important that these exercises and stretches are performed regularly and correctly. If you're not sure, ask a physiotherapist or a well-qualified exercise professional in the local gym. A personal Pilates instructor also qualified in cancer rehabilitation would be money well spent.

When to start?

A well designed multicentre trial from Holland looked at the benefits of a supervised exercise regimen adopted from the start of chemo. They randomised 230 patients undergoing chemo for breast or prostate cancer to receive either a standard or a supervised exercise regimen. The standard routine consisted of 30 minutes of activity every day but no weight training, while the 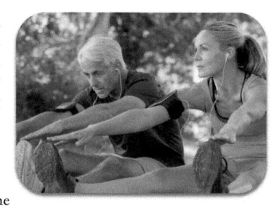 intense regimen consisted of 30 minutes daily of similar activity plus two sessions per week of 20 minutes of weight training and 30 minutes of intense aerobic exercise achieving 60-80% of the maximum heart rate. After 6 months, despite the burden of chemo, patients in the intense exercise regimen had less fatigue, less nausea and greater muscle strength.

A landmark trial from the USA, involving 355 patients with breast or bowel cancer receiving taxanes or platinum chemo, found that those randomised to a moderate-intensity, home-based, six-week progressive walking and resistance exercise programme, had significantly reduced peripheral neuropathy. The effect was greater if the participant was older and exercise is started from cycle one of chemo.

Formal rehabilitation programmes after cancer

Some oncology units have a list of local facilities or even offer exercise rehabilitation. The website cancernet.co.uk/exercise has tools which allow users to search for local exercise recreational facilities. There are over 5,500 community recreation centres in the UK, so most people have one in their area. A scheme exists which enables doctors to refer 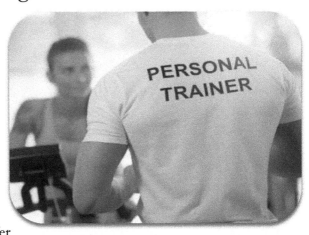 people for exercise rehabilitation, supervised by appropriately qualified exercise professionals. In addition, a course for exercise professionals was developed with the national body Skills Active, to allow exercise professionals to qualify in cancer rehabilitation. This qualification provides them with the knowledge of how cancer and its treatments affect an individual's ability to exercise, enabling them to design bespoke exercise programmes for their clients. Not all personal trainers have this Level 4 qualification, so if you are considering using the services of an exercise professional, it would be worth checking that they have it.

Tips to improve daily physical activity levels

Get prepared
- Buy a comfortable pair of training shoes and sports clothes
- Prioritise exercise sessions at least three times a week
- Tell your boss and family that this time must be protected
- Research the exercise facilities in your area
- Ask friends and family to exercise with you or invest in a personal trainer
- Ask your GP to refer you to a 12-week rehab programme

Join a local exercise group you could enjoy, e.g.
- Gym, walking group, swimming classes, cycling group, Tai Chi
- Walking football, table tennis, bowls, exercise class, Yoga, Pilates

Within your daily routine and social life
- Walk instead of using the car for short journeys
- Get off public transport one stop earlier
- Use the stairs instead of the lift, walk on the escalator
- Cycle to the shops – invest in a bike with a basket
- Meet friends in sports venues rather than the pub or cinema
- Consider an exercise retreat instead of a standard holiday

Sustain a regular exercise programme
- Find something you enjoy
- Keep an exercise diary – miss one day, do more the next

Plan your routine
- A warm-up followed by aerobic exercises and conditioning
- Include resistance training, as well as balance and flexibility exercises
- A cool down with general and specific stretching

Do more specific exercises for specific goals
- Weight control – exercise before breakfast on an empty stomach
- Stress and arthritis – yoga, Pilates
- Balance, cognitive function – Pilates, walking football
- Social – bowls, table tennis, golf, walking football
- Osteoporosis – Squat with weights

<table>
<tr><td>

Chapter 12

</td><td>

Smoking after cancer

</td></tr>
</table>

Smoking 25 cigarettes a day increases your chances of dying from cancer twenty-five-fold. Cigarettes are the number one cause of preventable death in the Western Word. In the USA alone it kills more people than HIV, heroin, crystal meth, cocaine, alcohol, motor vehicle accidents and firearms combined. The free radicals in cigarette smoke reduces a person's lifespan by at least 10 years. Although the relationship between cancer and smoking is no longer in doubt, its harmful effect during and after cancer therapies is less well known and include:

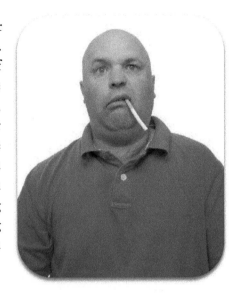

- Premature ageing and skin wrinkles
- Heart disease and stroke – smokers double their risk
- Arterial disease - peripheral vascular disease, aneurysms and gangrene
- Increased anxiety and risk of depression
- Cancer of the lung, mouth, nose, throat, larynx and oesophagus,
- Cancer of the bowel, breast pancreas, bladder, stomach and kidney
- Leukaemia, lymphoma, myeloma and other immune cancers
- Chronic bronchitis, emphysema and other lung diseases
- Stomach ulcers
- Tobacco amblyopia, macular degeneration (blindness)
- Increased risk of osteoporosis – brittle bones that are liable to fracture
- Infertility and earlier menopause
- Increased risk of erectile dysfunction and vaginal dryness
- Pregnancy, miscarriage and low birth weight
- Blood clots – deep-vein thrombosis, pulmonary embolism, strokes
- Dementia and memory loss

Smoking after cancer

Data obtained from thousands of patients with cancer reveals that the chance of cure is at least 10% lower in smokers compared to non-smokers. Patients with cancer of the bladder, kidney, and head and neck area, not only had a higher chance of their original cancer returning, but also an increased risk of the development of new cancers elsewhere. There is also an increased relapse rate of cancers not obviously related to smoking, including bowel, lymphoma, skin and prostate. Smoking during and after cancer treatments appreciably increases the risk of side-effects, particularly mouth ulcers, necrosis of the jaw, radiotherapy skin damage, fibrosis and long-term pain such as breast, prostate and bladder cystitis. Furthermore, it considerably exacerbates hot flushes and mood swings in patients on hormone therapies.

What makes smoking harmful?

Tobacco smoke contains over 4000 different chemicals, many of which are carcinogenic. The four components of smoke which are particularly damaging are the carcinogens, nicotine, carbon monoxide and tar.

Carcinogens include benzene, pyridine, ormaldehyde, ammonia, hydrogen cyanide, acetone and arsenic. These can directly damage the DNA of cells, causing locked cancer genes to become active. They can also damage the immune system, allowing early cancers to progress more rapidly. These chemicals are known to interact with the body's enzymes responsible for metabolising drugs used to treat cancer. For example, the biological agent erlotinib, used for lung cancer, is up to 25% less bio-available in smokers. The chemicals in smoke have also been shown to interact with the bile production pathway in up to 40% of cases, which in turn can interfere with the excretion of a chemotherapy drug called irinotecan used to treat bowel cancer. This makes it difficult for doctors to calculate the ideal dose of chemotherapy, usually leading to under-dosing and a worse outcome.

Nicotine is a powerful, fast acting and addictive drug. Most people who smoke are dependent on nicotine. When a smoker inhales, nicotine is absorbed into their bloodstream, and the effects are felt immediately.

- Increased heart rate
- Stimulates nerve impulses causing anxiety and tremors
- Constriction of the small blood vessels in the skin
- Increased blood pressure
- Adverse effects on mood and behaviour

Carbon monoxide is a poisonous gas found in high concentrations in cigarette smoke. It combines readily with haemoglobin, the oxygen-carrying substance in blood, to form carboxyhaemoglobin. It combines more readily with haemoglobin than oxygen does, meaning up to 15% of a smoker's blood may be carrying carbon monoxide around the body instead of oxygen. Oxygen is essential for body tissues and cells to function efficiently. If the supply of oxygen is reduced, this can cause problems with growth, repair and absorption of essential nutrients. Carbon

186

monoxide is particularly harmful during pregnancy as it reduces the amount of oxygen carried to the uterus and foetus. Carbon monoxide can also affect the 'electrical' activity of the heart and, combined with other changes in the blood associated with smoking and a poor diet, may encourage fatty deposits to form on the walls of the arteries. This process can eventually lead to the arteries becoming blocked, causing heart disease and other major circulatory problems.

Tar: When smokers inhale, 70% of the carcinogenic tar contained in the smoke is deposited in the lungs. Irritants in tar can also damage the lungs by causing narrowing of the bronchioles and damage to the small hairs (ciliostasis) that help protect the lungs from dirt and infection.

Other sources of smoke

Passive cigarette smoke: Studies have confirmed that breathing the smoke from other people's cigarettes is a Class A carcinogen which leads to a 20% increased risk of lung, bladder and kidney cancer. In the short term, it irritates the eyes and nose, increases respiratory infections and aggravates asthma and other allergies. In the long term, it can lead to chronic middle ear lesions (glue ear), while also increasing the risk of coronary heart disease and emphysema.

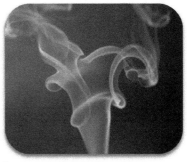

Candle smoke: Smoke does not just originate from cigarettes. Burning paraffin-wax candles can emit a multitude of toxic chemicals, including toluene and benzene. Researchers at South Carolina University found that frequent candle burning in tight, unventilated areas, can cause lung cancer, asthma, and skin rashes. Scented candles also increase atmospheric volatile organic compound (VOC) levels, contributing to general smog and xenoestrogenic pollution. It is best to either avoid their use entirely or use candles made from beeswax or soy wax which, although more expensive, are supposedly safer because they release less potentially harmful hydrocarbon pollutants.

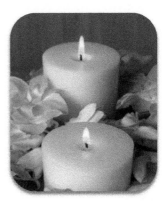

Tips to help you quit smoking

Each day without a cigarette is good news for your heart, your health, your family and your bank balance, but there is no quick and easy way to quit. Up to half of smokers continue to light up cigarettes after being diagnosed with cancer. Most smokers, however, do want to stop and, at any one time, one in six are trying to quit. Despite the highly addictive nature of cigarettes, more than 12 million people in Britain have successfully become ex-smokers. Deciding to quit and really wanting to succeed are the vital first steps to becoming a non-smoker, while having a detailed plan to stick to is also crucial. The following suggestions may help.

Deciding on a date to stop outright: Cutting down is less likely to work than simply stopping outright. Set a specific date.

Diet and physical activity: Both of these have an important effect on the body. Stopping smoking is a major change for the body to adapt to. A healthy diet and regular physical activity help facilitate this change and possibly even serve as a timely distraction.

Extra help: For those who have tried to quit but relapsed, there are other measures that can help, including products to help you quit smoking, joining a 'stop smoking' support group and alternative therapies such as hypnotherapy or acupuncture.

Products to help you quit

Nicotine replacement therapies help relieve some of the addiction associated with smoking. Many have been well-researched, and tests have shown that, if used correctly, they can double the chance of successfully quitting. If you smoke your first cigarette within 30 minutes of waking up, then it is particularly likely that you can benefit from them. Nicotine replacement products are generally safer than smoking, although if you have a heart problem, the nicotine can still cause issues. It is also important to use the product properly and to stop smoking completely when taking them, while the fact that nicotine replacement products are also known to potentially affect the action of certain drugs, such as warfarin and beta-blockers, should also be taken into account. Some manufacturers claim very high success rates, promising between an 80 to 90% success rate, but these claims are generally unfounded. Realistically, a smoking cessation aid can ease withdrawal, lessen the urge to smoke and boost your confidence and morale.

Nicotine patches and gum: The forms of nicotine replacement commonly available include patches, gum and nasal sprays, all of which are available from a pharmacist without requiring a prescription. While in use, the patch gives a continual supply of nicotine at a low dose, meaning it struggles to satisfy sudden cravings. The gum, nasal spray and inhalator deliver a higher dose quickly, which can respond to a craving with a 'quick fix', much like cigarettes. Side effects of nicotine replacement products include nausea, headaches, dizziness and palpitations.

E-cigarettes: These are made up of nicotine and flavourings dissolved in propylene glycol and glycerol. The e-liquid is superheated by a battery-powered vaporiser, converting it into a mist which is 'vaped' (inhaled). For individuals who smoke mainly in response to cravings or stress, and miss the 'hand to mouth' action of smoking, these can prove particularly 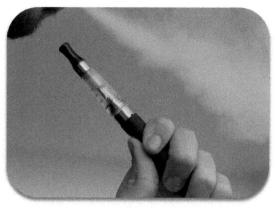 helpful. There remains some confusion regarding the health risks e-cigarettes pose, mainly because there exists very little data on the long-term health implications of 'vaping'. What information is available suggests E-cigarettes have a complex mix of potential harms and benefits. The one clear and obvious benefit with e-cigarettes, compared to regular cigarettes, is that they do not produce the tar or the toxic gases which are the source of much of the carcinogens found in cigarette smoke. However, it should be noted that the nicotine in e-cigarettes has the same negative health effects as the nicotine in cigarette smoke.

Early studies concerning e-cigarettes and the impact they can have on changing smoking behaviour show conflicting results, with some suggesting they are moderately helpful in kicking the habit, and others dismissing any link between e-cigarette usage and giving up smoking. Another study suggested that they actually encourage some young people to start smoking, as they naively believe e-cigarettes are safe. Furthermore, the nicotine content of many e-cigarettes is also problematic, with nicotine being linked to impaired prefrontal brain development and, in turn, attention deficit disorder and poor impulse control. Flavoured e-cigarettes may pose a further health threat as they often contain chemicals such as diacetyl, which can damage the lungs. Propylene glycol and glycerol, the major components of e-liquids, are not thought to be dangerous on their own but may decompose when heated by the vaporiser and transformed into toxic compounds such as formaldehyde. This is more common with vaporisers that use a high wattage. At least one study to date has reported a high incidence of cancer in people who, despite never smoking cigarettes, 'vaped' regularly.

Non-nicotine replacement products: These are many and varied, and include nicobrevin capsules, scented inhalers, dummy cigarettes, tobacco-flavoured chewing gum, herbal cigarettes and filters. Generally, there is not enough firm evidence to confirm how effective they are, and people should be wary of claims of very high success rates.

Complementary therapies: The two most popular tools for stopping smoking are hypnotherapy and acupuncture. There is some evidence for their success, but if you decide to try these therapies, it is important to find a registered practitioner.

Support groups: Joining a 'stop smoking' support group can help people feel less alone as they attempt to quit. Being with other people who are also trying can provide mutual support, a feeling of being understood and a sense of competition! They usually run over a period of several weeks and take you through the different stages of giving up smoking. Specialist smoker's clinics can improve an individual's likelihood of stopping three-fold.

Summary – Tips to quit smoking

- Cutting down helps initially, but set a date to quit completely
- Use aids and products initially, but make a date to stop these as well
- Keeping busy helps to take your mind off cigarettes.
- Discard ashtrays, lighters and unopened cigarette packets
- Drink plenty of fluids and keep a glass of water or juice close at hand.
- Get more active by joining a gym or fitness class.
- Thinking positively will help withdrawal mood swings
- Avoid places where you have smoked previously
- Distract yourself by doing something totally different
- Don't use good or bad news as an excuse for 'just one cigarette'
- Use the money that is saved to treat yourself
- Try not to snack on junk foods - try fruit, nuts or sugar-free gum

Chapter 13

Alcohol after cancer

Alcohol's role in facilitating social engagement is well known, and many of us who drink also appreciate the complex flavours and tastes various beverages offer. Red wine, in moderation, has been shown to be effective at counteracting heart disease and preventing certain cancers, with the natural antioxidant polyphenols it contains known to reduce inflammation and enhance healthy bacteria in the gut.

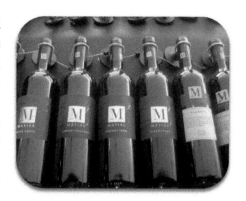

The most important polyphenol in wine is resveratrol, produced in grapes and several other plants as a response to invading fungus or sun exposure. Malbec, Sirrah and Pinot Noir, boast particularly high resveratrol contents. Dark red and purple grapes have higher concentrations, while the wine-making process used also has an influence. Traditional wine-making maintains a much higher concentration of resveratrol than the carbonic maceration process used in industrial wineries.

Why could alcohol be harmful?

Alcohol can be converted into acetaldehyde, a carcinogen, capable of damaging DNA repair mechanism. People who drink heavily have very high levels of acetaldehyde in their saliva. Other potential harmful attributes include:

- Generates reactive oxygen species and increases oxidative stress
- Damages healthy gut bacteria, leading to gut inflammation
- Alcohol drinks are calorific, often high in sugar contributing to weight gain
- Impairs ability to absorb essential vitamins and minerals
- In excess, causes cirrhosis which increases liver cancer risk
- Increases blood levels of oestrogen
- Encourages risky behaviour – smoking, eating late, unprotected sex

Head, neck, liver and oesophageal cancers: The data linking alcohol with head and neck cancer is confounded by the fact that many people who drink heavily also smoke, eat unhealthy and do not exercise. Nevertheless taking this factors in to account, people who consume >3 drinks per day have a 2-3 times greater risk of developing these cancers. Survivors of these cancers, who continued to drink excessively, have a 10% worse cure rate compared to those who give up.

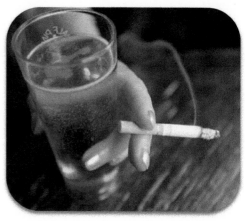

Breast cancer: The European Million Women Study estimated that for every 10g of alcohol drunk per day, there is a 12% increase in the risk of breast cancer. In term of relapse, the evidence is conflicting. One study, examining a group of 365 women with ER^{+ve} breast cancer, found that >7 drinks a week, obesity and smoking all increased the risk of cancer in the other breast. A study from the USA found that death from breast cancer was 30% higher in women taking >1 drink daily. On the other hand, a larger study from Cambridge University reported that a few glasses of wine a week actually lowered the risk of relapse slightly.

Bowel cancer: A meta-analysis of 57 studies concluded that people who regularly drank more than 50g alcohol per day (approximately 3.5 drinks) had 1.5 times the risk. For every 10 grams of alcohol consumed per day, there was a 7% increase in the risk of bowel cancer.

Prostate: One study suggested that light to moderate drinking reduced of prostate cancer risk. Another reported that drinking four or more glasses of red wine per week did not lower incidence overall, but did significantly lower the incidence of more aggressive types of prostate cancer. On the other hand, a study from the University of California showed that heavy drinkers (>50g of alcohol or four drinks daily) doubled their risk of prostate cancer compared to other men. What's more, the cancers they developed tended to be more advanced and have a poorer prognosis.

Other cancers: Studies suggest that about 4% of all cancer deaths are alcohol-related, particularly. There are links between alcohol consumption and uterus, sarcoma and skin cancer. Conversely, some trials have shown that consumption may reduce the risk of kidney cancer and lymphoma.

Safe limits for alcohol?

A safe alcohol limit is difficult to establish because its influence varies from person to person. People with any of the cancer susceptibility genes described in Part 1 will have a higher risk, as well as certain people with defects specifically in the genes that encode enzymes involved in breaking down alcohol. One way the body metabolises alcohol is through the activity of an enzyme called alcohol dehydrogenase (ADH), which metabolises alcohol into acetaldehyde rather than excreting it in the breath, skin and urine. Many people of Chinese, Korean, and Japanese descent carry a gene that codes for a superactive form of ADH. As a result, even after moderate alcohol intake, these individuals suffer a rapid buildup of acetaldehyde. A study from Japan has demonstrated how this leads to a higher risk of pancreatic cancer.

The Department of Health (DoH) have attempted to issue sensible guidelines based on available evidence, although these are largely related to heart, brain and liver-related damage. They currently suggest avoiding intake greater than 14 units per week for women and 21 units per week for men. To put this in perspective, a premium pint of lager, beer or cider (5%) contains 3 units, a standard 175ml glass of wine contains 2 units and a double shot of spirits contains 3 units. It is very easy to quickly exceed these limits, so it may be worth considering alternating with alcohol-free beers on a night out or trying the lower (2-3%) beers common in Scandinavia. Other tips to lower alcohol intake are summarised in the table below.

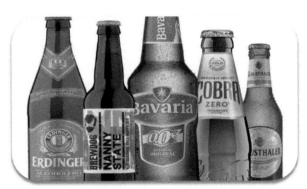

Other issues with alcohol during cancer treatments

Hormone therapies: Women on tamoxifen or other hormones and men prescribed injections which lower their testosterone, suffer from fatigue, abdominal weight gain, hot flushes, poor concentration and joint pains. All this adverse effects can be caused or exacerbated by drinking, the impact of which can last for several days.

Chemotherapy: Most people don't actually enjoy alcohol during chemo, so it's rarely an issue. The taste buds change, giving wine and other drinks an unpleasant metallic tinge. Already struggling with fatigue, nausea, headaches and poor concentration, people on chemotherapy often sensibly avoid substances which make these symptoms worse. The best advice is to give up alcohol completely during chemo.

Radiotherapy: One Italian study demonstrated that a glass of wine a day may cut the risk of treatment-linked skin toxicity by two-thirds in women undergoing radiation therapy for breast cancer. They evaluated the drinking habits of 348 women with breast cancer and found that patients who drank wine on the days they had their treatment had lower rates of acute toxicity than those who did not. This finding, however, failed to take into account the evidence that wine may reduce the effectiveness of radiotherapy in the first place. Although this is unlikely. Reducing effectiveness could increasing the local relapse rates so its best to what for more research before you consider red wine as an antidote to radiotherapy.

Sulphites: Most alcoholic beverages use sulphites as preservatives. These can cause flushing and nasal congestion, as well as increasing the severity of hangovers. Individuals on Herceptin often complain of a blocked nose, and this can be made worse by sulphites. The EU has designated an acceptable sulphite intake of about 50mg/day. A glass of white wine contains 25mg, making it very easy to exceed this limit. Good wines and champagne generally contain fewer sulphites, while sparkling wines and ciders typically have far higher levels. If you are sensitive to sulphites consider drinking better quality wines or search for low sulphite or organic varieties.

Gluten intolerance and gut health: Following chemotherapy, there may be an imbalance of gut bacteria. This may also trigger temporary gluten intolerance which may have not been present previously. In this case, it is worth avoiding beer, due to its gluten content and negative effect on gut bacteria, and switching to red wine which in moderation may improve gut health.

Tips for cutting down alcohol intake

- Keep an alcohol diary, set yourself an alcohol limit and stick to it
- Avoid drinking wines which smell strongly of sulphites
- Go for quality not quantity
- Consider Scandinavian type beers with 2-3% alcohol content
- Pace consumption by sipping drinks slowly
- Try not to choose export beers with higher alcohol percentages
- Red wines contain more antioxidants than whites and are less harmful
- German and organic UK beers have fewer chemicals and sulphites
- Alternate alcoholic drinks with soft drinks
- Try not to consume alcohol at home unless socialising
- Meet friends in alternative venues to the pub
- Look for alternative activities - a hobby or exercise class
- Have alcohol-free days
- When socialising meet people in alternative alcohol free venues:
    - Gym, walking groups, dance classes, cycling groups
- Consider holidays without alcohol such as health retreats
- Remember, you don't always have to drink to have fun

Chapter 14

Complementary therapies after cancer

with Jennifer Lenhart

There is no clear definition of what constitutes complementary medicine. Many believe that if a strategy helps a symptom or condition, it should be included in standard care guidelines. The lifestyle interventions described in this book have strong evidence for a benefit, yet it is not possible for them to gain a medical licence due to the barriers

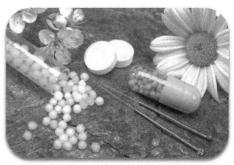

imposed by regulatory bodies. Unlicensed interventions tend to be grouped together, so the ones which offer a clear benefit stand alongside bogus products which prey on the vulnerability of patients. Consequently, it is very difficult for patients to decide whether interventions are worthwhile or not. Hopefully, this chapter will help.

Complementary therapies are popular with patients. Many formal surveys, including the Bedford Real World study, report that over 60% of patients have used one or more. This may reflect either an unmet need or simply a desire among patients to be more involved in the management of their own health. Ideally, all interventions should be evaluated in robust studies, ensuring that if they don't work, patients can look for more effective treatments. Furthermore, there may be overt or hidden risks which are only identified with formal evaluation and accurate data records. The subject of complementary medicine is incredibly vast, but a few the most notable practices are now outlined.

High dose vitamin C

The benefits of vitamin C have already been highlighted but they are worth summarising again as high dose IV infusions are an increasingly common complementary therapy. Therapists who advocate this treatment emphasise that case-control studies and epidemiologic evidence links inadequate consumption of fruit and vegetables and a higher

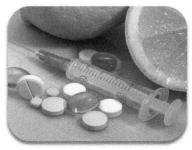

risk of most types of cancer. However, they often omit to mention that several cohort studies and at least three RCTs suggest that taking over the required amount of vitamin C does not reduce cancer risk but being deficient does increase the risk.

The evidence for high dose vitamin C has already been evaluated in detail in Chapter 15 (see pages 249-250). To summarise, the few studies which have suggested a possible benefit have been consistently undermined by a lack of controls, with many of the trial designs unlikely to pass an ethical committee using today's standards. The remaining evidence presented by studies is either inconclusive or points to no benefit at all. Despite this, some practitioners are still taking money off patients. For more information on high dose vitamin C, see (blog.cancernet.co.uk/vitamin-c).

Massage

Massage therapy works by stroking, kneading, tapping or pressing the soft tissues of the body. It can vary from light touching and stroking, to deep, intensive kneading and probing. It may cover the whole body or focus on a particular area and can be performed either with or without oils and lotions. There are many different types of massage depending on the country of origin, 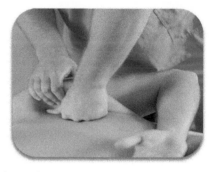 alongside a variety of different techniques such as deep tissue massage used for long-standing, deep muscular problems, sports massage to help heal sports injuries and neuromuscular massage to help balance the nerves and muscles.

Massage has been used for years to promote healing and well-being. Along with its relaxing and soothing properties, it can be a positive addition to conventional treatments and there is reasonable evidence to suggest that it helps:

- Reduce stress and anxiety
- Elevate mood and reduce depression
- Alleviate muscular pain

Is massage safe? There is an ill-informed urban myth that massage has safety issues in people who have had cancer. This stems from an idea that massage might increase the spread of cancer cells around the body. There is absolutely no evidence at all for this. On the contrary, people who have had radiotherapy, or surgical procedures such as mastectomy, greatly benefit from massage combined with stretching and exercise as this helps break down fibrous bands and adhesions which cause restriction of movement and pain. Furthermore, gentle massage for lymphoedema of the limbs can often relieve the discomfort and reduce the amount of fluid in the limb. Lymphoedema massage, known as manual lymphatic drainage (MLD), is best performed by an experienced professional. If you have just received radiotherapy and the skin is still red, avoid massaging this area. Also avoid massage to any part of the body where the skin is broken, bleeding or bruised.

Tips on finding a good masseur: It's important to have treatment with a qualified therapist. A few cancer centres in the UK now offer patients different types of massage therapy. If the massage is not available, they may have information on voluntary organisations that offer complementary therapies, free of charge or at a reduced cost. Currently, there is no single professional organisation that regulates the massage profession in the UK. Therapists can join several associations, but they do not have to finish any specific training. However, most reputable masseurs will belong to one of the recognised organisations. Before embarking on regular sessions, ask the therapist how many years of training they have undertaken, how long they have been practising and check they have indemnity insurance.

Homeopathy

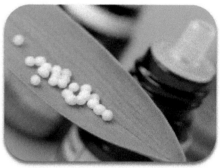

Homeopathic remedies are water (and sometimes alcohol) based solutions containing minute amounts of certain naturally occurring plants, minerals, animal products or chemicals. The term "homeopathy" comes from the Greek words "homoios" (similar) and "pathos" (suffering). Some practitioners claim homeopathy can help cancer patients by reducing pain, improving vitality and well-being, stopping the spread of cancer and strengthening the immune system. Some claim it can relieve certain side effects of radiation, chemotherapy and hormone therapy, such as infections, nausea, vomiting, mouth sores, hot flushes, hair loss, depression and fatigue.

What is the evidence? Two lab experiments published in 2006 found that homeopathic solutions had no effect on breast or prostate cancer cells growing in cultures. In a recent overview of all available clinical homeopathic trials conducted at the Royal London Hospital for Integrated Medicine, a number had reported psychological improvement including increased hope and optimism – which of course is a very good thing! No study showed an actual direct anti-tumour effect.

What does the treatment involve? During the first consultation, the homeopathic practitioner or physician will ask general questions regarding general health, medical history, lifestyle and diet. They might ask about your moods, emotions and sleeping patterns. All the gathered information about you will help them decide on the appropriate remedy for you. Homeopathic remedies come in the form of tablets, granules, powder or liquid. The therapist will explain how to take your remedies and when to come back for the follow-up consultation.

Side effects and risks Homeopathic remedies are completely safe, including when taken alongside conventional treatments. The main criticism of homeopathy is that a few misguided individuals rely on this type of treatment alone, and avoid or delay undergoing conventional medical care, a decision which may have serious health consequences. Another potential adverse effect is the price. It is a good idea to ask how much a homeopathy consultation will cost before you book it, while also getting some idea of how much the remedies are or whether the price is included in the consultation charge. You can get free treatment in one of the UK NHS homeopathic hospitals, but you will have to pay for the remedies.

Finding a practitioner The British Homeopathic Association, the Faculty of Homeopathy or The Council of Organisations Registering Homeopaths, can supply you with a list of registered professionals and hospitals that practice homeopathy. They can give you advice on how and where to get homeopathy treatment both privately and on the NHS. For more information see The Society of Homeopaths website (homeopathy-soh.org).

Reflexology

Reflexology originates in traditional Chinese medicine and consists of identifying and treating energy imbalances in the body through massage of reflexology points in specific areas of the feet or hands. The alternative theory is that reflexology enhances a relaxation response which has been shown to improve quality of life, reduce muscular tension and enhance mood.

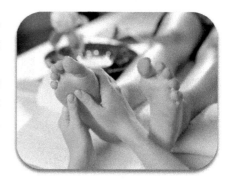

A small randomised trial showed that reflexology helped reduce anxiety before and during chemotherapy. Other studies have demonstrated a benefit for premenstrual syndrome including irritability and anxiety. The largest and best conducted trial of reflexology was published in the European Journal of Cancer in 2010 and involved 183 women with breast cancer. Post-surgery they were randomised to six weeks of either weekly reflexology, head massage or routine self-care. The results showed a significant benefit from both reflexology and head massage in terms of quality of life.

The reflexology appeared to benefit all groups of patients, including those receiving radiotherapy, chemotherapy, hormones and Herceptin.

Reflexology is not routinely available in oncology units, although some have volunteers from time to time. Perhaps with this benefit demonstrated in well-conducted trials, health care providers will eventually consider it an integral part of the management of breast cancer. In the meantime, there are numerous private reflexology practitioners available throughout the UK. For more information, see the Association of Reflexologists website (aor.org.uk).

Acupuncture

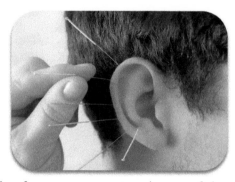

The term "acupuncture" describes a family of procedures involving the stimulation of anatomical points on the body using a variety of techniques. The acupuncture technique that has been most often studied scientifically involves penetrating the skin with thin, solid, metallic needles that are manipulated by the hands or by electrical stimulation. Practiced in China and other Asian countries for thousands of years, acupuncture is one of the key components of traditional Chinese medicine (TCM). In TCM, the body is seen as a delicate balance of two opposing and inseparable forces, the *yin* and the *yang*. The yin represents the cold, slow, or passive principle, while yang represents the hot, excited, or active principle. According to TCM, health is achieved by maintaining the body in a "balanced state", while disease is due to an internal imbalance of yin and yang. This imbalance leads to blockage in the flow of vital energy along pathways known as meridians. These can apparently be unblocked by using acupuncture at certain points on the body that connect with these meridians. There is some evidence that acupuncture may help the following conditions.

Hot flushes: More recently. there was a study published in the well respected Journal of Oncology which demonstrated a benefit for women with hot flushes. The study involved 50 women and compared a standard treatment for hot flushes called venlafaxine, an antidepressant, with acupuncture. In the acupuncture group, women received treatment twice a week for 12 weeks. They were analysed for a year. Although at two months there was no difference in the number or severity of hot flushes and night sweats, by three months there was a significant reduction from baseline. There was no variance between the two groups, suggesting that acupuncture was at least as effective as the antidepressant. There was, however, a significant difference in other symptoms between the two groups. Sex drive, fatigue, energy levels, clarity of thought and a sense of well being were all better in the acupuncture group. What's more, acupuncture was safe and had no side effects in this group of women. Results of the study suggest that, alongside the measures suggested in the "Tips for hot flushes" section of this book, it may be worth considering a course of acupuncture before considering antidepressants.

Chemotherapy-induced nausea: There have previously been some small studies which have shown that acupuncture minimally helped nausea associated with chemo. More recently, a study from the University of Rochester involving 586 patients receiving chemo randomly evaluated the effect of acupressure wrist bands which stimulate the P6 acupuncture point. Overall, there was a moderate benefit.

Dry mouth (xerostomia): A Canadian study evaluated 46 patients who had radiotherapy to the head and neck area and were suffering from a dry mouth, a common side effect if the salivary glands are included in the radiotherapy fields. They used an acupuncture point stimulation device twice a week for six weeks and found that dry mouth symptoms significantly improved over the 3-6 month trial. No adverse effects were reported.

Advice when considering acupuncture

Check a practitioner's credentials. Most countries require a licence to practice acupuncture, but education, training standards and requirements to practice vary. While a license does not ensure quality of care, it does indicate that the practitioner meets certain standards. Usually, acupuncture requires payment unless you are receiving cancer treatments at one of the UK Genesis Health private hospitals, it is included as standard care. Alternatively, ask your GP if they can refer to the Royal London Hospital for Integrated Medicine,. For more information, see the British Medical Acupuncture Society website (www.thwbmas.com).

Aromatherapy with Rhiannon Lewis

We have 1,000 different smell receptors in our nose and mouth, allowing us to distinguish between millions of different odours. Any odour which evokes a happy memory has the potential to increase positive emotions, decrease negative moods, disrupt cravings, lower stress, reduce nausea, increase appetite and even decrease

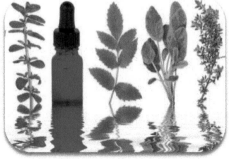

inflammatory immune responses, thereby having a generally beneficial effect on psychological and physiological wellbeing. An odour memory of a successful sporting event has been shown to trigger greater alertness and less fatigue.

Aromatherapy, along with massage and reflexology, is one of the most popular complementary therapies accessed by people with cancer in the UK. It uses fragrant essential oils that are extracted from aromatic plants for their beneficial effects on the mind and body. Common essential oils used in cancer care include frankincense and citrus essential oils such as lemon and sweet orange. The six oils associated with anti-nausea are lavender, ginger, peppermint, spearmint, cardamom and fennel.

They may be used in conjunction with body massage or via inhalation, diffusion, baths and topical products such as creams. They are also available in commercial devices which make them more convenient to self-administer (e.g. Quease Ease). They can accompany progressive relaxation and guided imagery. As essential oils are concentrated, they are diluted prior to use and, therefore, the doses are very low.

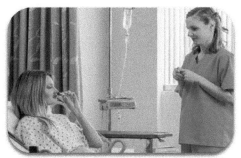

Aromatherapy can accompany a cancer patient from diagnosis, through treatment and into survivorship or palliative care. It is primarily used to help cope with the stress of the cancer experience, reduce anxiety, promote relaxation and sleep, as well as generally improve well-being. It is a pleasant, non-painful intervention that focuses on the whole person rather than the cancer itself and provides the opportunity for self-care. Many cancer support hospices now offer aromatherapy free of charge to people affected by cancer. Most aromatherapists working in cancer care have attended special training that helps them adapt their techniques to the specific needs of someone with the disease. As essential oils are concentrated substances, it is recommended that you seek professional advice rather than self-administering at home without guidance. See the international Journal of Clinical Aromatherapy website (www.ijca.net).

Hypnotherapy with Cathryn Woodwood

The use of hypnosis in a medical setting is nothing new; it has been used since Egyptian times. In 1955, the British Medical Association suggested that students should be trained in hypnosis. However, because clinical hypnosis sessions are usually individualised, rather than scripted, it has been difficult to carry out RCTs. As clinical hypnosis deals with medical problems and can raise deep emotions, it is very important to choose a practitioner who is properly trained and has a clinical background. Members of The British Society for Clinical and Academic Hypnosis are all qualified professionals (bscah.co.uk).

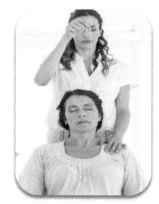

Cancer and treatment-related symptoms: Clinical hypnosis has been reported to reduce, and in some cases even eliminate, early and late onset nausea and vomiting in adults who have already experienced severe chemo-induced vomiting, particularly anticipatory nausea. Hypnosis does need to be continued for each session of chemo but, with time, patients can learn to hypnotise themselves. A meta-analysis concluded that there was such a beneficial impact on post-treatment depression, anxiety and emotional adjustment that many recommended it should be introduced as a standard aspect of treatment. Likewise, NICE guidelines in 2005 stated that for children and young people with anticipatory nausea, management should include behavioural therapy including hypnosis.

Scan related anxiety (Scanxiety): Scan-related claustrophobia and needle phobia are common. Hypnosis can effectively help deal with the phobia, enabling patients to tolerate the scans or needles required for their treatment with no more than the usual dislike and discomfort.

Procedure-related anxiety: Pain and distress can be reduced with the use of hypnosis for procedures such as biopsy insertion of stents in adults and children.

Menopausal symptoms: Hypnosis has been shown to be at least as effective as medical interventions at reducing menopausal symptoms, with a study reporting up to a 68% improvement. Another audit of personal outcomes in 2013 showed an 81% improvement after an average of only 2 sessions, a similar impact to the drug Megace.

Repurposing drugs for cancer

Drugs should, on the whole, be used solely for the purpose they are developed for. Furthermore, oncology drugs have been specifically developed to fight cancer and they should always be considered first. That said, main stream oncology practice is not averse to using drugs for different purposes. Thalidomide, designed (albeit incorrectly with devastating consequences for nausea) is used in multiple myeloma and bone hardening drugs for preventing breast cancer

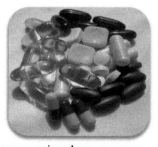

relapse but these are used under strict medical supervision. Other drugs are available over the counter or can be easily obtained and there is a lot of reference to repurposing some of these in online resources and complementary circles. The more well-known drugs used because of their supposed anti-cancer effect include:

- Bisphosphonates
- Salicylates and aspirin
- Non-steroidal anti-inflammatory pain killers
- Anti-histamines
- Anti-helminths
- Metformin

Bisphosphonates (Bone hardening drugs)

These are drugs that interfere with the cells which break down bone (osteoclasts), thus increasing bone density and reducing the risk of fractures. They have been shown to help age-related osteoporosis and prevent bone loss caused by hormonal therapy and other cancer treatments. They are also used to prevent or treat cancer that has spread to the bone and recently it has been discovered via a number of robust, well conducted medical trial that it adds a small but significant reduction in relapse after breast cancer. This is probably because they have anti-angiogenic properties (stopping metastasis taking hold by forming new blood vessels to feed themselves). A rare side effect of bisphosphonate treatment is osteonecrosis of the jaw which is when the jaw bone begins to starve from a lack of blood. This rarely happens with oral tablets or bi-annual administration used after breast cancer – which incidentally also has a small but significant benefit in reducing relapse. It frequently occurs with 3-4 weekly IV administration, especially if there is another disease of the jaw including cancer itself or dental caries. It's usually necessary to take calcium and vit-D supplements whilst on these drugs otherwise the calcium will drop in the blood.

Aspirin and salicylates

Lifestyle factors which reduce inflammation include eating polyphenol-rich fruit and vegetables, ensuring a healthy gut flora, taking regular exercise and avoiding pro-inflammatory foods and smoking. Over the last few years, salicylate has also attracted increasing attention due to its apparent effectiveness at reducing inflammation. Salicylates within aspirin and anti-inflammatory drugs can block COX-2. Many cancer cells have been shown to over-express COX-2. What's more, the more aggressive the cancer cells get, the higher the expression of the protein. Laboratory studies have found that COX-2 is integrally involved in pathways which promote the formation and spread of cancer, particularly by enhancing apoptosis of the cancer cell and reducing proliferation, invasion and angiogenesis. A number of population studies have reported that people who take aspirin regularly seem to have a lower incidence of cancer. The most notable of these was the HPFS, which reported a decreased risk of advanced prostate cancer among men taking regular aspirin.

An observational study published in the reputable JCO in 2010, evaluated 4,164 women who had been diagnosed with early breast cancer and found that those women who just happened to be taking 1-5 aspirin per week had a significant reduction in the risk of dying of the breast cancer. Two RCTs involving individuals with polyps and bowel cancer evaluated the benefits of aspirin. The first involved participants who had polyps removed from their bowel. The half randomised to take aspirin had a significantly lower number of polyps after two years compared to those given a placebo. The same benefit was found in a second study involving patients who had actually had bowel cancer. Not only did aspirin reduce the incidence of subsequent polyps, but it also reduced the incidence of new secondary cancers in the bowel. Excitement over the apparent anti-cancer effect of aspirin was tempered somewhat by a 2018 trial which combined aspirin with omega 3 oils and reported no reduction in the risk of polyps.

The problem with aspirin is that it can cause indigestion and increase the risk of bleeding from stomach ulcers. Ongoing studies such as the Add-Aspirin study are trying to determine whether the apparent anticancer properties outweigh its negative effects. In the meantime, it must be remembered that many vegetables and some fruits contain salicylates and enhance gastric health at the same time. One study of vegetarian Seventh Day Adventists found they have levels of salicylates in their bloodstream equivalent to taking 75mg of aspirin a day.

Anti-inflammatory drugs

The newer nonsteroidal anti-inflammatory drugs (NSAID) have more selective COX-2 inhibition properties and were originally thought to have less unwanted gastrointestinal side effects. However, the reduction in gastrointestinal side effects of pure COX-2 inhibitors was not as strong as expected when tested clinically, and indigestion and gastric damage remains high. Moreover, pure COX-2's have been shown to adversely affect blood pressure, increasing the cardiac risk, while long-term use causes kidney damage in some individuals. The largest RCT of highly selective NSAIDs had to be stopped prematurely as there was an increased death rate.

Antihistamines

Histamine is a protein, synthesised and released by mast cells, which acts as a vasodilator in response to infection or allergy. Anti-histamines offer relief for red eyes, nasal congestion and wheeze in hay fever and asthma suffers, while they also play an important role in dampening allergic reactions to insect bites and acute drug and food allergies. Many cancer cells have histamine receptors which, when activated, can signal metabolic pathways and stimulate growth. By blocking these receptors, anti-histamines are thought to reduce growth rates. There is also evidence to suggest that anti-histamines have an effect on inflammatory cytokines. Studies to date have been conflicting, with some showing antihistamines promote cancer cell growth and others showing they inhibit it. Laboratory studies specifically looking at a category of antihistamines called cationic amphiphilic drugs (CAD) reported that they promoted apoptosis (death) in lung cancer cells. Another lab experiment showed they sensitised lung, breast and prostate cancer cells to chemo and reverted multidrug resistance. A clinical study from Denmark involving patients with metastatic lung cancer showed that loratadine use was associated with better outcomes compared with use of non-CAD antihistamines or no anti-histamines. The effect was stronger among patients receiving chemo, a finding which supported the lab data.

Cimetidine is an antihistamine designed to target the H2 receptor commonly found in the stomach and which is responsible for reducing stomach acid and helping ease indigestion. A study published in the *Journal of Cancer* reported that cimetidine given before colorectal surgery improved lymphocyte levels in more than half of subjects. It also has been shown to block receptors which regulate cancer cell stickiness. This stickiness acts a bit like "Velcro", allowing cancer cells to creep along vessels without being washed away and killed. The first report of cimetidine being used to counteract cancer appeared in an article in The Lancet in 1979, and since then small studies have appeared in other journals which have reported improved survival if the drug is given before and during surgery. However, in a Danish study where it was started three weeks after surgery there was no benefit, so timing appears to be important.

Other studies have looked at prostate cancer and reported similarly improved survival. There is some concern, however, that Cimetidine has estrogenic properties and should not be used with, say, ER+ breast cancer. Despite this, Swedish researchers looked at women who had ER+ Breast cancer and those who simultaneously took a second generation antihistamine. When comparing users with non-users, a significant survival improvement was seen for the users of the anti-histamines. The same benefits have not been reported with newer anti-indigestion remedies such as proton pump inhibitors (PPIs), which block the secretion of stomach acid. This has the effect of reducing heartburn and nausea, but it also blocks one of the body's main defences against bacteria and viruses.

Anti-helminths

Mebendazole, a well-known anti-helminthic drug in wide clinical use, It is commonly prescribed to treat a range of parasitical worm infections, including threadworm,

205

tapeworms, roundworms, and other nematode and trematode infections in humans and domestic animals. A number of cell line and animal experiments in have concluded there is a an growth inhibition effect on cancer cells due to its action as a microtubule-disrupting agent. In helminths this prevents the polymerisation of tubulin in the gut, causing the parasites to die. Tubulin is vital to cell division and is therefore a cancer target for several widely used chemotherapy drugs. This suggest there could be synergy with some chemotherapy agent.

In humans, two case reports claim a moderate response in a man with bowel cancer and a women with breast cancer but monitoring was not robust. One ongoing phase one trial, involving children with brain tumours but to date, no trial trials in humans have been conducted so no clinical benefit can be concluded.

Metformin

Numerous epidemiologic studies have repeatedly indicated that T2D patients receiving metformin, compared to those taking other anti-diabetic medications, have a 30-50% decreased risk of the occurrence of various types of cancers. In the UK, a total of 62,809 patients with diabetes were found to have a higher risk of pancreatic cancer, particularly if also obese, but a lower risk if they were taking metformin as opposed to gliclazide or insulin. This finding was substantiated by a pooled analysis of 108,161 patients which reported that metformin treatment was associated with a significantly lower risk of colorectal cancer. Data from 3,837 patients obtained from several Canadian databases highlighted how a longer duration of metformin treatment after diagnosis of prostate cancer was associated with a significant decrease in all-cause mortality. In the USA, 68,019 postmenopausal women with diabetes participating in the Women's Health Initiative clinical trial had a lower risk of breast cancer if taking metformin.

One proposed indirect mechanism behind metformin's benefit lies in the fact that it improves cellular sensitivity to insulin and thus reduces IGF levels in those developing insulin resistance. Other studies have demonstrated a direct anticancer mechanism via inhibition of the mammalian target of rapamycin complex 1 (mTOR), a protein complex which plays a pivotal role in hormone resistance as well as the metabolism, growth and proliferation of cancer cells. Although prospective randomised trials confirming the protective benefits of metformin have yet to be completed, the existing data is very convincing, especially as studies involved such large numbers and were developed and carried out by independent prestigious organisations. It certainly would be common sense, if diabetic, to ask your doctor to take metformin as opposed to Glyclazide if medically feasible.

Fasting with chemo and other cancer treatments

The effect of fasting on chemotherapy has been evaluated in a number of small laboratory studies involving mice and dogs. Most reported that fasting for 24 hours, before and after chemotherapy, reduced side effects such as organ damage, toxic features, immunosuppression, reduced body weight and

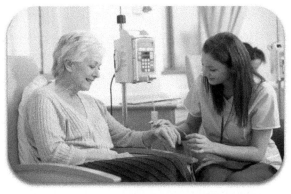

chemotherapy-induced death. Moreover, it appeared to enhance the effectiveness of chemotherapy by suppressing tumour growth and spread. The reason for this benefit is thought to be because when normal cells are deprived of glucose and nutrients after short-term fasting, they down-regulate cell growth, diverting energy from growth to maintenance and ultimately slowing their proliferation, protecting them from chemotherapy. Conversely, dividing cancer cells continue to expend energy while starving, making them more susceptible to chemotherapy because they are still dividing rapidly, especially if dose intensity is maintained or even increased. Some researchers have termed this phenomenon "Differential Stress Resistance (DSR)" and harnessing it could, in theory, help chemo outcomes.

The results of radiotherapy were likewise improved in mice with mammary tumours fed an alternate day fasting regimen. The authors hypothesised this was due to enhanced oxidative stress and DNA damage within cancer cells during short-term fasting. Biological treatments including the tyrosine kinase inhibitors (TKIs), such as erlotinib, gefitinib and lapatinib, slow cancer cell growth by inhibiting grow signalling pathways. Laboratory studies, involving mice with implanted cancers, have shown that combining short-term fasting with TKI's significantly enhanced their effect.

Human studies: While these lab studies are interesting, convincing clinical evidence is lacking. In one uncontrolled case report involving 10 patients, those who fasted for a day before chemo, and up to 24 hours afterwards, reported greater tolerance to treatment and less fatigue, weakness, and nausea. Authors commented that fasting did not appear to prevent chemo-induced tumour shrinkage or affect tumour markers, although it is not possible to make this conclusion definitive with such a small group. There were complaints during fasting of minor dizziness, hunger and headaches, as well as slight weight loss which was quickly recovered. Another study evaluated the safety of fasting (<200 kcal calories/day) in twenty patients receiving platinum-based regimens 48 hours pre and 24 hours post-chemotherapy. They were instructed to consume only non-calorific beverages such as water. There were no grade 3 toxicities attributed to fasting and laboratory studies revealed no evidence of malnutrition. The researchers excluded patients with more than 10% recent weight loss, a body mass index of less than 20.5 and diabetes mellitus. Another small study from Holland involved a group of 13 women being instructed to either follow a standard diet or fast the day before and after chemotherapy. There was no difference in nausea, other symptoms, white blood cells levels or infection rates, but platelets and red cells (haemoglobin) were statistically higher in the fasting group. They also measured levels of γ-H2AX phosphorylation in blood lymphocytes, a protein which indicates the presence of DNA damage and is thought to serve as a marker for chemotherapy toxicity in healthy cells. After seven days this was significantly lower in the fasting group, suggesting that fasting may promote the recovery of chemotherapy-induced DNA damage in cells.

Effects of dexamethasone (steroids): Due to their anti-sickness capabilities and effectiveness at curtailing hypersensitivity reactions, corticosteroids are often administered before and after chemo. The metabolic effects of steroids, however, are likely to significantly affect the influence of fasting as they raise blood glucose and insulin levels. Most of the studies summarised above do not mention steroids, but many of the subjects taking part would have had them prescribed, particularly those containing taxanes. Perhaps clinical studies of fasting should investigate chemo regimens which do not require steroids.

Fasting mimicking

Given the nutritional concerns most patients with cancer have regarding fasting and chemo, there is increasing interest in manoeuvres which may trigger similar biochemical pathways, particularly those which decrease blood sugar, reduce tumour-associated inflammation or increase metabolic stress in cancer cells. Several alternative measures have been considered, including exercise, but studies so far of 'fasting mimickers' have used drugs. Those under investigation so far include everolimus, metformin and hydroxycitrate. The use of natural polyphenols in fasting mimicking is also gaining some traction.

Everolimus is an mTOR inhibitor, already licenced for ER$^+$ advanced breast cancer, which has been shown in mice to be capable of mimicking the anticancer effects of fasting by sensitising certain cells to chemo and radiation therapy. In humans, a number of phase I and II clinical trials are aiming to determine the effect of combining everolimus with chemo for various cancer types including breast, sarcoma, pancreas and myeloma.

Metformin is a biguanide commonly used to reduce glucose and insulin levels in T2D by restoring insulin sensitivity and inhibiting gluconeogenesis. As a monotherapy, metformin suppresses tumour development and growth in multiple experimental cell lines. Humans with treated cancer who have been taking metformin, as opposed to other diabetic drugs, have significantly lower relapse rates. Several phase II trials evaluating the potential efficacy of combining metformin with chemotherapy are currently underway.

Hydroxycitrate is an over-the-counter weight loss drug which encourages acetyl-CoA to enter the Krebs cycle. Its effectiveness for weight loss has been questioned, and it does not affect systemic glucose or insulin levels. One small lab study showed enhanced anticancer effects when combining it with chemo, although this was not confirmed in subsequent trials. Despite this weak data clinical studies are underway, but it's best to avoid in the meantime.

Polyphenols and chemotherapy: There have been some concerns that polyphenols may interfere with oncology treatments via their antioxidant properties. However, they also slow glucose absorption and reduce insulin resistance and excess inflammation, much like short-term calorie restriction. This results in direct anticancer properties by inhibiting cell proliferation, de-differentiation, cell adhesion and metastasis, enhancing apoptosis. Lab studies have actually reported that 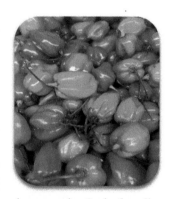 polyphenols reduce damage to normal tissues by enhancing repair. It is hardly surprising that several studies have actually found that polyphenols enhance the cytotoxic effects of chemotherapy. Curcumin has been shown to significantly improve the efficacy of docetaxel, with one laboratory study involving prostate cell lines demonstrating that a combined treatment of curcumin and docetaxel inhibited proliferation far more effectively than when docetaxel was used alone. Curcumin has also been found to enhance the effectiveness of cisplatin by helping to reduce cell proliferation in an in vitro laryngeal carcinoma cancer stem cell model, while another study highlighted how it can help to overcome cisplatin resistance. Beetroot extract has been shown to both help promote apoptosis of breast cancer cells after exposure of the cells to doxorubicin, while also protecting normal cardiomyocytes (heart muscle cells) from the toxic effects of doxorubicin. Resveratrol, found in grapes, berries and red wine, has also been under consideration as a CR mimetic, and several studies have indicated that resveratrol can enhance anti-cancer treatments.

Not all laboratory studies, however, have shown such positive effects on chemo. One cell line study suggested resveratrol interfered with paclitaxel, while another suggested high levels of turmeric may have blocked apoptosis. Moreover, while many human studies have been encouraging, data is still relatively limited and more trials need to be conducted for us to develop a more complete understanding of their role.

Cannabis and CBD oils

Hemp, marijuana, cannabidiol (CBD) oils and medicinal cannabis are separate varieties of the same plant, *cannabis sativa*. Cannabis oil, if extracted by cold pressing, contains 80% omega-3 and omega-6 fatty acids. It is rich in vitamin E and phytochemicals which have numerous reported health benefits. Scientists have recently been focusing on cannabinoids, 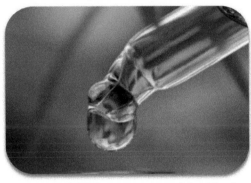 its biologically active components. There are over 100 known cannabinoids in cannabis, but the two best known are delta-9-tetrahydrocannabinol (THC) and CBD, the former having the psychotropic effects responsible for the plant's popularity. THC can help nausea and stimulate appetite, but most of the health benefits of cannabis stem from its CBD oils, the properties of which include:

- anti-inflammatory
- anti-convulsant
- anti-psychotic
- anti-oxidant
- neuroprotection
- immunomodulation

Cannabinoids can either be made synthetically or extracted from the plant, in which case they are referred to as phytocannabinoids. The ratio of ingredients depends on the variety of plant, it's sex, growing conditions and what part is used for the extract. THC is produced largely by female plants and is found mainly in the resin secreted by glands located around the reproductive organs (flowering buds). CBD is found in the seeds, leaves and stems. The dried buds, seeds and leaves of cannabis have been used in herbal remedies for centuries. Recently they've been developed as a nutritional supplement and, from 2018, a medicinal product:

Medicinal cannabis

A clear definition of what constitutes a cannabis-derived medicinal product has been developed by the Department for Health and Social Care for England and the Medicines and Health Products Regulatory Agency (MHRA). Only products meeting this definition have been rescheduled under the UK's misuse of drugs legislation, otherwise the directors of these companies would have faced jail time. Synthetic cannabis has had a medical licence since 1982, while natural extracts gained a licence in autumn 2018, largely due to the research and development efforts of the UK company GW Pharma. All other products containing THC remain illegal in the UK and many other countries.

Nausea: Dronabinol and nabilone, both containing man-made THC, are approved for cancer-related nausea. A Cochrane meta-analysis of 23 randomised RCTs concluded that, either on their own or in combination with other anti-emetics, individuals were more likely to report a complete absence of nausea and vomiting when they received them compared with a placebo. Participants were, however, more likely to withdraw from the studies because of adverse events such as sedation, drowsiness, dizziness, dysphoria, depression, hallucinations, paranoia or hypotension. Since these studies, new and highly effective anti-emetics are available, namely ondansetron and aprepitant. These have fewer side effects, so are generally used over synthetic cannabis.

Multiple sclerosis: Sativex contains the principal cannabinoids THC and CBD in a 1:1 ratio, as well as other minor cannabinoids. It has received regulatory approval in twenty-one countries to help relieve the muscle spasticity, spasms, bladder dysfunction and pain symptoms associated with multiple sclerosis.

Epilepsy: Epidiolex gained a medical licence for the treatment of rare epilepsies associated with Lennox-Gastaut syndrome and Dravet syndrome in patients two years of age and older. It contains a mixture of THC and CBD.

Conditions under investigation

Appetite stimulation: Small studies have shown increased appetite in patients off their food, much like Megestrol, a progesterone with appetite stimulator properties. Trials conducted in the 1980s reported better appetite in healthy subjects inhaling cannabis, although most of these calories were via unhealthy foods.

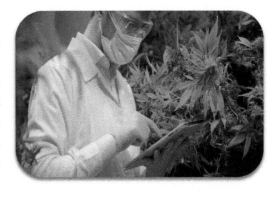

Analgesia, anxiety and sleep disorders: Cannabinoids have been reported to provide substantial analgesic effects, relaxation benefits and appetite stimulation. In one study, 10mg of THC produced analgesic effects for 7 hours, comparable to 60 mg of codeine. Another study reported that patients experienced improved management of pain, nausea, anxiety, as well as increased quality of sleep and relaxation. It also resulted in decreased use of opioids, anti-inflammatory drugs, anti-depressants, gabapentin and anti-sickness drugs.

Peripheral neuropathy (neuropathic pain): Two RCTs, looking at the impact of cannabis in patients with peripheral neuropathy or neuropathic pain of various aetiologies, found that pain was reduced. Two other trials demonstrated a benefit for HIV-associated neuropathic pain.

Hot flushes: CBD is thought to help by increasing an enzyme called fatty acid amide hydrolase (FAAH) which falls as oestrogen falls. Formal trials are lacking, but there are anecdotal reports of benefit so it may be worth a try if other measures fail.

Aarthritis: Numerous lab studies have found that CBD reduces inflammation, which can trigger joint pains. Anecdotal reports of improved pain in humans are numerous, and it is routinely prescribed to dogs with arthritis. One study, involving 58 patients with arthritis, reported a significant reduction in pain compared to placebo.

The evidence for cannabis in cancer management

There is enormous interest in the anti-cancer properties of cannabinoids. Most of this interest is based on effects seen on cancer cells in the laboratory and anecdotal reports of responses and cures in humans, but there are very few robust RCTs substantiating its use for several possible reasons.

First and foremost, its illegal status has established substantial bureaucratic barriers to designing trials. Secondly, as a plant product, it is difficult to conform to the rules of the MHRA and FDA, who require precise levels of active ingredients. For most plant-based products, sourced from various farms across the world, it is difficult to achieve this. Companies such as GW Pharma, grow their crops in heavily guarded hermetically sealed biospheres. The seeds, soil, nutrients, water and light have to be identical for each crop. This level of technology is beyond the capabilities and budgets of most companies. Finally, cannabis itself cannot be patented or intellectually protected, meaning companies are reluctant to invest millions of dollars into development when the results could just be copied and made by rivals. Some clinical research into the relationship between cannabis and cancer has been undertaken, the results of which are now outlined.

Can smoking cannabis increase the risk of cancer?

Most studies have not reported an increased risk of lung cancer associated with cannabis smoking. Likewise, another study of 64,855 American men found that it was not associated with mouth, throat or oesophageal cancer. Chronic marijuana use can affect the endocrine and reproductive systems, which explains why three population-based case-control studies reported a slightly elevated risk of testicular cancers. This included a study which looked at 49,343 Swedish men enrolled in the military over 40 years. Although it did not affect infrequent users, heavy cannabis use (more than 50 times in a lifetime) was associated with a 2.5-fold increased risk of testicular cancer.

Can cannabis use reduce the risk of cancer?

In animal studies, cannabis has demonstrated anticancer properties via stimulation of apoptosis, inhibition of tumour angiogenesis and restriction of cancer cell migration and invasion into adjacent tissues. The California Men's Health Study followed 84,170 participants for 16 years and found that cannabis users had a slightly lower than expected rate of bladder cancer. One small pilot study gave intra-tumour injections of THC to patients with a recurrent brain tumour called glioblastoma multiforme (GBM), but there was no significant clinical benefit. A number of other ongoing trials are giving CBD to patients with recurrent solid tumours in combination with chemo, but at the time of writing they had been recruiting slowly and results have not been reported. There is particular interest in the use of THC:CBD oils with temozolomide chemo in patients with recurrent GBM, as synergy has been found in lab studies.

Some published case studies have reported good responses after topical application of cannabis oil for a type of skin cancer called basal cell carcinoma, but further long-term randomised studies are required before this becomes confirmed and added to routine management. The future of cannabis as an anti-cancer treatment lies in the discovery of two major endocannabinoid-specific receptors. These are known as anandamide and 2-arachidonoyllglycerol (2-AG). These receptors are increased (overexpressed) in certain cancers, including GBM and some higher grade prostate and colon cancers.

In regards to safety, cannabinoids are known to potentially interact with the liver enzyme cytochrome P450, but in one small study of patients the addition of cannabis tea did not significantly influence exposure to and clearance of the chemo.

Smoking or eating recreational cannabis

This goes by many names including marijuana, pot, grass, weed, hemp, hash and ganja. Usage, while illegal across much of the world, is widespread. When whole cannabis is eaten, between 6-20% of the cannabinoids become bioavailable with 1-6 hours and can stay in the body for up to 30 hours. Inhaled cannabis has

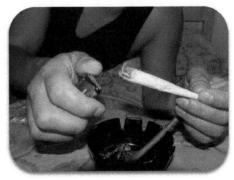

a peak serum level within 2-30 minutes, declining rapidly within an hour and generating less psychoactive metabolites. The either pleasant or detrimental effects of cannabis vary from person to person.

Cannabis products as a food supplement

Oils and extracts can be sold legally as nutritional supplements in most countries and do not require a medical licence, provided they contain <0.2% THC. They include Hemp oil and cannabinoid (CBD) oils. Oils containing higher THC are illegal in the UK but not in Canada and some USA states.

Difference between CBD oils, hemp oil and THC containing oils: Hemp oil is rich in short-chain omega-3, omega-6 and vitamin E but has no THC and very little CBD. It is usually a by-product of industrial hemp production, grown for rope, clothes and insulation. The seeds are then crushed and the oil extracted for either biofuel or supplement use. CBD oil is found in the seeds, leaves and stems of plants which have been grown specifically to enhance their CBD levels. As previously mentioned, THC oils include extracts from the flower and resin from the adjacent glands.

There has been an enormous interest in the potential efficacy of CBD oils in cancer management. It has potent anti-oxidant, anti-inflammatory and immunomodulation properties, while they also have exhibited direct anti-cancer mechanisms in some laboratory experiments. Significantly, they are free of the often unwelcome psychotropic and sedative properties associated with THC. They usually come in an oil containing between 5-12% cannabinoids, which is dropped into the mouth under the tongue. They are regarded as safe with few drug interactions.

The best CBD oils are derived from organically grown plants. It takes a lot of plant to produce a small amount of oil, so if it is sprayed with pesticides and herbicides, significant amounts will make their way through to the oil. It is also important to buy from a reputable source as the supplement industry is not as well-regulated as the pharmaceutical industry. Reports of bogus product with contaminants and inadequate levels of CBD are rife. Finally, it is worth noting that the law allows a very small amount of THC within the oil, something which many supplements do not contain. However, this small amount will not cause any negative psychotropic effects and is in fact very likely to add to the potentially beneficial effects. The keep-healthy.com site has links to one of the best organic, high-quality CBD.

Chapter 15

Issues with vitamins and mineral after cancer

Vitamins and minerals are chemicals which are essential to the normal biochemical function of the human body. They cannot be made internally, so have to be consumed via a varied diet. There are several notable historical examples of vitamin deficiencies. In the eighteen century, scurvy plagued British sailors until the surgeon James Lind discovered it could be corrected by consuming vitamin C through eating limes. In South and Central America, the reliance

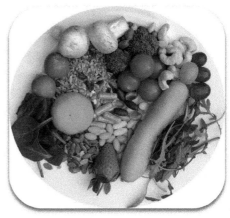

on corn as a main carbohydrate caused a deficiency in vitamin B_6, resulting in a disease called pellagra until it was discovered that adding limes to corn enabled the vitamin B_6 to be absorbed – hence the propensity to include limes with tortilla and other corn dishes to this day. In the Far East, overdependence on processed rice, low in thiamine, caused vitamin B_1 deficiency, resulting in nerve damage and a disease known as Beriberi. In the UK and other northern countries, Asians arriving in the 1960s, particularly women and children, had a high incidence of the bone diseases osteomalacia and rickets due to vitamin D and calcium deficiency, brought on by the lack of sunshine and low dairy diet. Around the world, vitamin A deficiency remains the main cause of blindness.

In modern western society, and food shortages are rare, so full-blown syndrome deficiency syndromes are unlikely. However, intensive farming and sterile food processing are blamed for reduced essential nutrients in the human diet. Alarmingly, as countries get richer, the diversity of the typical diet actually shrinks. Today, 75% of the world's food supply comes from only twelve

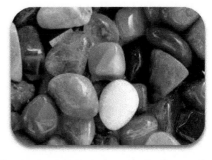

plants and five animal species. This can contribute to immune, metabolic and hormonal imbalances such as infertility, hypothyroidism, osteoporosis and menopausal problems. Minerals are also needed for protein formation, muscle repair and energy utilisation, so elite sports men and women have constant monitoring to ensure adequate levels. Sub-clinical deficiencies, may also impair the body's ability to fight cancer and lead to an increased risk of chronic degenerative diseases. Vitamins, especially A, E and C, and minerals such as iron, copper, zinc and selenium have a vital role in the healthy functioning of oxidative stress so deficiency leads to impaired antioxidant enzyme production, and impaired immunity due to the restricted formation of enzymes that play a role in immune function protection from carcinogens and regulation of chronic inflammation Chronic subclinical mineral deficiencies can also contribute to hormonal imbalances such as hypothyroidism, osteoporosis, menopausal problems and infertility. Minerals are also needed for protein formation, muscle repair and energy utilisation, so elite sportsmen and women have constant monitoring to ensure adequate levels.

It is clearly very important to avoid deficiencies of mineral and vitamins with a well-balanced diet. Numerous studies have investigate a benefit of mineral and vitamin supplements as a way of boosting their intake. In general only those studies which corrected a pre-existing, deficiency reported a benefit. Other studies have shown that overcorrecting levels, especially with mega-doses of a single vitamin, may carry a number of risks including cancer itself. The difficulty is knowing whether an individual has adequate levels or without a blood micronutrient test (see later), but this chapter highlights the importance and sources of vitamin and mineral rich foods

Vitamin A and carotenoids

Vitamin A is a fat-soluble pigment, found in fish and dairy food in three main isoforms: retinol, retinal and retinoic acid found in oily fish, cod liver oil, other fish oil, beef, pork, lamb, chicken liver and kidneys, eggs, milk, cream, yoghurt and some cheeses. It can also be made in the body from carotenoids, which are pro-vitamins (alpha, beta and gamma carotene) of vitamin present in fruits and vegetables with red, orange or yellow colours such as sweet potato, carrots, apricots, pumpkin, kale, peppers, guava, mangoes and papaya. Carotenoids also have direct health benefits of their own via anti-oxidant and anti-proliferative mechanisms. Vitamin A plays a role in a variety of functions throughout the body.

A summary of several large population trials demonstrated that women who consumed higher amounts of carotenoids had a significantly reduced risk of breast cancer. Other studies based on questionnaires, but also blood levels of dietary carotenoids, have likewise demonstrated associations between high intake and lower risks of ovarian and pancreatic cancers. An investigation of men and women who had been treated for squamous cell carcinoma of the skin found that higher carotenoid intake reduced their usually high risk of developing further skin lesions. A similar study from Australia examined this association in more detail, finding that two specific carotenoids present in leafy green and yellow vegetables, lutein and zeaxanthin, had the greatest benefits on skin cancer relapse.

A deficiency of vitamin A in the west is rare, but suboptimal levels are thought to lower immunity which can increase cancer risk. In laboratory studies, carotenoids had direct anti-cancer effects by triggering apoptosis and reducing proliferation. In genetically susceptible mice, carotenoids reduced the incidence of prostate cancer. In humans, numerous large cohort studies have linked low intake of carotenoid-rich foods with a higher risk of breast, prostate, bowel, head and neck, oesophagus and lung cancer. Despite the anti-cancer benefits of having adequate vitamin A, caution must be taken with taking extra pro-vitamin A (carotenoids) in supplement form.

Carotenoid supplements have been shown to slow the progression of macular degeneration via a supplement containing beta-carotene, Vitamin E, Vitamin C and Zinc. This RCT, called the Age-Related Eye Disease Study (AREDS), has prompted ophthalmologists to recommend this supplement to people suffering from the early stages of the disease. Interestingly, the study did not demonstrate protection against other degenerative eye diseases such as cataracts, unless participants had a deficiency of these foods in their pre-trial diet.

In terms of cancer, a landmark European study (The CARET Study) revealed that individuals who had a previous cancer of the throat or were heavy smokers, given beta-carotene and vitamin E (alpha-tocopherol), had an increased risk of lung and prostate cancer compared to those given a placebo. Another large, human dietary prevention study combined beta-carotene with retinol (The ABTC study) and showed complex but fascinating results which provide further insight into the impact of supplements. People who started the trial with naturally low blood levels of beta-carotene had lower levels of prostate cancer after years of supplementation. However, those who had either high or normal initial levels of beta-carotene to begin with, eventually ended up with a higher risk of cancer, particularly prostate. This trial provides a clear take-home message – correcting a natural or acquired deficit is beneficial, but over-supplementing just for the sake of it can be harmful.

Vitamin B and folic acid

These are water soluble vitamins which have several subtypes, including vitamin B_1 (thiamine), folic acid, and vitamin B_6 found in grains and pulses Vitamin B has an important and complex relationship with cancer risk. A well-known EPIC study reported that people deficient in folic acid had an increased risk of cancer. A Swedish research group reviewed data from 13 dietary studies and concluded that

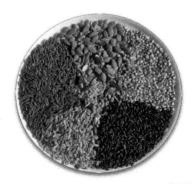

individuals with adequate blood levels of pyridoxal-phosphate (PLP), the main active coenzyme form of vitamin B_6, had a lower incidence of colon cancer, whereas those with low levels had a higher risk. On the other hand, those who had elevated levels because they took vitamin B_6 supplement had a higher risk of cancer.

A study from Norway compared a folic acid supplements with placebo to 6,837 patients following a heart attack. After three years, there was no cardiac benefit but a significant increase in lung cancer in those who received folic acid. These results were confirmed in a separate post heart-attack study which reported that although prostate cancer incidence was slightly lower in men who had adequate amounts of folate in their diet, men who took folic acid were more than twice as likely to develop prostate cancer compared to men who took a placebo.

Vitamin B12 deficiency can lead to anaemia, causing symptoms such as fatigue, pallor, shortness of breath and chest pain, as well as neurological symptoms such as numbness in the hands and feet, poor balance, a smooth red tongue, depression and confusion. There are several causes of B_{12} deficiency, including an autoimmune condition called pernicious anaemia in which the body attacks the cells responsible for B_{12} absorption, alongside surgical removal or damage by Crohn's disease of part of the stomach or terminal ileum. Vegans are at risk of B12 deficiency unless they take specific precautions as meat is the best source. Chlorella and nori seaweed may contain some useable vitamin B12 supply, but this is not produced by the algae itself but rather by microorganisms which live within the plant or soil it is grown in. This means it's only found in the natural wild form and not the farmed varieties. Although vitamin B12 does represent a problem for health, no study has associated B_{12} deficiency with an increased risk of cancer or relapse. Vitamin B_{12} is found in meat and, to a lesser extent, legumes and seaweed. The other B vitamins are found in grains such as wheat, barley and oats, so sources in western diets come from bread and cereals. Folic acid id found in leafy dark green vegetables such as kale and spinach.

Vitamin C

Vitamin C is an essential water-soluble nutrient which humans need on a daily basis as it cannot be made and only lasts for a short period of time in the bloodstream. Fortunately, it is present in a wide variety of citrus fruit, vegetables, herbs and nuts. Vitamin C is a cofactor for several enzymes and plays an important role in the synthesis of collagen, which is vital for the growth and repair of skin, bones, teeth, cartilage, tendons, ligaments and blood vessels. It also helps the body absorb iron from non-haem sources such as lentils

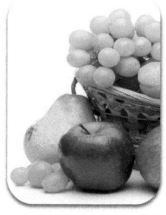

Along with vitamin E, beta-carotene, and other plant-based nutrients, vitamin C has important antioxidant abilities. More specifically, vitamin C is involved in the mechanism that enables DNA to 'sense' the damage done by free radicals produced from carcinogens. This is an important factor in the first stage of cancer development, as it prevents mutation and gene rearrangement as the cells divide. Vitamin C has also been shown to protect DNA from toxic products such as hydrogen peroxide via inhibition of gap-junction intercellular communication. It also limits the formation of nitrosamines, formed from meat.

In today's society, scurvy is rare, although it can still be found among elderly people in social isolation or those with mental illness, especially if they smoke heavily. Having chronically suboptimal levels has been linked with an increased risk of degenerative conditions such as high blood pressure, macular degeneration, gallbladder disease, atherosclerosis, heart attacks and stroke. Most case-control studies and epidemiologic evidence suggest that higher consumption of fruits and vegetables is associated with lower risk of most types of cancer including lung, breast, colon or rectum, stomach, oral cavity and oesophagus. This may, in part, be due to their high vitamin C content, although fruit also contains other healthy components including fibre, other vitamins, minerals and polyphenols.

Low vitamin C levels are thought to increase vulnerability to the common cold, but taking high amounts, especially after a cold has developed, has not been shown to reduce its effect. In terms of cancer, a recent meta-analysis reported that women who, after their breast cancer diagnosis, either took vitamin C supplements or increased their dietary intake of vitamin C by >100 mg/day, had significantly reduced risks of both breast cancer-specific and total mortality. Likewise, in the Nurses' Health Study, consumption of an adequate (>200 mg/day) intake of vitamin C from food, compared with below normal consumption (< 70 mg/day), was associated with a lower risk of breast cancer, especially among premenopausal women with a family history. On the other hand, two large cohort trials found an increased risk of cancer if individuals consumed less than 87mg/day, but no reduction if they consumed over 200mg/day. It therefore appears that taking more than the required amount of vitamin C does not reduce cancer risk, but being deficient does increase the risk. The issues with high dose vitamins C are described in the in complementary section.

A warning about fruit juices and smoothies While these are a reasonable way to increase your fruit intake, they also increase the effect of the sugar by speeding up how quickly it is absorbed into the bloodstream (glycaemic index). Most juice and smoothie aficionados counterbalance this by mixing them with plenty of vegetables. Moreover, if you do make fruit juices, they should ideally be drunk fresh. After squeezing, juice changes its chemical composition, quickly becoming more acidic and losing its nutritional content. Juices within cartons have generally been heavily processed, which means an increased sugar content and often a lack of vitamin C.

Fruit intake and indigestion

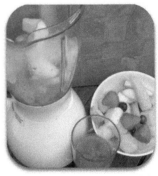

People often say – "I can't eat fruit because I have indigestion or heartburn". Although it's true that fruit can cause a little irritation in vulnerable individuals, it is not the root cause of the problem and, in the long term, fruit will improve the health of the stomach and oesophagus (gullet). The underlying cause is usually an unhealthy balance of fat, meats and sugar which the stomach has to work harder to digest – i.e. produce more of its own hydrochloric acid. To make matters worse, sufferers often turn to antacids for immediate relief. The stomach then senses a more alkaline environment and responds by producing yet more acid, perpetuating the problem. On the other hand, consumption of mildly acidic fruit sends signals to the stomach lining to produce less of its own acid. After a while, with perseverance, eating fruit and other less gastric-irritating foods will reduce acid levels and improve the health of the gastric lining, thus preventing indigestion.

Vitamin D

As described above, chronic low levels of vitamin D increase the risk of bone loss (osteoporosis) in adults. In addition, lower levels of vitamin D have also been linked to infertility, dementia, heart disease and arthritis. There is also data to suggest that adequate vitamin D helps reduce joint pains related to certain breast cancer hormone drugs such as aromatase inhibitors.

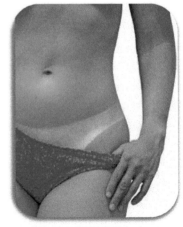

The national RDA of vitamin D is 800iu, but recent studies have shown that this dose rarely corrects an established deficiency, especially among those living in the Northern Hemisphere. In this case, doses up to 3000iu are required initially, before being followed by regular does of 1000iu once normal levels have been achieved. In terms of cancer, vitamin D has links with several crucial biochemical pathways. It inhibits activation of the pro-inflammatory cytokine IL6, implicated in the initiation and progression of many cancers. Laboratory studies have also shown that, when added to cancer cells, calciferol reduces proliferation, inhibits invasion, prevents loss of adhesion and promotes apoptosis. Furthermore, it interacts with the androgen-signalling pathway, inhibiting the production of factors which stimulate growth and new blood vessel formation (angiogenesis) in prostate cancer models. This may explain a paper published in 2018, which showed that men with prostate cancer on surveillance had faster cancer progression if deficient then correcting this with 4000iu of vitamin D3, subsequently slowed PSA progression.

Vitamin D deficiency can negatively impact immune function and increase inflammation, resulting in higher cancer risk and reduced cardiovascular health. In one study involving healthy women, increased concentrations of serum TNF-α, an inflammatory marker, were found in women who had insufficient vitamin D levels. This could explain the vitamin's role in the prevention and treatment of inflammatory diseases, including heart disease, multiple sclerosis and rheumatoid arthritis.

Two retrospective studies have highlighted the benefits of vitamin D after cancer. The first showed that survivors of bowel cancer with regular exposure to sunlight had a lower incidence of subsequent relapse. A study involved people who had been treated for melanoma skin cancers. Obviously, as the risk of this disease increases with sun-burning during adolescence, patients are told to keep out of the sun after their diagnosis. However, those patients who ignored this advice and continued to have regular sun exposure actually had a lower risk of the melanoma spreading to another part of the body. This data was confirmed by another observational evaluation of men with jobs involving exposure to high levels of sunlight. They found that they were 30% less likely to develop kidney and prostate cancer than those with little or no sunlight exposure at such as sedentary, indoor desk jobs. Advise on how to increase vitamin D levels with diet and sensible sun bathing have already been highlighted in the bone health section.

Vitamin E

Vitamin E is fat-soluble vitamin with eight forms (4 tocopherols and 4 tocotrienols). The two most significant forms for humans are alpha and gamma tocopherols. It's found in pistachios, lmonds, hazelnuts, spinach, Swiss chard, cruciferous vegetables, extra virgin olive oil and is often added to fish oils as a preservative against oxidation.

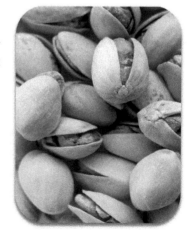

These have anti-inflammatory properties and are important for a healthy immune system. It also has some enzymatic activities which help smooth muscle growth, have a role in eye and neurological functions and inhibit platelet clotting. Along with vitamin A, C and carotenoids, they are direct antioxidants. Unlike polyphenols, which are anti-oxidants because they increase anti-oxidant enzyme production, vitamin E's have direct antioxidant properties because of their ability to donate a hydrogen atom to reactive oxygen species formed when tissue undergoes oxidation.

Severe vitamin E deficiency is rare and is usually caused by malabsorption of fats caused by bowel surgery, disease of the bowel or diseases of the pancreas (which produce the enzymes required to absorb fat). Severe deficiency can cause neuromuscular problems such as loss of balance and poor movement (ataxia), muscle damage, anaemia, impaired immunity, eye damage and infertility. Moreover, suboptimal vitamin E levels over long periods of time may increase our susceptibility to mutagenic carcinogens. In laboratory studies, tocopherols have been shown to prevent less aggressive tumours changing to more aggressive types (differentiation). As mentioned earlier, while a French-based RCT studying a combination of low dose antioxidants (ascorbic acid, vitamin E, beta-carotene, selenium and zinc) found a reduction in cancer after 7.5 years in men, these changes were thought to be due to pre-existing dietary deficiencies. In another interventional trial, four different combinations of mineral and vitamin supplements were administered to 29,584 adults in Linxian, China, at a time when its population was known to have widespread micronutrient deficiencies. After five years, the study found a reduced risk of oesophageal cancer for the group receiving supplementation with beta-carotene, vitamin E and selenium.

Concerns with vitamin E supplementation: While correcting deficient levels of vitamin E is clearly both appropriate and advantageous, there are concerns regarding over-correcting serum vitamin E levels with supplements. The Alpha-Tocopherol, Beta-Carotene cancer prevention trial (ATBC) involved 29,133 male smokers taking vitamin E (alpha-tocopherol) and vitamin A (Beta-carotene), or a placebo. After 7 years, the treatment group had a statistically significant reduction in the risk of prostate cancer, yet the incidence of lung cancer in smokers, the main trial endpoint, was higher. The relationship between smokers, the risk of prostate cancer and vitamin E was confirmed in the Cancer Prevention II (CPII) Nutrition Cohort study. As well as a dietary history, this study also measured participant's blood levels of vitamin E, which were lower in smokers and that there was a correlation between low blood vitamin E levels and a higher incidence of prostate cancer. This correlation was particularly high with the isoform of vitamin E, gamma-tocopherol, which is the main vitamin E found in health foods, as opposed to the alpha-tocopherol found in man-made supplements. A further trial involving 5000 patients with diabetes or heart disease in women (The Women's Health Study) showed alpha tocopherol provided demonstrated no reduction in cancer, and the incidence of heart disease was slightly worse. Likewise, in the ATBC study, cerebral haemorrhage risk was also higher in smokers with hypertension who took alpha-tocopherol.

A study from Australia, analysed individuals who had been treated for skin cancer. The risk of a further cancer was reduced if individuals ate foods rich in vitamin E and other antioxidants, but individuals who took supplements of vitamin E actually had a higher rate of recurrent skin cancers. The Selenium and Vitamin E Cancer Prevention Trial (SELECT), randomised 43,887 men to one of four groups; selenium pills alone, vitamin E pills alone, a pill containing both or a placebo. It demonstrated a significantly increased risk of prostate cancer with vitamin E pills, compared with the other groups after a seven-year period. Finally, a detailed Cochrane meta-analysis in 2011, summarised 78 trials involving 296,707 participants and concluded that vitamin E, as well as other antioxidant vitamins and minerals (beta-carotene, vitamin A, C, E, and selenium), led to no reduction in mortality and may, increase it.

This published data suggests that vitamin E is an important antioxidant vitamin, deficiency of which increases the risk of chronic diseases including cancer. Levels are lower in smokers, who should take extra care to eat more vitamin E-rich foods or even take a low dose supplement. Higher dose supplements, particularly if serum levels are adequate to start with, are likely to be harmful and will increase the cancer risk. It is best to concentrate on sensible vitamin E-rich dietary measures or, better still, measure serum levels and correct accordingly.

Zinc

Zinc is required for the formation and activity of over 100 enzymes that play a role in immune function, protein formation, wound healing and DNA synthesis. It is one of the minerals required to make the superoxide dismutase (SOD) enzyme, an important enzyme defense against dangerous free radical producing carcinogens. Very low levels are linked with 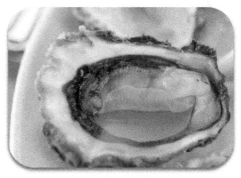 poor skin, reduced wound healing, poor nail and hair health, diarrhoea and an impaired taste and smell. Trials have linked zinc deficiency and increased cancer risk, although no RCTs have confirmed this.

The RDA of zinc for women is 8mg/day, while men require a bit more (11mg/day), especially if sexually active as zinc is lost in semen. Regular intake of zinc is required to maintain a steady state as the body doesn't store it. Zinc rich foods include oysters, clams, obster, crab, dark bird meat, seaweed, hummus, pumpkin seeds and nuts

Blood results from over 500 people who ordered the Cancer Risk Nutritional Profile (CRNP) have revealed that nearly 40% had zinc levels below the normal range, with only 2% having higher than normal levels. This does imply that, as a UK population, we need to eat more zinc containing foods or even take a low dose supplement three days a week such as 20mg of zinc gluconate. High doses may be required if marked deficiencies are seen, but caution is required as in the HPFS, men who regularly took extra zinc at levels of more than 100mg/day were more than twice as likely to develop advanced prostate cancer. Taking a supplement of >40 mg per day may also interfere with the absorption of copper, another important essential mineral.

Phytic acid, common in plant foods, can prevent zinc absorption by attaching to zinc in the gut. This could be a problem for vegetarians or people who eat a lot of high phytate sources such as quinoa, whole grains, legumes, nuts and seeds.

Selenium

Selenium is incorporated into many proteins (selenoproteins) and enzymes which have important regulatory functions in the body. It is also required to make SOD and glutathione, both of which are important antioxidant enzymes. Other selenoproteins help regulate thyroid function.

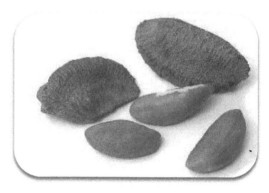

Health benefits of selenium: There is no doubt that maintaining adequate selenium levels has long-term benefits for health and immunity. Two major studies in 1980 and 1990 showed that a low selenium status was associated with an increased risk of developing cancer. The HPFS, for example, linked low selenium status with higher rates of aggressive prostate cancer. Finnish and Taiwanese studies have linked lower blood levels of selenium with higher rates of lung and liver cancer. In China, where the incidence of liver cancer is high, the inhabitants of one village were supplemented with selenium while other villages were given simple salt. After six years, there was a 35% reduction in cancer in the selenium-supplemented village.

This data prompted the design and initiation of an excellent double-blind randomised trial in the USA called the Nutritional Prevention Study. It recruited 1,312 individuals with a history of skin cancer and prescribed either a placebo or 220 micrograms of selenium a day. The primary aim was to see if dietary selenium supplementation could reduce the risk of recurrent skin cancer. There was no difference in the number of skin cancers between the selenium and placebo groups. However, when the data was analysed in more detail, a lower level of lung, bowel and prostate cancer was seen in the selenium group. Following this came the SELECT study, which gave either selenium pills alone, vitamin E pills alone, a pill containing both or a placebo to a large group of healthy men. After many years, the rate of prostate cancer was slightly higher in the vitamin E alone and vitamin E and selenium groups. It was felt that the vitamin E caused the increased risk, although researchers could not be certain. No measurements of underlying selenium or vitamin E levels were recorded in this study. Many suspect, however, that the people who would benefit from selenium supplements are those with a dietary deficiency in the first place, such as those living in areas with low levels in the soil, although this needs to be confirmed in further research.

What foods provide selenium?

The recommended daily amount is 55 mircog/day. Serum levels are optimum between 1.0–1.9 micromols/L. Soils in the high plains of northern USA have high levels of selenium, whereas those in Asia, central Europe and China tend to have low levels of selenium. Animals that eat grains or plants that were grown in selenium-rich soil have higher levels of selenium in their muscle. Selenium rich foods include Brazil nuts, soybeans, tuna, lobster and other seafood

Vegetarians, especially those with a nut allergy, may be deficient and, in this case, a low dose supplement would be advised (50 micrograms/day). Taking more than needed does not have any benefits and may have some risks, especially if combined with Vitamin E. If you are concerned about having too little or too much selenium in your body, consider a micronutrient test.

Magnesium

Magnesium (Mg) is the fourth most abundant mineral in the body and is important for health. About 50% of total body magnesium is found in bone. The other half is found inside cells of body tissues and organs. Only 1% of magnesium is found in blood. This is why serum levels (measured routinely) are not a good indicator of body levels.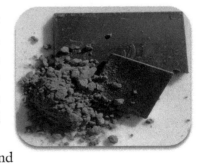
Magnesium helps to maintain normal muscle and
nerve function, supports a healthy immunity by helping make the antioxidant enzyme glutathione, and helps keep bones strong. Mg also helps regulate blood sugar levels, promotes normal blood pressure and is known to be involved in energy metabolism and protein synthesis. Mg deficiency can impact on the bioavailability of vitamin D and other vitamin function.

Specific deficiency syndromes are rare in humans, but lower than normal levels are commonly seen on micronutrient testing. Low levels, unless caused by recent illness or medications such as diuretics, antibiotics, painkillers and steroids, or increased renal excretion, can be an indicator of chronic poor intake of green vegetables, nuts, beans and fish.

A number of oncology agents can deplete magnesium, particularly cisplatin and erbitux (cetuximab) – if you are receiving these drugs, it's advisable to make an extra effort to eat more foods rich in Mg. Very low levels can cause fatigue, insomnia, poor memory, muscular cramps, tremor, fasciculations, muscle weakness and an increased risk of nausea, low mood and peripheral nerve damage during chemotherapy. Moderate deficiency can cause muscle spasms and prolongation of the QT interval, leading to abnormal heartbeats (arrhythmia), something which is particularly important if taking chemotherapy drugs such as oxaliplatin and biological agents which also prolong the QT interval such as ribociclib.

The RDA is between 320 – 420 mg/day. Cocoa beans in real dark chocolate are one of the best sources of magnesium. The problem is that most chocolate products have a high sugar content. Even dark chocolate varieties have a lot of added sugar, but there are some 100% chocolate brands available with no added sugar which can be bought on the internet from single plantations. These are very bitter, but to make them palatable they can be broken up and mixed with fruit, making them both delicious and healthy. Fish, such as halibut, and other seafood are good sources. Green vegetables such as spinach, kale, seaweed and spirulina are rich in Mg because the centre of the chlorophyll molecule (which gives green vegetables their colour) contains mg. Some legumes (beans and peas), nuts and seeds, and whole, unrefined grains are also good sources of magnesium. Refined grains are generally low in Mg because white flour is refined and processed, stripping it of its Mg-rich germ and bran content. Whole grain, wheat flour contains far more magnesium.

Calcium

Dietary calcium intakes of 1000mg/day for women and 800mg/day for men are recommended. In people with established osteoporosis, between 1,000 to 1,200mg a day is advisable. Many regard dietary calcium greater than 1500mg per day as excessive.

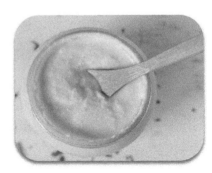

This complex arrangement between calcium, vitamin K2, osteoporosis an dheart disease has already been described above, so will not be repeated here. In terms of cancer, the EPIC study found that one pint of milk a day was linked to a 20% reduced bowel cancer risk. Calcium in milk was thought to inhibit the formation of nitroso-compounds from heterocyclic amines. Moreover, other naturally occurring omega fats in milk include sphingomyelin and butyric acid, both of which have been shown to directly reduce colon cancer in laboratory animals. Several trials have tried to evaluate the effects of calcium supplementation, but a meta-analysis of them all concluded no reduction in bowel cancer risk. It is likely that other ingredients in milk products were responsible for the benefits, including its Vitamin D content and the lactobacillus bacteria which can contribute to gut health.

Four prospective cohort studies relating to calcium and prostate cancer have been published. Two giving between 1330-1840 mg/day, showed no benefit or increased risk of cancer. Two others, one involving 86,404 men in the CP II Nutrition cohort who were recording >2000 mg/day intake from food and supplements, actually showed a significantly higher rate of prostate cancer. Further questionnaire surveys found an increased risk of prostate and breast cancer with a high intake of dairy food, but this data was complicated by the fact that a diet high in dairy products was associated with high fat intake. The detrimental effect of excessive calcium is thought to lie in the finding that high dietary calcium can reduce blood and cellular vitamin D levels. Calcium supplements, on their own, may well have a detrimental effect on cancer, but when combined with vitamin D are useful to treat and prevent bone loss. To get enough calcium daily, it is advisable to eat foods that are rich in calcium, such as milk, cheese, yoghurt, kefir, seaweed, tinned oily fish with the bones

Individuals eating a dairy-free diet should ensure a higher intake of non-dairy foods that contain calcium. Some foods can upset the calcium balance in the body. These include caffeine, red meat, salt and fizzy drinks that contain phosphates, such as cola. With dwindling fish stocks and global climate change, we should be developing a taste for seaweed as a viable stable food. Sea kelp is a natural source of calcium as well as vitamins A, B1, B2, C, D and E, and minerals including zinc, iodine, magnesium, iron, potassium, copper and calcium.

Copper

The estimated safe and adequate intake for copper is 1.5 – 3.0 mg/day. Many survey studies show that in the West we tend to consume 1.0 mg or less of copper per day. Copper is involved in the absorption, storage and metabolism of iron, and the formation of red blood cells. It also helps supply oxygen to the body. The symptoms

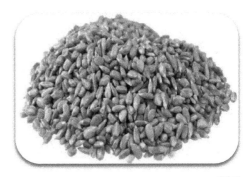

of a copper deficiency are similar to iron-deficiency anaemia. A study which removed copper from the feed of cows showed an excess of cancer and function of the enzyme SOD. Dietary sources include: avocados, bananas, beans, brussels, sunflower seeds, dark chocolate and grains.

Manganese

The estimated adequate intake for manganese is 2.0-5.0 mg/day for adults. The functions of this mineral are not specific as other minerals can perform in its place. Manganese does function in enzyme reactions concerning blood sugar, metabolism and thyroid hormone function. It is worth measuring, if thyroid deficiency occurs during or after completion of cancer therapies such 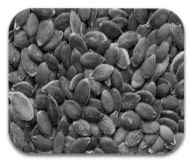 as chemotherapy. Deficiency is rare in humans, and good food sources include pumpkin seeds. kiwi, avocado, blackberries and artichoke.

Iron

Iron is needed to form the haem part of haemoglobin, which carries oxygen around the body. In the blood, iron is mainly carried bound to a protein called transferrin. Prolonged deficiency will lead to anaemia. Symptoms of anaemia include fatigue, pallor, breathlessness on exertion, feeling dizzy upon standing, mood changes and depression. A chronic low iron 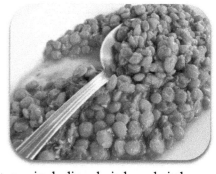 level is also associated with a range of other symptoms including; hair loss, brittle nails, Plummer-Vinson syndrome (painful mucous membrane covering the tongue, mouth and throat) and reduced immunity. Blood loss is the most common cause of excess iron loss so unexplained iron deficiency should be investigated. Other causes include inadequate diet, malabsorption (Crohn's disease, bowel surgery) or prolonged fever. Sources include red meat, liver, lentils, beans, chickpeas, black-eyed peas, tinned sardines, tuna, swordfish, leafy green and cruciferous vegetables

Iron in meat (haem iron source) is more easily broken down and absorbed than iron in grains and vegetables ("non-haem" iron source). Oxalates form insoluble complexes which bind iron in the gut before it can be absorbed. Oxalate is found in spinach, Swiss chard, sorrel, rhubarb, buckwheat, quinoa and star fruit. Leaves of the tea plant contain oxalic acid, however, the infusion beverage typically contains only low to moderate amounts of oxalic acid per serving. Phytic acid forms insoluble complexes which can also impair absorption. Phytic acid is used as a preservative labelled E391. Cadmium encourages the transformation of vitamin C into oxalic acid, reducing iron absorption. This can be a problem for people exposed to high levels of cadmium in their diet, at their workplace or, most commonly, through smoking.

Vitamin C as well as being healthy in its own right, reduces the effect of phytic acid and enhances iron absorption. Probiotics such as lactobacilli can create a more favourable PH and environment for oxalic acid excretion, increasing iron absorption.

Caution with iron supplements: Free iron is needed for pathogenic (bad) bacterial growth, which is one reason why iron is protein bound with transferrin in the blood. It is possible that iron supplements adversely affect bacterial growth. Some suggest it is sensible to stop iron supplements in the presence of a systemic bacterial infection. The haem iron by facilitating the conversion of nitrites to carcinogenic nitrosamines, has been implicated with an increased risk of bowel cancer.

Summary – Advice to ensure adequate trace mineral intake

- Diversify your foods as much as possible
- Alternate your carbohydrate sources:
    - Different potato varieties
    - Brown or wild rice, as well as white
    - Couscous, quinoa, buckwheat
    - Different types of pasta, especially wholemeal
- Alternate your daily snacks
    - Snack on pumpkin, sunflower and sesame seeds
    - Mixed nuts
    - Fresh unsalted peanuts
- Try to eat organic fruit, veg and nuts
- Alternate brands and countries of origin
- Eat seafood such as crab and shellfish once or twice a fortnight
- Alternate fish between oily, freshwater and sea varieties
- Alternate water sources – tap, filtered and different mineral waters
- Think about growing your own vegetables
- Avoid taking extra mineral supplements unless deficient
- Consider measuring your mineral levels to avoid deficiency or excess

---

Micronutrient testing

The evidence summarised, so far shows that chronic deficiencies in vitamins, minerals, healthy fats, essential proteins and polyphenols can put a strain on metabolic pathways and oxidative stress, leading to an increased risk of many chronic illnesses. The solution eagerly suggested by the supplement industry would be to take a mineral and vitamin pill. These pills would 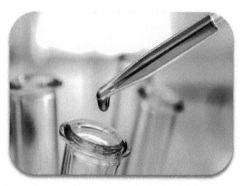 help if it happened to contain a nutrient which an individual specifically needs. It is very unlikely, however, that an individual would be aware of a deficiency or an excess of one or more individual nutrients. Also, even if a deficiency is present, the levels of nutrients in a standard pill may be inadequate and offer false reassurance.

Apart from the expense, most supplements, in moderation, are harmless and may help in the short-term when someone is off their food or hasn't been eating well after surgery or medical treatments. Taking prolonged high doses of minerals and vitamins, without knowing underlying levels, however, could just as easily contribute to excess levels. This is why the WCRF and Memorial Sloane Kettering Hospital have issued statements that taking long-term mineral or vitamin supplements, without a recognised need, is not required and could do more harm than good.

Many cancer survivors are turning to nutritional testing in order to give themselves an understanding of their underlying micronutrient status. Empowered with this knowledge, individuals can modify their diet by eating more of the foods they need and less of those they don't, while they can also identify ideal selective food supplements if required. One of the UK's most comprehensive is available via the website **cancernet.co.uk**. After payment a pack is sent to the individual with instructions how to get the blood taken and sent back to the laboratory is designated air sealed containers suitable for the normal post. The lab then measures over 50 micronutrients, levels of antioxidant enzymes, candidate polyphenols omega 3,6,7 and 9 fats most relevant to the cancer process. These results, together with a report and series of advice recommendations is written by oncologist is written by a consultant oncologist. At the moment this test is only available in the UK.

Chapter 16

Phytochemicals after cancer

Phytochemicals are gifts from nature, found mainly in plants and responsible for their colour, taste, and aroma. They reduce chronic inflammation and act as prebiotics for gut bacteria enriching gut health and improving immunity. They enhance sports performance by improving oxygenation, muscle repair and preventing joint damage. Their regular intake have been shown to lowering the risk of

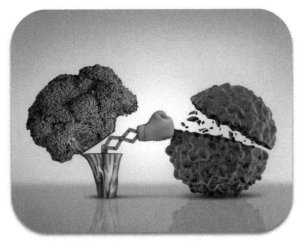

chronic illnesses such as dementia, high cholesterol, skin ageing, heart disease, atherosclerosis, osteoarthritis, and macular degeneration. They even slow the transfer of glucose through the gut wall reducing the risk of diabetes and aiding weight loss programmes.

In terms of cancer, they protect us from environmental and ingested carcinogens by arming antioxidant enzymes, enhancing DNA repair pathways and reducing the epigenetic expression of cancer promoting genes. One of their many mechanisms of action being via their anti-inflammatory properties as they help inhibit upregulation of NF-kappa B signalling which is responsible for triggering excess inflammation. Even after cancer has formed they have been shown to reduce proliferation (growth) rates, block angiogenesis (new blood vessel formation in cancers), reduce invasion into adjacent structures and distant blood born spread (metastasis) It is no surprise then that the World Cancer Research Fund, and many other academic bodies, advise that eating foods rich in phytochemicals will lower risk of cancer, slow its progress and lower the risk of relapse after treatments.

How to ensure adequate polyphenol intake

Asian and Mediterranean diets are typically abundant in polyphenol-rich vegetables, salads, herbs, spices, teas, nuts, fruits, seeds and legumes. Typical western diets, on the other hand, are dreadfully deficient in polyphenols, meaning we need to eat a lot more of them with every meal of the day. Health magazines often use the expression "superfoods" to describe foods which contain high levels of phytochemicals, vitamins, fibre and vitamins, although there is no official definition. Great emphasis is also placed on new foods from distant sources, yet polyphenol-rich foods are all around us and readily available in most local supermarkets.

Tomatoes and lycopene: Unlike other phytochemicals, beta-carotenes such as lycopene are not destroyed by the cooking process. This means that while they are only found in relatively small quantities in tomatoes, higher concentrations can be found in tomato sauces and pastes. An analysis of the HPFS indicated that men with diets rich in tomatoes and tomato sauces had a lower risk of prostate 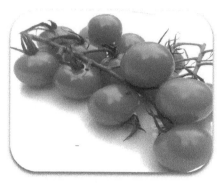 cancer. This finding has been confirmed in other population studies. This benefit was attributed largely to lycopene, but it should be noted that tomatoes have other polyphenols, vitamins, fibre and removing the lycopene and concentrating it has not resulted in an enhanced benefit. In terms of the impact on prostate health, a laboratory study randomly gave either a pure lycopene extract or whole tomato powder to mice with implanted prostate tumours. It was only the whole tomato powder which triggered some shrinkage. A study published in 2002 involving 26 men with localised prostate cancer gave subjects either a tomato extract or a placebo for three weeks prior to prostatectomy. Despite the tiny numbers involved, the study reported significant differences in PSA and tumour volume in the lycopene group. The study was well reported in the media and is often quoted by manufacturers of lycopene supplements, but many doctors argue that these results were unreliable considering the short intervention period. A larger, study in 2017, involving 81 men from Tobago, showed no benefit of lycopene supplements. In 2008, a German study randomised 40 men with benign prostatic hypertrophy (BPH) to receive either a lycopene supplement or a placebo. After six months they reported a difference in PSA, prostate symptoms and prostate volume, but critics of this study pointed out that this benefit could not be established conclusively with such small numbers. In terms of prevention, a prestigious Cochrane meta-analysis in 2011 found no benefit between lycopene supplements and prostate cancer incidence. This lack of evidence for a benefit was the reason lycopene was not included in the pomi-T trial.

Cruciferous vegetables

This ubiquitous group of vegetables have long been hailed for their myriad of health benefits. Sources include broccoli, cabbage, bok choy, kale, cauliflower, asparagus, Brussels, mustard, horseradish, wasabi, watercress, radish and garden cress. As well as offering a strong and unique flavour, they contain fibre, vitamins and other healthy nutrients. They are particularly rich in glucosinolates such as isothiocyanates (sulforaphane), and indoles such as Indole-3-carbinol. In lab studies, these phytochemicals, when added to prostate cancer cells, inhibited growth and promoted programmed death. Human studies have found that people who eat cruciferous vegetables regularly have a decreased risk of prostate and breast cancer, and the cancers they develop tend to be less aggressive and less likely to spread.

A study from the British Institute of Food Research sheds further light on the underlying anti-cancer mechanisms of cruciferous vegetables. Men with pre-cancerous lesions in their prostate were randomised to consume either a broccoli-rich diet or a standard diet. After six months, future prostate biopsies revealed over a hundred, epigenetic changes in gene expression among the men eating broccoli 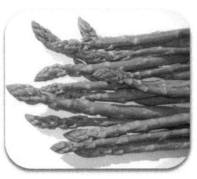 but not the standard diet. The most notable improvements in gene expression related to androgen signalling and insulin signalling. Another, lab experiment confirmed that dried cruciferous vegetable extracts also blocked histone deacetylase (HDAC), an enzyme, which encourages the epigenetic expression of pro-inflammatory genes. Another clinical study from Singapore reported a correlation between increased consumption of cruciferous vegetables, rich in indole-3-carbinol, and decreased urinary levels of 8-hydroxy-2'-deoxyguanosine, a marker of oxidative stress.

More specifically, the isothiocyanates in cruciferous vegetables promote the formation of one of the main anti-oxidant enzymes, Glutathione S-transferases (GST). This important enzyme, normally located in the liver, is particularly valuable in dealing with environmental pollutants such as dioxins and PCBs, food additives, hydrocarbons, and pesticides. GST neutralises these toxins, so they don't damage cells and cause cancer. It is a strange quirk of nature that up to 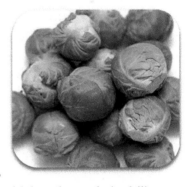 40% of the population have defects of the GST gene, which reduces their ability to produce GST. These people have a higher risk of cancer because carcinogens stay in the body for longer. Broccoli particularly helps these people because the isothiocyanates also stay in the body for longer. The antioxidant properties of extra isothiocyanates after broccoli intake more than compensate for the lack of GST. Those who don't eat broccoli as part of their diet fail to reap these benefits and have an increased vulnerability to pollutants.

Radish, mustard and cress: As members of the cruciferous vegetable group, radish, mustard and cress are high in GST. Because they are usually eaten raw, they also have particularly high levels of the enzyme myrosinase. This enzyme is required to convert GST into the bioactive sulforaphane form. Although present in other cruciferous vegetables, it is partially damaged by heat. Even though GST itself is heat resistant, the longer it is cooked for, and the higher the temperature used during cooking, the less sulforaphane is formed. This is one good reason to blanch broccoli or even try some raw in salads. Studies have shown that adding some radish, mustard or cress to the plate will enhance the formation of sulforaphane, even from cooked vegetables. Other factors which influence the availability of myrosinase include:

- It's released from foods by chewing or mashing
- It starts degrading at cooking temperatures over 60° C
- The longer the cooking time the more degradation
- Cooking under moderate pressure helps retain its levels
- Healthy gut bacteria can also supply some myrosinase

Herbs

The strong aroma, taste, and colour of herbs and spices are due to their high phytochemical content. They are usually taken in small amounts, but nevertheless, in countries such as Japan and India, where they are used extensively in everyday cooking, they represent major sources of intake. This is one of the reasons why these populations have a lower

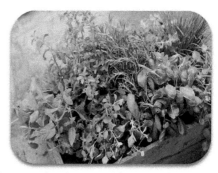

cancer risk. In general, they are fairly robust to heat and other cooking processes. In fact, drying and grinding herbs increases their phytochemical content 5-fold. It's a good idea when cooking spicy foods to add as many herbs as possible such as paprika, chilli, black pepper basil, rosemary, oregano, marjoram, coriander, sage and parsley. For desserts, do not hold back on real cinnamon, raw cocoa powder and vanilla. Although most are beneficial, three herbs are worth emphasising:

Chilli pepper

Chilli peppers, the fruit from the genus Capsicum, are used worldwide and are considered an indispensable ingredient within a diverse range of culinary cultures. In lab studies, capsaicin, the polyphenol responsible for its famous heat, was found to trigger suicide (apoptosis) in prostate cancer cell lines but not normal cells. Data gathered from a large

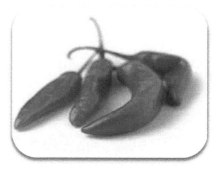

population study in China highlighted how people who ate spicy food once or twice

234

a week had a mortality rate 10% lower than those who ate spicy food less than once a week. Risk of death was reduced still further among those who ate spicy food six or seven days a week. There are also reports that, in moderation, it is associated with a reduced risk of stomach cancer, while chillies have also been identified as helping improve many other conditions relevant to cancer survivors.

Cholesterol, weight and blood sugar: A study from the University of Adelaide found that the receptors in the stomach that interact with capsaicin play a role in creating a feeling of fullness, something which can be instrumental in helping promote weight loss. In 2012, a team of nutritionists working with animals at the Chinese University of Hong Kong found that capsaicin helped reduce LDL (bad) cholesterol. Another study from the University of Tasmania demonstrated that after eating chillies, the amount of insulin diabetics required to lower their body's blood sugar level following a meal was significantly reduced.

Peripheral neuropathy: This is an uncomfortable condition in which the sensory nerves are damaged in the hands and feet. It causes numbness, pins and needles and even hyperaesthesia (burning like sensation). If severe, it can affect walking, balance, and a range of activities essential to daily living. Sometimes there is no obvious cause, but it is often associated with diabetes, alcoholism (B1 deficiency) and chemotherapy drugs such as Taxotere and platinum agents. Topical creams containing capsaicin cream have been shown to provide significant relief for diabetic neuropathy, and some relief for post-herpetic neuralgia, but trials investigating a benefit for chemotherapy-induced neuropathy are yet to be performed. As it is otherwise well tolerated, it is certainly worth a try as very little has been shown to help this nasty side effect.

Localised joint pains: Capsaicin binds to the pain receptor which interferes with pain thresholds. In the extensive overview of the evidence for plant products and joint pains published by the UK charity Arthritis Research, creams containing capsaicin (chilli) had the strongest evidence of benefit. The greatest relief was reported for osteoarthritis and psoriasis-related arthritis. Despite the evidence on offer, very few of the topical joint relieving creams available on the market today contain capsaicin.

Black pepper (piperine)

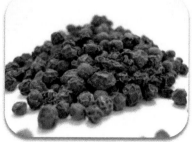

Black pepper, from black and long pepper plants (Piper nigrum and Piper longum), is used as a spice and a herbal medicine. Pepper is packed with minerals including potassium, magnesium and calcium, plus vitamins such as B1, B6, riboflavin, C and E. Its high polyphenol content provides anti-inflammatory, antioxidant and anti-ageing properties. It also supports the bioavailability of other phytochemicals by inhibiting their breakdown and excretion from the body. This allows higher levels of other polyphenol-rich herbs such as turmeric to remain in the body for longer. It has been estimated that in one study on humans, 20mg of piperine, given concomitantly with 2g curcumin, increased serum curcumin bioavailability 20-fold.

Curcumin (Turmeric)

Curcumin, which gives turmeric its yellow colour, has often garnered positive attention in the media. Turmeric is a rhizomatous herbaceous perennial flowering plant of the ginger family, Zingiberaceae. Aside from contributing a vibrant taste to curries and casseroles, it is rich in fibre, vitamin B6, C, magnesium and iron, alongside polyphenols 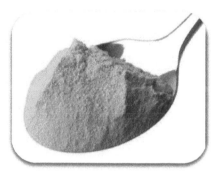 called curcuminoids. In the laboratory, curcumin has been shown to stop or delay the progression of breast cancer cells by promoting apoptosis of cancer cells, blocking mechanisms which encourage cancer cells to spread, blocking new blood vessel formation (angiogenesis), and inhibiting mTOR which helps restore sensitivity to hormone drugs such as the aromatase inhibitor anastrozole. It also reduces the formation of cancers by minimising chronic inflammation, reducing oxidative stress by enhancing anti-oxidant enzymes. Research conducted at the University of Michigan found that turmeric halted the growth of stem cells that give rise to breast cancer, without harming normal breast cells. Numerous studies have also highlighted its impact on inhibiting prostate cancer cell growth by blocking the S/G2M phase of the cell cycle. Interestingly, in a similar experiment, green tea extract slowed growth by blocking another phase in the cell cycle (G1). When added together, because of this different mode of action, the benefits of turmeric were found to be synergistic with teas, leading to both these ingredients being included in the UK Pomi-T study.

On the safety side, curcumin has been shown to inhibit platelet aggregation. This is an advantage for most people as it could reduce the risk of thrombosis, but could be a potential problem for those already on anticoagulation therapies. That said, neither of these issues have been found to be present in humans, even after doses of up to 4g a day, an amount regarded as safe by the FDA.

Pomegranate

This is a fruit-bearing shrub or small tree originally from the Middle East but now grown across the world, particularly in warm climates. Pomegranate has been a source of traditional remedies for thousands of years. The rind of the fruit and the

236

bark of the pomegranate tree are a traditional remedy for diarrhoea, dysentery, and parasites. Pomegranate juice is a reasonable source of vitamin C, B5 (pantothenic acid), potassium and the phytochemicals; ellagitannins, pelargonidin, punicalin, punicalagin, anthocyanin, cyaniding and ellagic acid. The seeds and skin contain a variety of natural chemicals including; punicotannic acid, gallic acid, mannite, pelletierine and n-methylisopelletierine, which is why the ground and dried seed is more effective than the juice.

These polyphenols have been shown to inhibit proliferation and markers of migration, while also inducing apoptosis and cell adhesion in breast and prostate cancer cell lines. In humans, although studies of pomegranate juice were not consistently significant, three phase II studies of dried pomegranate powder demonstrated a reduction in PSA progression and reduced markers of oxidative stress. Its 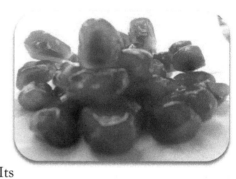 influence on prostate cancer was not via the hormonal route, as it affected both androgen-sensitive and resistant human prostate cancer cells, and clinical studies have shown no change in testosterone levels following regular intake.

Furthermore, pomegranate was found to inhibit the process by which breast cancer cells are attracted to and spread to the bone. Bacteria are known to metabolise ellagic acid into ellagitannin, which has demonstrated oestrogenic activity in some lab studies. However, even at high concentrations, no increased growth of oestrogen-sensitive breast cancer cells has ever been seen – instead, it slows growth via its anti-proliferative effect which far out-weighs any stimulatory effect on the oestrogen receptor. Some studies suggest pomegranate is particularly helpful for prostate health, as there is a tendency for their metabolites to accumulate in the prostate gland. A small North American phase II study, sponsored by the Pomegranate Growers Association, reported that men with prostate cancer given pomegranate juice to drink every day had a slowing of PSA progression. This has not been substantiated in subsequent studies, and two reasons for this have been proposed. Firstly, juices tend to be quite sweet, and some even have added sugar which mitigates any benefit. Secondly, the juice only contains a small proportion of the polyphenols in pomegranate, which are predominately found in the seeds and pulp. A number of studies using dried whole prostate powder, however, did show it affected PSA progression and also improved baseline oxidative stress. Most notably, a randomised study carried out at Johns Hopkins Hospital USA found that men taking pomegranate extract supplement for 18 months, experienced a significant reduction in progression of PSA levels compared to the baseline PSA progression rate pre-treatment. This was the reason ground pomegranate seed and rind was included as one of the ingredients in the successful Pomi-T study.

Green tea

It may surprise some people that both green tea, and the black stuff we've been drinking in the UK for several hundred years, come from the same plant. When the leaves of the Camellia Sinensis plant are dried, they are fermented and oxidised to form the black tea we are familiar with. Green tea is unfermented and is merely steamed. Reassuringly, both variants contain good quantities of the active polyphenol, epigallocatechin gallate (EGCG).

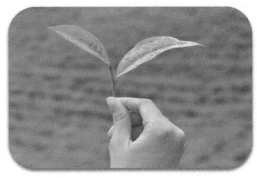

By blocking the G1 phase of the cell cycle, while concurrently blocking de-differentiation and angiogenesis, tea has also been reported to reduce growth of breast and prostate cancers. EGCG has potent antioxidant activities which are 25 times greater than vitamin C and plays a key role in promoting the formation of anti-oxidant enzymes. It has also been shown to block an enzyme called ornithine decarboxylase which tells cells to proliferate faster and bypass apoptosis. Green tea polyphenols also impede the effect of harmful oestrogenic pollutants, which explains why in one population study on humans, regular tea drinkers had a significant reduction in breast, prostate and ovarian cancer risk. This was confirmed in a further study in 2009, which showed that regular green tea consumption was associated with a 40% reduced risk of breast cancer, especially if women also tended to eat mushrooms on a daily basis. Green tea was also shown to reduce breast cancer relapse after initial treatments in another large study. The Mayo Clinic in the USA found that green tea decreased the abnormal white cell count in up 30% of patients with chronic leukaemia, although further confirmatory trials have yet to be done. Further research from Perth University highlighted how drinking just one cup per day reduced ovarian cancer risk by half, while a year later the same group suggested that tea consumption reduced prostate cancer risk by a third. A small study of men with prostate cancer, scheduled for radical prostatectomy, reported that daily administration of a green tea concentrate supplement containing 800 mg of EGCG (and a total of 1300 mg of tea polyphenols) for several weeks, from initiation of the study until the scheduled prostatectomy, caused a significant reduction in the serum levels of PSA and several cancer-promoting growth factors when compared to pre-study baseline levels.

As well as cancer, the polyphenols in green tea have also been shown to protect against heart disease by preventing the oxidation of LDL into cholesterol. Moreover, researchers from the University of Pennsylvania and Boston have shown that EGCG helps protect the brain from the build-up of amyloid proteins and, in turn, the possible development of Parkinson´s and Alzheimer's. Researchers from the American College of Nutrition found that regular consumption may also prevent colds and flu, improve skin tone, smooth out wrinkles and even help with weight loss programmes. EGCG is also known to help good bacteria in the intestine flourish.

Other factors to consider when drinking green tea: Most teas contain some caffeine so be careful not to drink it in the evening. Tremors and agitation can occur following high levels of consumption and side effects such as diarrhoea and stomach irritation have been reported. There exists a whole range of soft drinks based on green tea, but avoid those with added sugar. Green tea can discolour the teeth, so it would be a good habit to swill the mouth out with water after drinking.

Phytoestrogenic foods - Lignans and Isoflavones

These unique polyphenol groups have multiple healthy attributes of their own, but they share a common ability to weakly bind to oestrogen receptors. Because of this, for years, women with breast cancer have missed out on the wonderful benefits offered by these foods, as doctors were concerned that their oestrogenic properties could stimulate breast cancer cells. The previous chapter has 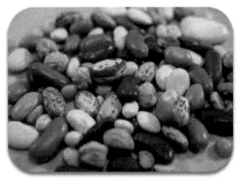 already highlighted that research has shown the opposite effect – they actually reduce the risk of breast and prostate cancer as well as decreasing the risk of relapse after radical treatments.

Lignan polyphenols are found in many healthy foods, particularly in the outer layers of whole grains and seeds. People who only eat refined grains and seeds with the outer husks removed are likely to have an inadequate intake. Lignin-rich foods include:

- Flaxseeds and sesame seeds, pulses such as beans, lentils and peas
- Pumpkin, sunflower, poppy seeds, quinoa and buckwheat
- Unrefined whole grains such as rye, oats, barley

Isoflavone polyphenols such as genistein and daidzein are found in soya products and pulses, both of which are eaten in considerably higher quantities in the Far East. Typical isoflavone foods include:

- Fermented soya produce - miso, natto, tempeh
- Unfermented soya produce - tofu, soy milk, soybeans (edamame)
- Peanuts, chickpeas, fava beans, alfalfa, kudzu tea

Several observational studies have reported an association between a regular intake of plant lignans and isoflavones, and a lower risk of developing lifestyle-related diseases such as cardiovascular disease, osteoporosis and cancer, as well as lower menopausal symptoms such as hot flushes. After cancer, soya products, particularly those which are fermented 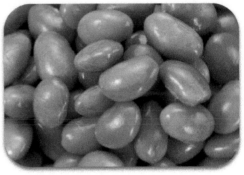 (miso, tofu, tempura) and more easily digested, are also beneficial because they reduce the risk of osteoporosis, relapse rate and improve the chances of overall survival. As mentioned above, in sensible amounts, phytoestrogens in these foods attach to the oestrogen receptor (ER) but only have weak activity. They consequently dilute the effect of the body's own oestrogen by blocking the receptor. Genistein (from soya) attaches to the ER in the same way as tamoxifen – inhibiting the oestrogen effect on tumours but at the same time stimulating the bones and uterus.

Women with breast cancer who had the highest serum lignan levels, reflecting good intake of legumes, cereals, cruciferous vegetables, and soya, were reported to have better overall survival after established cancer than those with the lowest levels. This effect was further supported by a major study conducted by the Roswell Park Cancer Institute, which found that as well as a lower overall breast cancer incidence in regular lignan food consumers, there was a particularly low incidence of the worst types of breast cancers, all of which require more intensive treatments and carry a poorer prognosis. Dietary lignans can also help non-hormone sensitive cancers. Regular intake was found to decrease the risk of adenocarcinoma of the oesophagus junction in one case-control study. Another study linked lignan-rich diets with a lower colorectal cancer relapse rate.

Lignan polyphenols also appear to protect patients from the adverse effects of radiotherapy. A laboratory study found that dietary lignans reduced radiation, thus decreasing inflammation, lung injury and eventual fibrosis in mice with cancers. Research is now exploring whether enterolactone or other lignan polyphenols may be used to mitigate the adverse effects of radiation in individuals who suffered incidental exposure. Patients receiving to the rectum have been reported to have a lower than expected toxicity if they consumed lignan-rich foods. It's better to avoid foods which produce gas during prostate cancer radiotherapy, as this could change the shape of the rectum and reduce accuracy. Therefore, consider foods such as quinoa and flaxseeds rather than pulses and grains.

In terms of what soya products to eat, a large cohort study in 2009 linked a lower risk of prostate cancer with higher consumption of both soya products and non-fermented products such as tofu, soy milk and whole soybeans (edamame), but not fermented products such as miso, natto, and tempeh. Since then, another large meta-analysis 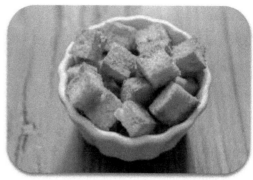 concluded that soya and total isoflavone intake was associated with a lower prostate cancer risk among Asians but not men from Western populations. Two large cohort studies, from China and the USA, demonstrated that women with the highest intake of phytoestrogenic polyphenols, isoflavones and flavanones, found in soya and other beans, had a significantly reduced risk of breast cancer recurrence and death from any cause, compared to those with the lowest intake at a median follow-up of 4 years. Similar findings have been observed following a high intake of green tea (containing small amounts of isoflavone) after breast cancer and colorectal cancer.

As also highlighted in the previous chapter, the results are not all consistent. One analysis of a dataset from California linked a higher total isoflavone intake with a higher prostate cancer risk, yet this data is likely to be influenced by the use of cheap soya products, phytoestrogenic supplements and highly sugared ice tea, which the authors included in the questionnaire as a recognised isoflavone source.

Concerns with phytoestrogenic food supplements
Although phytoestrogenic-rich foods are generally healthy, their benefits are not replicated by phytoestrogenic foods supplements. These supplements were previously promoted by some enthusiasts to help hot flushes and improve prostate health. Well-conducted placebo-controlled studies involving patients with breast cancer have shown no reduction in hot flushes with phytoestrogenic-rich food supplements. More worryingly, the oestrogenic effect can become overpowered, leading the oestrogen receptor to become stimulated rather than weakly blocked. This was highlighted in an experiment with monkeys which, after being given a high dose of phytoestrogen extract, began to experience a thickening of the uterus after several months, indicating a negative oestrogenic effect. Likewise, a RCT from the

241

Memorial Sloan-Kettering Cancer Centre in New York gave a group of women with early-stage breast cancer either a supplement containing high-dose genistein (the main isoflavone in soya) or a placebo for a period of 30 days prior to surgery. The supplementation was found to induce changes in the expression of 21 genes, potentially leading to increased signals for elevated growth rate. Furthermore, blood serum obtained from women in the supplementation group, added to laboratory tumour cells, caused the tumour cells to proliferate faster.

In men, the data for phytoestrogenic supplements is conflicting. One small crossover RCT found that a dietary supplement containing isoflavone-rich foods, including 60 mg of soya and 15 mg of lycopene among other phytochemicals and antioxidants, administered 4 times a day for treatment periods lasting 10 weeks, significantly delayed PSA progression among men whose PSA relapsed after radical therapies. A subsequent larger study of men with prostate cancer on active surveillance, using mixed isoflavones and other nutraceuticals, reported no effect on PSA. Of some concern, a study involving men with rising PSA after prostate radiotherapy reported no slowing after taking a supplement with high dose genistein, while IGF levels actually went up (a chemical often associated with cancer development).

Saw palmetto: Supplements containing the liposterolic extract from Saw Palmetto are widely rumoured to help prostate health, based on the hypothesis that it has anti-androgenic properties via inhibition of 5α-reductase. However, there are no clinical studies that show any decrease in serum testosterone or prostate-specific antigen after taking saw palmetto extracts. Its efficacy in the treatment of lower urinary tract symptoms has also not been conclusively proven. While several small commercially sponsored studies suggest that Saw Palmetto may help symptoms relating to benign prostatic hypertrophy, larger trials found little or no evidence that it affects prostate enlargement or symptoms. This includes a robust study sponsored by the prestigious National Cancer Institute. This is why this organisation and many others do not recommend supplements containing phytoestrogenic foods and was one of the principal reasons why they were not included in the Pomi-T trial.

Allium Vegetables - Onions, Garlic and Leeks

These are particularly rich in the antioxidant polyphenols quercetin, gallic acid and kaempferol. Their regular intake is linked with a reduced incidence of cancers of the lung, oesophagus and pancreas, especially among smokers and alcoholics. These polyphenols are damaged somewhat by heat, so it's better to introduce raw onions in salads. The red Spanish varieties are

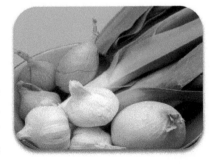

particularly beneficial, but their strong taste and smell do put some people off. In this case, try using smaller spring onions or marinating them in extra virgin olive oil before mixing with lettuce and other ingredients in a salad.

Cohort studies have correlated consumption of garlic and raw onions with a lower need for drugs to treat high blood pressure (BP). A summary of 25 RCTs, published in 2008, compared garlic and onions with a placebo and found sizable effects on lowering BP, allowing some individuals to avoid using anti-hypertensive drugs. Another study, involving patients with poorly controlled BP, reported that a 1g garlic supplementation resulted in a significant reduction in BP 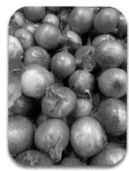 levels and better control even in those on medication. This action is thought to be due to garlic's polysulfides which have a vasodilatory action on blood vessels.

Berries and Fruit

Virtually all edible berries and fruit are an excellent source of vitamin C, fibre and minerals, and are abundant in many categories of polyphenols, carotenoids, non-carotenoid terpenoids and other phytochemicals. Wild varieties have higher levels compared to their cultivated cousins, while also having the additional advantage of not being sprayed 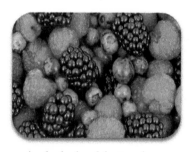 with pesticides and herbicides. Wild blackberries are particularly healthy and grow widely in the UK between July and September. Berries are also a rich source of healthy plant nitrates which improve sports performance and reduce blood pressure.

With the exception of grapefruit (highlighted below), fruit and berries should be eaten liberally, but be careful with smoothies which break down the pulp and increase the glycaemic index. Drying fruit is a useful way to preserve it for longer, yet the process can damage some of the nutrients and, more significantly, concentrate the fructose content. Some manufacturers also add extra sugar and sulphites in order to improve taste and preservation. It would be particularly wise to avoid consumption on an empty stomach, such as first thing in the morning, despite their popularity in breakfast cereals.

The other issue with fruit and berries to consider is that many are now intensively farmed and are sprayed with large amounts of pesticides and herbicides. Intensive farming methods may change from country to country or over time. A prime example is the much-loved goji berry which became popular in the early 2000s after it was discovered to be one of the world's richest sources of vitamin C, lycopene and other polyphenols. It originates from Tibet, where it was traditionally hand-picked from pesticide-free, wild trees which grew in pollutant-free, high-altitude soils. Unfortunately, widespread popularity drove up the commercial price, leading to mass production across lowland areas of China where intensive farming techniques which entail the use of herbicides and pesticides are commonplace. In 2007, the FDA calculated its antioxidant capacity at over 25,000 units/g. By 2010 the capacity among commercially produced berries had fallen to 3,500 units/g, less than an apple.

Grapefruit

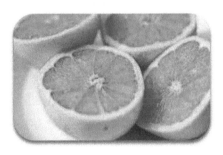

The idea that fruit can increase the risk of breast cancer seems almost implausible. Yet there is significant evidence to raise concerns. Grapefruit is known to inhibit an enzyme in the gut called cytochrome P450 or CYP3A4, which is integral to the metabolism and excretion of alcohol, drugs and endogenous oestrogen. Their inhibition can occur after a single glass of grapefruit juice, with the peak effect approximately 24 hours after consumption resulting in increased blood levels of alcohol, drugs and oestrogen. Unlike phytoestrogens such as soya which lower the amount of oestrogen in the body, grapefruit actually increases oestrogen levels. It was hardly surprising then that a study, which evaluated a population of 50,000 post-menopausal women, found a 20% increased risk of breast cancer among those who consumed more than ¼ of a grapefruit a day on average. This went up to almost 40% in high grapefruit consumers (>60g/day). Lean women (BMI< 25) also had a slightly higher risk. This was because oestrogen levels are already higher in overweight women, so a further increase has less of an effect on the risk of breast cancer. For the same reason, pre-menopausal women (with naturally high oestrogen levels) had no increased risk after grapefruit consumption. As grapefruits also contain many healthy substances such as vitamins, antioxidants and fibre, it would a shame for men, pre-menopausal women and overweight post-menopausal women to avoid the fruit. However, for post-menopausal, thin women its best to avoid regular intake.

Red wine – Resveratrol

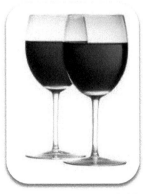

The chapter on alcohol describes the evidence for and against the complex array of alcoholic drinks which many people enjoy. While beer, cider and white wine contain some polyphenols, red wine is particularly rich in the pigmented polyphenol resveratrol. It's a class of compounds produced as part of a plant's defence system against invading fungus or ultraviolet irradiation disease. Spanish wines have the highest levels among the red wine variety, followed by the

Pinot Noir varieties. Although wine takes the limelight in the resveratrol discussion, it is also found in grapes, blueberries, raspberries, as well as exotic fruit such as white hellebore and Japanese knotweed. It has strong anti-oxidant properties and has demonstrated growth inhibition of cancer prostate, breast and bowel cells in culture experiments. Evidence also suggests that it can reduce inflammation via inhibition of the COX-2 pathway, improve gut health and boost immunity.

In humans, there is conflicting evidence surrounding the alleged health benefits of red wine. Some research has highlighted that in low amounts it can reduce the risk of bowel cancer, although this is countered by the fact that as soon as alcohol intake reaches higher levels the risk of bowel cancer increases. Likewise, head and neck, oesophageal, lung and stomach cancers are more common in those with a higher alcohol intake, although data is contaminated by the association with smoking. Research published in the International Journal of Cancer shows that drinking a glass of red wine a day may cut a man's risk of prostate cancer in half, with the protective effect appearing to be strongest against the most aggressive forms of the disease. Likewise, according to a comprehensive Cambridge University study, a few glasses of red wine a week reduces breast cancer relapse rates.

Chocolate

The earliest evidence of chocolate consumption dates back to 1900 years BC in South America, where the drinking of fermented chocolate beans as part of ceremonial events was practiced widely. In its natural form, cocoa has many nutritional benefits and is a valuable source of essential 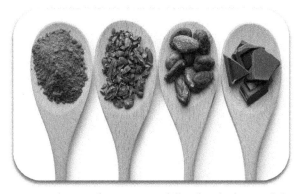 minerals including magnesium, manganese, zinc and copper, while also being a rich source of polyphenols, particularly the flavonoids epicatechin, catechin and procyanidins. In one laboratory study, a chocolate-enhanced diet significantly improved total antioxidant capacity (TAC) by promoting antioxidant enzymes such as superoxide dismutase (SOD) and catalase. A further study demonstrated how women who had consumed a dark chocolate, flavanol-rich drink before being exposed to UV light, had significantly lower erythema and skin damage than those who had not consumed the drink. Another large cohort study showed that the anthoxanthins in dark chocolate lowered the risk of colon cancer.

In controlled studies, cocoa powder significantly decreased LDL cholesterol in men and reduced insulin resistance. The Zutphen Elderly Study found that people who regularly eat dark chocolate tended to have lower BP. The effect on BP was also confirmed in a recent Cochrane review. A pilot study showed that a cup of flavanol-rich cocoa increased blood flow to the brains grey matter, suggesting a role in helping prevent dementia and strokes. It should be noted, however, that these studies used unadulterated cocoa free from

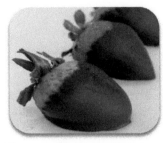

processed sugar. In reality, most chocolate products available to ordinary consumers are alarmingly high in sugar content. Chocolate contains alkaloids such as caffeine, theobromine and phenethylamine, which in sensitive individuals may cause nervousness, increased urination, sleeplessness, a fast heartbeat, sweating, trembling and severe headaches. In fact, the presence of theobromine renders it toxic to some animals, including dogs and cats. Cocoa beans can also absorb heavy metals from the soil, particularly cadmium, lead and mercury. These minerals in excess can be harmful. One bar of dark chocolate could represent the safe limit for cadmium for an entire week. The EU has a set a cadmium limit of 0.8mg/kg in chocolate consisting of >50% cocoa concentration. So, although, chocolate offers an array of health benefits in small amounts but avoid added sugar or excess quantities. To make it less bitter, try melting dark chocolate with coconut milk and pouring over fruit, nuts and berries for a delicious, polyphenol rich, snack or dessert.

Coffee

In 1981, a much-publicised Harvard University study linked coffee intake to a higher risk of pancreatic cancer. This prompted the state of California to put a cancer warning on coffee cups, a move subsequently considered inappropriate after the authors of the study later admitted that the association may have been largely down to the fact that coffee drinkers were more likely to smoke. Coffee has several healthy

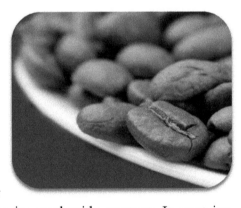

ingredients which more than compensate for its acrylamide content. It contains essential minerals such as magnesium and calcium, alongside numerous healthy polyphenols such as chlorogenic acids (esters of quinic and cinnamic acids). More recently, an international review of 66 studies found that coffee drinking had little if any effect on the risk of developing cancer. Another review in 2008 suggested that coffee drinkers, compared with people who do not drink coffee, had half the risk of liver cancer. In 2010, an observational study suggested that regular coffee consumers had a lower incidence of prostate cancer, while a paper presented at the 2013 ASCO conference sent the Starbucks share-price soaring after it revealed that more than three cups a day significantly reduced the risk of bowel cancer. A further study presented in the same conference showed higher intake reduced risks of both non-melanoma skin cancers and melanoma, even after controlling for confounding factors such as ultraviolet radiation exposure, BMI, age, sex, physical activity, alcohol intake and smoking history.

Coffee and heart disease: The US-based Centre for Science in the Public Interest published a comprehensive appraisal of coffee. They analysed 10 studies of more than 400,000 people and found no increase in heart disease or raised BP among daily coffee drinkers, whether their coffee contained caffeine or not. Even more reassuringly, a recent study suggested that two polyphenols in coffee, caffeic and ferulic acids, help reduce blood cholesterol levels. Several studies have also linked coffee with a reduced risk of T2 diabetes. Animal studies confirmed the polyphenol responsible was trigonelline, a nicotinic acid commonly present in the coffee.

Coffee and bone loss: Some observational studies have linked caffeinated beverages to bone loss and fractures. Human physiological studies found that a slight reduction in calcium absorption was mainly in consumers of caffeinated sugary drinks. Coffee and tea drinkers who consume the currently recommended amount of calcium, and add a little milk to the drink without sugar, need not worry about caffeine's effect on their bones.

Mental ability and fatigue: Coffee drinkers are all too aware of the immediate 'lift' after their morning brew. Researchers have confirmed this with studies that show that coffee has an immediate ability to enhance mood, mental and physical performance, and to foster a sense of well-being, happiness, energy, alertness and sociability. The trouble is that, like all additive drugs, there is an upside and a downside. In excess, it can cause anxiety and the "shakes". Furthermore, when the positive 'lift effect' wears off, there may be a drop in "energy levels" caused by the withdrawal of caffeine from the bloodstream, leading to fatigue. Individuals suffering from fatigue may be advised not to drink strong coffee as this withdrawal may cause more problems over the course of the day. For those who have trouble sleeping, remember that the caffeine in coffee can stay in the bloodstream for 6-7 hours, so it should be avoided from mid-afternoon.

Tree nuts and peanuts

These are a great example of complete functional foods, packed with healthy macro and micronutrients. They contain bioactive compounds which work in synergy to prevent and delay age-related chronic conditions. Tree nuts are low in carbohydrates, contain good quality fatty acids and are an ideal source of proteins. vitamin E and minerals.

They are a rich source of polyphenols, particularly flavanols, which protect individuals from environmental carcinogens, UV radiation and photoaging. They help reduce the chronic inflammatory response by down-regulating the NFхB system and inhibit COX-2. They are good prebiotics and enhance healthy gut microbiota. The phytosterols in nuts and peanuts are responsible for their ability to lower total cholesterol, which explains the link with lower vascular disease and heart attacks. Nut consumption, particularly pistachios, lowers systolic BP and, to a lesser extent, diastolic BP within formal randomised trials.

Given their multitude of health benefits, it's hardly surprising that the HPFS, as well as the comprehensive EPIC study, argued that the consumption of nuts lowered the risk of cancer, particularly prostate, breast and bowel. The most dramatic support for their anti-cancer benefits was presented at the ASCO conference in 2017. Researchers announced that a handful of tea nuts (almonds, walnuts, hazelnuts, cashews, pecans) a week reduced the risk of bowel cancer relapse and death from bowel cancer by 40% - a greater impact than chemotherapy.

It's a good idea to buy large bags of nuts and plain (unroasted) peanuts, and add them to your breakfast cereals or snacking on them regularly. It is important to remember that the stability of the nutrients in nuts can be influenced by cooking techniques, temperature of storage and post-harvest processing methods. Rancid nuts should be altogether avoided as the fatty acids can degenerate into toxic oxygenative products via lipoxidation. Likewise, peanuts stored in warm, humid conditions can contain aflatoxin, a natural toxin produced by certain strains of the mould Aspergillus.

Mushrooms

The edible varieties of mushrooms include Chanterelles, Cremini, Morels, Portobello, Enoki, Shiitake, Oyster and the ubiquitous white button. Most varieties provide a broad range of vitamins, minerals and phytochemicals. As they contain no cholesterol or fat, they represent a useful food for those wishing to lose weight or lower cholesterol. The vitamins commonly found in mushrooms include niacin, 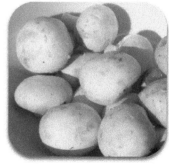 riboflavin and pantothenic acid; while the minerals contained can include calcium, copper, potassium and selenium. Mushrooms are an excellent source of protein due to the fact that they typically contain many essential amino acids, including ergothioneine, which is required for nail, skin and lens production.

Their high concentration of many phytochemicals enhance their health benefits but are also responsible for the hallucinogenic or poisonous effects in the non-edible varieties. Many mushrooms, including the commonly consumed "white button" variety, contain polyphenols such as flavones and isoflavones which are able to inhibit aromatase, an enzyme responsible for producing oestrogen in peripheral fat. In doing so, mushrooms could negate the excess oestrogen effects of being overweight in post-menopausal women. Although this has been reported in animal studies, it has yet not been proven in clinical studies involving humans.

Mushrooms contain beta-glucans, a soluble fibre and a source of prebiotics which help gut bacteria. They also promote a healthy gut flora as they contain natural antibiotics such as penicillin, streptomycin, and tetracycline. Because they are in their natural form, they do not cause antibiotic resistance but do help to discourage pathogenic *Firmicutes* (bad) bacterial growth, while encouraging the growth of *Bacteroidetes* (good) bacteria.

Plants rich in nitrates

The benefits of plant nitrates and nitrites have already been highlighted in the chapter outlining the pros and cons of meat. But to recap, plant nitrates provide a natural means of increasing blood nitric oxide (NO) levels. Many vegetables contain nitrates, notably:

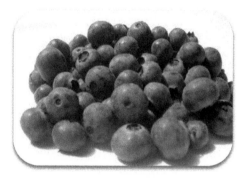

- Herbs – Turmeric, ginger, green tea
- Beetroot, apples, strawberries, cherries, pomegranate, blackberries
- Spinach, kale, cress, rocket, lettuce, radish, celery and broccoli

The microflora in the saliva and upper gut convert nitrates to nitrites, which are then metabolised to nitrogen oxides by a variety of reductase enzymes. This process is enhanced by vitamin C and polyphenols, which also prevent nitrites in meat being converted to carcinogenic nitrosamines. After being absorbed by endothelial cells lining the arteries, NO penetrates the underlying smooth muscles and acts as a potent vasodilator that relaxes the arteries. It plays a critical role in controlling BP and enhancing overall circulation, while also improving the oxygenation of the heart, muscles and brain during exercise. Studies in humans have demonstrated that the NO-generating properties of nitrate-rich foods are likely to be responsible for improvements in cerebrovascular blood flow, alongside improved cognitive and erectile function. Other studies have found that higher intake of nitrate-rich foods such as turmeric, broccoli, pomegranate and green tea, enhance athletic performance due to improved muscle blood flow, accelerated muscle recovery, reduced joint pains and absorption of free radicals produced by strenuous exercise.

Beetroot (*beta vulgaris rubra*) is rich in plant nitrate as well as bioactive compounds including ascorbic acid, carotenoids, phenolic acids and flavonoids. It is also one of the few vegetables that contain a group of phytochemical pigments known as betalains. These are categorised as either betacyanin pigments which are red-violet in colour, or betaxanthin pigments which are yellow-orange in colour. A number of investigations have 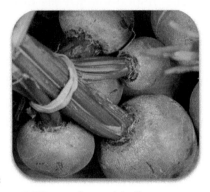 identified betalains as having high antioxidant, NO and anti-inflammatory capabilities. This suggests beetroot may have a role in the nutritional management of clinical pathologies characterised by oxidative stress and chronic inflammation, including arthritis and even cancer.

Incorporating polyphenol-rich foods into a daily routine

Healthy eating is often regarded as a novelty rather than a necessity. Some people pat themselves on the back because they have had a salad or eaten some broccoli once or twice a week, in the meantime binging on hot dogs, crisps and fizzy drinks. To achieve the level of polyphenols and other healthy nutrients we need to maintain or enhance our wellbeing, they should be included in every meal. For many people, this requires substantial innovative changes to their cooking and eating habits which may require some extra help and supervision. Here are some tips to help achieve this.

Getting help

Not all of us possess the culinary skills, time or motivation to change established eating habits. A commonly heard expression is "everything in moderation", which is usually nonsense if the norm for that individual is a bacon sandwich washed down with a sugary instant coffee. For most people, the dietary change advocated in this book, if aiming for long-term improvement, may initially seem alien and unsatisfying. However, with time and perseverance, such change will prove to be extremely fulfilling. When starting you should not be embarrassed to look for or ask for help.

Online cooking tips: There are countless online resources describing healthy meals. Blog.cancernet.co.uk has a series of guest chefs and nutritionists who provide regular meal options, including a description of the ingredients required, an explanation of the health benefits and videos showing how they are prepared and cooked.

Qualified nutritionist or dietitian: Although more expensive, an appointment with an experienced nutritionist may represent money well spent. They can advise on how to add more phytochemicals to every meal within a sustainable diet plan tailored to the individual's needs and tastes.

Nutritional programmes: It is well-known that a formal dietary intervention programme has a greater chance of changing eating behaviour. Most successful programmes take place in groups which provide a social element, and the most beneficial are stimulating and enjoyable, encouraging participants to keep going in the long term. It is worth doing some searching to find a good one in your area. It's often the first step which is most difficult, and many encourage participants to attend with a friend or relative until they find their feet.

Polyphenols may enhance some chemotherapy regimens

There has been some concern that polyphenols may interfere with oncology treatments, via their antioxidant ability. This property is, however, only one of the many mechanisms of action wielded by polyphenols. Moreover, unlike other nutrients such as vitamins A and E, polyphenols mainly enhance the production antioxidant enzymes, as opposed to having a direct impact on free radical absorption. Most importantly, the direct anticancer properties of polyphenols completely outweigh any negative effect on chemotherapy. It is not surprising then that several studies have actually found that polyphenols enhance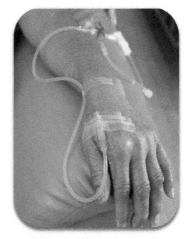
the cytotoxic effects of chemotherapy, rather than impede it. For example, a transplanted xenograft mouse model of lung cancer highlighted how docetaxel, a chemotherapy drug, was twice as effective when used in tandem with curcumin. Remarkably, these sensitising effects are not found on normal, healthy cells, so they remain protected during treatment. Curcumin has also been found to enhance the effectiveness of cisplatin, another chemotherapy drug, by helping to reduce cell proliferation in an animal model of laryngeal carcinoma cancer. Studies in humans are limited or ongoing but, in the meantime, it is worth referencing an interesting case. A man receiving Taxotere in our oncology unit for metastatic prostate cancer, initially had a good response but after 8 cycles, as is commonly the case, the disease started progressing. He then began taking turmeric and started, fairly dramatically, responding again. He is still received low dose taxotere and turmeric an unprecedented 2 years later!

Another study reported that beetroot juice promoted apoptosis of breast cancer cells after exposure to doxorubicin, while at the same time protecting normal heart muscle cells. In view of the synergy of cannabis with a chemotherapy for brain tumours seen in animal studies, there is particular interest in the investigation of cannabinoid extracts, particularly the legal CBD, in conjunction with temozolomide in patients with recurrent glioblastoma. So far, there have been some anecdotal reports of better than expected results and results of the RCT are awaited.

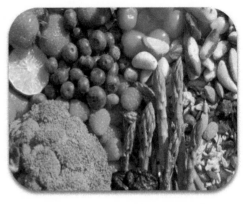

How to boost polyphenol intake

While new approaches to everyday eating can undoubtedly enhance polyphenol intake, specific techniques are useful in situations where normal diets may be inadequate, or when higher levels of polyphenols are required during periods of illness, physical and mental stress, vigorous exercise or even after cancer. Research is now suggesting that we need a much higher intake of polyphenols than previously thought, a discovery which prompts a complete rethink of the government's recommended 5-a day message. A recent study found that breast cancer survivors who consumed more than five portions of polyphenol-rich fruit and vegetables a day, and participated in regular physical activity, had a significantly lower risk of breast cancer recurrence.

This section highlights the foods and meals which help boost polyphenol intake, including tips on how to make them or links to quality commercial products. It should be noted that when manipulating foods in order to boost their phytochemical or vitamin content, care has to be taken not enhance the negative elements along with the good elements. That is why good quality nutritional research in this field is so important. Some of the research on individual foods or extracts has already been explained, but this chapter provides more detail on the benefits of whole food nutritional supplements, most notably the world's largest RCT in humans with cancer (the Pomi-T study), as well as techniques which can boost the daily intake of polyphenols and other healthy phytochemicals which include:

Juices and smoothies: Many of the fruit juices available on the market today aren't actually 'real' fruit juices. They consist of water mixed with concentrate and extra sugar. Even real fruit juice has a high concentration of fructose as so many fruits are used to make them. There is also little chewing resistance to slow down consumption, making it very easy to drink a large amount of sugar in a short period of time. Lack of pulp significantly speeds up gastric emptying and glycaemic index. Juicing, where the whole fruit has been put in the blender, is more effective at maintaining the pulp and fibre, yet the use of just fruits still leads to a high fructose content. To overcome this, smoothie aficionados add avocado, vegetables such as kale or spices such as ginger, lowering the sugar content while improving the polyphenol intake.

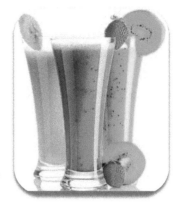

Soups: Most polyphenols survive a degree of cooking, making soups an ideal way to guarantee an effective intake. Tomato soup significantly increases lycopene intake, making it perfect for those not keen on raw tomatoes. A vegetable broth flavoured with extra spices and herbs and consumed before a meal tends to fill the stomach, helping with weight loss regimens, while broccoli, onion and pea soup, with a sprinkle of turmeric and a generous twist of fresh ground pepper, constitutes the perfect superfood mix. The case report chapter highlights the amazing response one man with metastatic prostate cancer had to broccoli soup.

To get the most out of soups, eat them with a fresh salad containing raw onions, lettuce or radish, all of which contain the enzyme myrosinase which is required to convert the sulforaphane in cooked cruciferous vegetables into the bioactive antioxidant enzyme Glutathione. Also add pepper liberally, as the peperine it contains helps bioavailability of the polyphenols in both the vegetables and other spices.

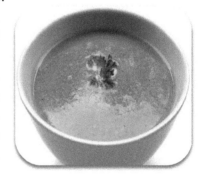

Shots: Some more forward-thinking food outlets are offering healthy shots (around 50ml) of polyphenol-rich ingredients. The fact that they are not heated means they preserve their nutrient and polyphenol content. Common shot blends include ginger with apple, and turmeric and chilli with orange juice. These provide a quick boost but are usually not cheap. It is possible to make your own shot by grating fresh ginger into a small apple juice and adding a twist of lemon. If you have the time, it is also possible to make ginger shots with a high-powered blender, a technique which gets much more out of the root. Roughly chop ginger and add a few tablespoons of water or lemon juice to the blender. Blend until the ginger is broken down and then, if you don't like the bits, pour the blend through a fine mesh. For a

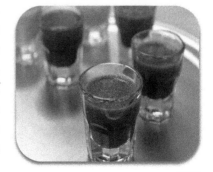

green shot, try combining a 2cm length piece of fresh-scrubbed clean ginger with 1/2 small green apple, 1 cup of packed spinach leaves and half an avocado, before adding the juice from 1 large lemon and a small pinch of cayenne pepper.

Blending grains and seeds: Although individual foods can be very healthy, mixing them together is a fantastic way to provide your body with a great variety of essential nutrients. Most health food shops, now sell mixed grain and seeds, either ground in bags or in the form of health bars, cereals or drinks. They tend to be expensive and still have to be processed in some way. You can, however, make your own superfood grain mix very easily with the help of a blender.

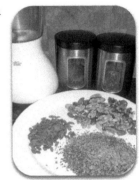

Linseeds (also known as flaxseeds) tend to pass through the system untouched, unless crushed. When broken down, their valuable omega-3 fatty acids, proteins and polyphenols are released and made available for absorption. They can be mixed with seeds, nuts, and berries for extra taste and nutritional value. They are an excellent source of fibre – a tablespoon of this mix a day will displace the need for laxatives and help bring down blood cholesterol and BP. A batch can be placed in an airtight container and used over several weeks. The mix can then be added to cereals, porridge, live yoghurt, milk, smoothies or soups. Remember to clean the container thoroughly before adding the next batch in order to avoid moulds. The mix can be altered each time depending on your nutritional needs. If more omega is needed add more walnuts, if more roughage required include more grains. If you are looking to add more vitamin E, include shelled pistachio nuts. The trick is to be organised to ensure your supplies do not run out. Maybe invest in a rack of storage tins or jars for the various ingredients, and buy in bulk to reduce the cost.

Whole food polyphenol-rich supplements

The two chapters above have already highlighted the concerns over supplements which remove and concentrate specific chemicals from foods or contain concentrated phytoestrogenic plants. The next two chapters will highlight similar concerns with extracting specific minerals and vitamins. On the other hand, with the exception of

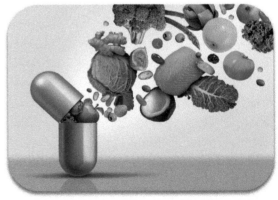

phytoestrogenic plants, food supplements made from concentrated whole foods can have a useful role to play. They can overcome polyphenol deficiencies in people with poor diets and enhance seemingly adequate diets, especially during times of oxidative stress or inflammation. It is reassuring to note that, thus far, no scientific study of non-phytoestrogenic whole food supplements have shown any detrimental effects on cancer outcomes, while an increasing body of research has demonstrated considerable benefits.

Well-made whole food supplements are essential for interventional studies as they provide a more objective, scientific answer compared to dietary questionnaire. Many people considering dietary interventions after cancer are attracted to the benefits of some supplements. Several studies, including our own from the UK, show this figure to be 60%, and even higher if they have an ongoing symptom. It vital however that if supplement are considered they have been investigated in robust scientific studies. The world's largest and probably most impactful trial will now be described:

The UK Pomi-T Trial

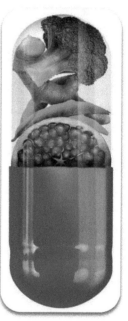

This study evaluated the impact of a whole food nutritional supplement containing green tea, pomegranate, turmeric, and broccoli. The results were announced at the world's biggest and most prestigious medical conference, the American Society of Clinical Oncology (ASCO). This conference is where most substantial cancer breakthroughs are revealed each year, so to be included as a full oral presentation in the main prostate section in 2014 was a powerful reflection on the significance and impact of this intervention. In 2015, the full study was published in an esteemed 'Nature' journal and received global media attention.

Background to the study

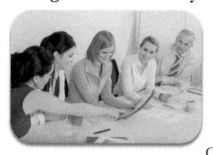

In 2012, a UK government committee was set up to design and encourage robust double-blind, randomised controlled trials evaluating complementary and supportive therapies. The RCT is the gold standard for clinical research, excluding bias from outside sources and proving decisively whether an intervention works or not.

One of the key remits of the committee (supported by the National Cancer Research Institute) was to investigate nutritional supplements, in light of their popularity among patients with cancer. The committee felt it was especially important to investigate polyphenol-rich foods, given the growing body of evidence linking their increased intake with a lower incidence of cancer and cancer relapse following radical treatments.

The study committee set out to examine over 200 polyphenol-rich natural foods and whittle the search down to four prime candidates (the maximum which would sensibly fit into a single capsule). Their remit was to establish those which did not have a significant hormonal action but had an established laboratory and clinical evidence of benefit;

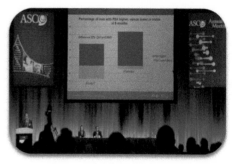

had a wide range of different polyphenols from different food sources; had ingredients with varying modes of action likely to be synergistic. After an 18-month development period, the panel of an oncologist, nutritionists, plant scientist, medical researchers and, above all, interested patients, devised the combination of green tea, pomegranate, broccoli and turmeric. Their phytochemical components, their mode of action and evidence of benefit have been summarised in the section above.

Synergy between ingredients: It was no coincidence that the committee chose extracts that originated from different food groups (fruit, herb, vegetable, and leaf), each with their own unique profile and concentration of polyphenols. Although they had some over-lapping modes of action, notably reducing chronic inflammation, their other anti-cancer mechanisms differ and were deemed likely to be synergistic if combined. An example is the

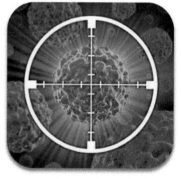

inhibition of cancer cell proliferation. All cancer cells go through a cycle in order to duplicate (M, G1, S, and G2). They may only be in each phase for a short period of time, so if you can inhibit more than one phase, growth is more likely to be reduced. Tea is known to block the G1 phase of the cancer cell cycle, turmeric the G2 phase and broccoli both G1 and G2, making their combination particularly damaging to cancer cells. As these foods do not have inhibition effects on normal cells or even normal stem cells, it makes them ideal for the specific targeting of cancer cells.

Avoiding too much of one polyphenol: Another advantage of combining lower quantities of four separate foods is that their variable composition avoids over-consumption of one particular phytochemical. Previous trials involving high concentrations of one food, or extracting a specific chemical from foods, have been unsuccessful and produced unwelcome side effects.

The making of Pomi-T

In order for Pomi-T to be put forward for investigation in a medical trial, it needed to be produced with a quality assurance rare in the food supplement industry. Fortunately, a company was found which could guarantee:

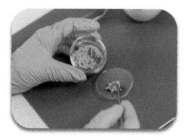

- EU and international Good Manufacturing Practice
- Traceably pure 'grade A' sourced ingredients
- Ingredients with very low levels of herbicide and pesticides
- Exclusion of heavy metal contaminant
- Authenticity of ingredients

On top of these requirements, detailed chemical analysis of the blend using mass spectrometry procedure was conducted at Newcastle University. This confirmed its purity by excluding other chemical contaminants which may have affected trial results. There are no other nutritional supplements which have undergone this level of scrutiny, a key factor differentiating Pomi-T from any other available supplement.

Why were men with Prostate cancer chosen for the study?

The trial committee was initially researching foods which had a general anti-cancer effect, but convention dictates the study had to be narrowed down to one disease. Men with early or relapsing prostate cancer were ideal because:

- Prostate cancer is the most common disease in men
- Men with early disease do not require initial medical intervention
- Men with PSA relapse after radiotherapy can also be watched initially
- PSA and MRI can monitor the disease accurately
- They are generally very interested in nutritional interventions

Funding, trial structure, and quality assurance

This was a non-commercial academic trial designed with the NCRI Complementary Therapies Research Committee. It received peer-reviewed funding from the charity Prostate Action. Research staff and nursing support were provided by the National Cancer Research Network, who also independently audited the trial to ensure it adhered to National Ethics committee requirements. The randomisation process was outsourced and the trial methodology, collection, and storage of data were verified and independently audited to ensure adherence to European

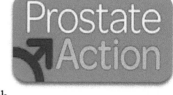

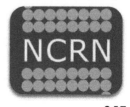

Good Clinical Practice. At the end of the trial, data was externally audited for a second time to ensure that there was no deviation from the trial design, before the database was sealed and sent for blinded analysis by independent statisticians at Cranfield University.

How was the trial conducted?
The researchers recruited 203 men aged 53 to 89 years with prostate cancer proven by biopsy. 59% of the men had not yet undergone any treatment and were being followed closely with periodic PSA tests (Active surveillance), while 41% had already

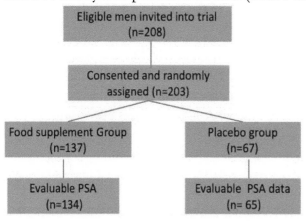

had a radical intervention (radiotherapy or surgery and radiotherapy) but had relapsed with significantly climbing PSA levels. Men were randomly assigned to receive either the twice-daily oral capsule containing a blend of purified, polyphenol-rich whole foods, or a similar looking placebo for 6 months. At baseline, there were no significant differences between the two groups. Neither the doctors supervising the trial, the men involved or statisticians analysing the data knew which men were taking a placebo or the Pomi-T.

What did the trial discover? In the placebo group, PSA levels rose by an average of 78.5% by 6 months. In the Pomi-T group, it rose by an average of only 14.7%, a 64.8% difference. The statistician produced a p-value of P<0.001, which meant that there was a less than 1:1000 probability that the results occurred by chance.

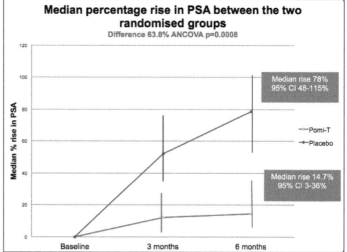

Furthermore, 46% of men in the Pomi-T group had a stable or lower PSA by the end of the study, versus 14% within the placebo group. Again, a significant difference which suggested that in nearly half of the treated men, their cancers had, in all likelihood, stopped growing or even regressed.

Of further clinical relevance, just 7.4% of men taking Pomi-T required a change to their management, compared to 26% on placebo. Simply put, the supplement directly supported the decision to defer, or avoid altogether, interventions such as hormones, radiotherapy or surgery. Notwithstanding the cost, hormones can cause adverse effects such as hot flushes, weight gain, fatigue, joint pains, while radical interventions can lead to incontinence, erectile dysfunction and bowel damage.

Other positive effects of Pomi-T

As this was a formal clinical trial, a whole host of other factors were measured by blood tests and questionnaires. Fortunately, none of these threw up any unexpected adverse events. As anticipated, as the supplement did not contain any phytoestrogenic ingredients, there was no effect on average serum sex hormones, including testosterone. Green tea does 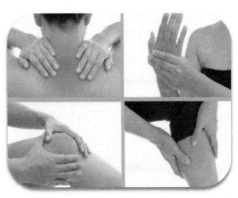 contain a small amount of caffeine but within one capsule of Pomi-T this only amounts to a quarter of an average cup of coffee. Nevertheless, it was reassuring to see that no man in either group reported central nervous system symptoms such as agitation, insomnia or tremors. The pomegranate, like many fruit juices, is a weak inhibitor of cytochrome P450. There is, therefore, a small potential risk of reducing the metabolism and thereby increasing serum levels of warfarin anti-hypertensives

such as captopril, Ramipril, or anticonvulsants such as carbimazole. For the doses in Pomi-T, this would have been extremely unlikely, and it was encouraging that none of the 30 men on warfarin reported any unexpected change in the international normalized ratio, nor did the 43 men taking ramipril report an unexpected change in their blood pressure.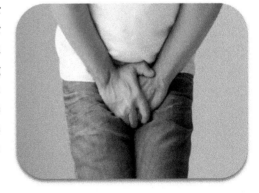

General well-being: It was interesting to note that, although not powered for significance, a summation of all adverse events was 10% lower in the Pomi-T group than the placebo group.

Joint pains: Troublesome symptoms (mainly joint pains) were reported in 3.4% of the Pomi-T group, versus 13.4% in the placebo group. After study, the trials unit has received numerous reports that Pomi-T helped with joint pains. A further trial with joint pains as a primary endpoint is now underway (see below).

Urinary function: In terms of flow, frequency, urgency or prostate discomfort, 12% of men recorded improvement on Pomi-T versus 4.6% in the placebo group. A further trial with urinary symptoms as a primary endpoint is now planned in Finland.

In conclusion: This capsule represents a breakthrough in nutritional research. It appears to work by targeting a number of biological pathways crucial to cancer initiation and progression. These are likely to involve reducing chronic inflammation, improving oxidative stress and enhancing gut health. In this tightly controlled clinical trial, putting four purified polyphenol-rich foods together in a single capsule was shown to be effective at slowing the growth of existing prostate cancers and preventing surgical and other side effect-prone procedures. Many regard this as a potential game-changer in the management of low-risk prostate cancer and trials examining the impact on other cancers are eagerly awaited. In the meantime, while Pomi-T cannot currently be prescribed by doctors, people have the option to obtain it themselves online as part of an evidence-based, self-help lifestyle strategy (see Pomi-T.com).

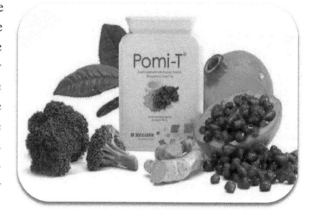

Follow up studies involving polyphenols

One further study has been completed and published in the International Journal of Lifestyle Medicine in 2015. Two are in progress, and a series of others are planned over the next 10 years. These will now be summarised.

The MRI-PSA follow up study

A potential limitation of the first Pomi-T study was that PSA was the only primary endpoint. This was chosen because PSA and PSA kinetics are useful markers to follow disease progression in men with known cancer, and a number of previous pharmaceutical trials which resulted in medical products gaining licences used PSA as their primary endpoint. Furthermore, PSA is more than just a marker; we now realize that it is an enzyme that degrades the matrix proteins holding cells together. The higher the level, the more likely it is that cancer invades other organs and spreads.

That's why physicians and patients should monitor PSA levels carefully once a prostate tumour has been discovered. Therapies that lower PSA are therefore not just producing an encouraging marker response but are demonstrably slowing disease progression and lowering the patient's risk of dying.

Since the availability of sophisticated MRI scans in most hospitals, men on active surveillance receive an MRI once a year as part of their routine management. That is why a further study was designed which involved men who received annual MRIs and had either begun taking or were continuing to take Pomi-T.

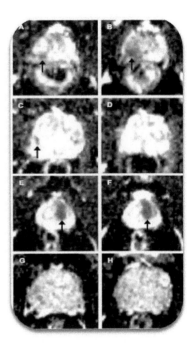

In this follow up study, men were included if they had histologically confirmed prostate cancer, were being managed with active surveillance and had received at least two consecutive diffusion-weighted MRI's of their prostate. They were split into four groups depending on the size and change of disease within the prostate between at least two annual MRI scans - disease worse, disease better, no change, no disease seen. The changes in PSA were then correlated with MRI disease.

Encouragingly, the results confirmed the findings from the main Pomi-T study, with the progression rate in men taking Pomi-T remaining very low (<4% rise at a median of one year). The new data from this analysis indicated a 100% correlation between disease on MRI and PSA changes. In other words, no man whose PSA was lower after one year had a worse disease on MRI, and no man with an improvement seen on MRI had a higher PSA after a year. As most men in the evaluation were taking Pomi-T, this provided reassurance that the supplement was very unlikely to have affected the level of PSA without impacting the underlying disease.

The polyphenols in cancer prevention study

Following the success of the Pomi-T study, many people have enquired whether this supplement could have a cancer prevention role. The only way to know for sure is by conducting a large RCT of the general public, comparing Pomi-T with a placebo and monitoring the numbers of cancers in the years to come. This would require thousands of participants, take up to ten years to complete and be very expensive. This is certainly

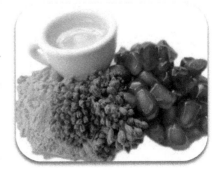

beyond the means of the Primrose Lifestyle Research Unit. It is also outside the budget for the Swiss Company who now make the supplement, bearing in mind that between searching for Grade A ingredients, excluding pesticides and the extra quality assurance tests required for Good Manufacturing Practice (GMP), the profit margin is just over €1 per unit. The only hope for funding is from a major national charity or government body at some point in the future. In the meantime, the best way to investigate whether regular intake of the ingredients of Pomi-T reduces the cancer risk is to analyse a large database which has recorded dietary pattern and cancer incidence over many years. The Primrose Oncology Unit are conducting such an analysis in partnership with the biostatistics department at Glasgow University, the University of California and the National Cancer Institute.

The study is currently analysing the dietary habits of 155,000 men and women recorded within the Prostate, Lung, Colorectal, and Ovarian (PLCO) cancer screening trial obtained

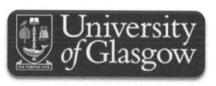

from screening centres across the USA between 1993 and 2001. The aim of the study is to determine whether people who are in the highest quartile of broccoli, tea, turmeric and pomegranate consumption have fewer cancers (after 10 years follow up) than those in the lowest quartile of consumption. The result of this study swill appear by early 2019 and a peer-reviewed journal later in the year.

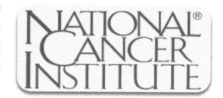

Future prevention studies

Although the NCI cohort analysis described above will be interesting, only a double-blind RCT will provide definitive conclusions. To be achievable, these trials must address situations where the time between the start of the intervention and cancer development is likely to be short. This would involve participants with a high risk of early second cancers who are also being monitored closely. In this time frame, a comparison of a nutritional intervention or placebo would be eminently feasible. The scientific committee and now considering funding opportunities to design such trials involving people with resected bowel or bladder polyps; Barret's oesophagus; premalignant cells in a prostate biopsy; resected non-melanoma skin; lung cancer and pancreatic cancer

Sports enhancement

It is well established from studies conducted with athletes that polyphenols in beetroot, berries, tea and turmeric, reduce the oxidative stress caused by strenuous exercise while also improving muscle recovery. These factors, coupled with the protective effect they have on joints and their reassuringly legal status, make these foods attractive to cyclists, rowers and runners who regularly put their bodies under intense physical

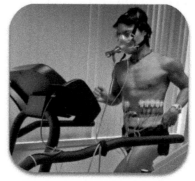

strain. As Pomi-T contains these foods and has the added benefit of being purified and authenticated, this supplement is now becoming an attractive option for both

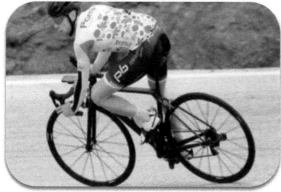

elite sportsmen and weekend warriors. Enthusiasm for studies examining the link between athletic performance and Pomi-T were triggered by comments on the blog of Tom Davies, the youngest person to cycle around the world in 200 days:

"Halfway across the USA, with 500 miles to go, I ran into issues with knee pain. A week after taking Pomi-T, the pain resolved and I was able to continue."

Since then Team Pomi-T cycling has been established, winning numerous sportifs across the UK and Europe. Further plans for measuring elite athletic outcomes are planned but, in the mean-time, measures of exercise performance and fitness are being included in the arthritis and exercise study, monitored by the Exercise Scientists at the Bedford University.

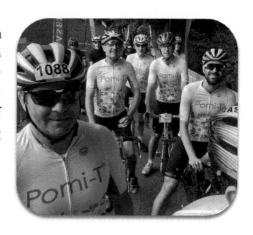

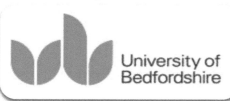

University of
Bedfordshire

Summary – increasing phytochemical-polyphenol intake

Eat more of the following foods:

- Spices – Chillies, paprika, cinnamon, cumin, turmeric
- Green vegetables – Cabbage, kale, spinach.
- Colourful vegetables - Carrots, red and yellow peppers
- Cruciferous vegetables – Broccoli, asparagus, brussels sprouts, radish
- Allium vegetables - Onions, spring onions, leeks, garlic
- Salad – Lettuce, celery, cucumber
- Fruits (especially ripe) – Plums, apples, apricots, pears, oranges, grapes
- Tropical fruits – Pomegranates, kiwis, oranges, nectarines, bananas
- Mushrooms – White and wild varieties
- Dried fruits are good but only after a meal e.g. raisins, prunes, apricots
- Berries – Cherries, blueberries, strawberries, cranberries, goji berries
- Legumes – Beans, peas, lentils, quinoa, chickpeas
- Nuts – Hazelnuts, almonds, walnuts, peanuts, cashews, brazils
- Herbs – Parsley, mint, coriander, thyme, sage, rosemary
- Chocolate (no sugar) and freshly ground coffee in moderation
- Tea - Green and black varieties
- Red wine in moderation
- Soy products – Tofu, soy milk, yoghurt, miso soup
- Legumes – Soya, lentils, red kidney bean and pinto (baked beans)
- Seeds and grains – Flaxseed, linseeds and cereals
- Consider an evidence based whole food polyphenol supplement (pomi-T)

Immunity and chronic inflammation

An intact, functioning immune system protects us from daily attack form pathogens. It is vital to kill the thousands of early cancer cells which form every day. For established cancers, a healthy immune system can slow its growth and spread. On the other hand, a chronically overactive dysfunctional inflammatory response can increase the risk of cancer and enhance its progression.

If cells carrying cancerous mutations progress into early cancer cells, they still have to get past the body's immune system before they become full-blown cancers. It has been estimated that every day, there are 3000 genetically dysfunctional cells which could go on to form cancer, but are usually dealt with efficiently by the immunity killer cells. The cancers which make it past this defence have developed intricate ways of hiding from the immune killer cells as summarised in the diagram below:

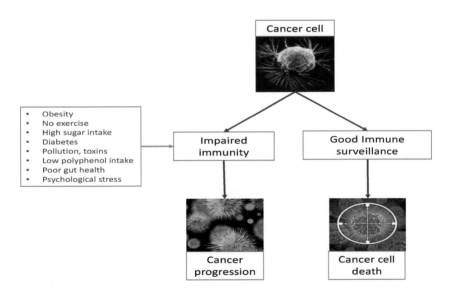

Factors which affect immune function

The importance of the immune system in cancer progression cannot be stressed enough. You only have to look through a microscope at tumours to see thousands of immune cells such as macrophages, neutrophils, mast cells, myeloid-derived suppressor cells, dendritic cells, natural killer cells and adaptive immune cells. In fact, the cancer cells themselves only form half the number of cells in a cancerous lump.

A healthy immune system detects and destroys thousands of cancer cells every day before they get a chance to establish a foothold. Even after cancerous lumps have formed, the immune system helps to contain the lumps by forming physical barriers around them and killing off metastases in the bloodstream. It is not a surprise then that deficiencies in the immune system lead to increased cancer progression and cancer relapse. One theory of why there are more cancers in the elderly is that the performance of the immune system deteriorates with age although, that said, lifestyle can also have a strong influence on how fast or slow immunity deteriorates.

People with advanced cancer experience a tipping point from which cancer begins to overwhelm the immune system. To do this, cancers have learnt to change their appearance to the immune system in a process called immune-editing. Some cancer cells are able to dissolve the proteins which identify them from the cell surface. Others have managed to go a step further and actually hijack immune pathways (known as hedgehog pathways) to help them invade adjacent tissues, or even piggyback on circulating immune cells to help them spread around the body. A very important recent discovery involves immune checkpoint pathways. Normal tissues are able to signal checkpoint molecules on immune cells to be activated (or inactivated) and start (or stop) an immune response. Some cancer cells have found ways to manipulate these checkpoints and avoid being attacked by the immune system. PD-1 is a checkpoint protein on immune cells called T cells. When PD-1 binds to its receptors (PD-L1), it tells the T cell to leave the cell alone. Some cancer cells have large amounts of PD-L1 which allows them to evade immune attack.

Fortunately, amazing new immunotherapies have been developed which inhibit PD-L1 allowing to immune to recognise and kill cancers celled such as Pembrolizumab (Keytruda). For these immunotherapies to work well, a health immunity is essential. This was eloquently demonstrated in a study from the famous MD Anderson Cancer Hospital in Texas. While investigating the PD1-inhibitor drugs in patients with melanoma, skin, non-small cell lung cancer, kidney cancer, bladder cancer, head and neck cancers, and Hodgkin lymphoma. They noticed that there was a 40% better response rate in patients with a healthy immune system, and in particular a diverse and optimal gut flora. This is a massive difference in outcome compared to people with poor gut health and explains why pharmaceutical companies and academic bodies are looking in much greater detail at lifestyle strategies designed to promote strong immunity. In fact, both ASCO, the world's largest cancer organisation, and Cancer Research UK have announced that major funding initiatives related to lifestyle, immunity and gut health will now be launched.

Other immunotherapies have been used for some time in oncology. In one of the earlier forms dead tuberculosis bacteria, is put into the bladder via a catheter. The immune reaction against it then triggers an attack against the cancer cells. Trying to achieve this response for the whole body has been attempted with interleukin and interferon, but they usually cause severe allergic responses and distressing side effects meaning they are rarely used now. Monoclonal antibodies (MABs) can be made outside the body and then concentrated and injected into a patient. They are made to recognise specific proteins which are different on cancer cells than normal cells. Once attached, some MABs, such as Herceptin block the receptors, switching off growth, while others, such as Avastin, used to treat bowel cancer, slow the formation of new blood vessels. Other MABs have been conjugated with poisons or radioactive elements which kill the cells directly. Certain kinds of leukaemia or lymphoma feature an overexpression of protein (antigen) on the outside of the cancer cells called CD19. The T-cells used in CAR T-cell therapies are changed in the lab to spot specific cancer cells by adding a man-made receptor. This helps them better identify specific cancer cell antigens. The patient's own T-cells are used to make the CAR T-cells. Results have been encouraging in many patients and the race is on to expand this technique for other cancers.

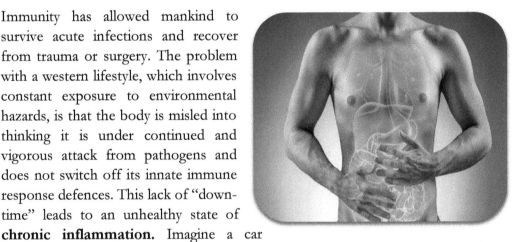

Immunity has allowed mankind to survive acute infections and recover from trauma or surgery. The problem with a western lifestyle, which involves constant exposure to environmental hazards, is that the body is misled into thinking it is under continued and vigorous attack from pathogens and does not switch off its innate immune response defences. This lack of "down-time" leads to an unhealthy state of **chronic inflammation.** Imagine a car being driven with a foot on the accelerator the entire time – over-heating and will soon wear out and go wrong.

The swelling and redness produced by the local (innate) response protect the body from the spread of infection, but can trigger uncomfortable symptoms which affect quality of life and can cause collateral damaged to normal tissues. If this happens over a long period of time, it can damage cartilage, ligaments and other soft tissues, leading to arthritis, premature ageing, Amyloidosis and other degenerative diseases. Inappropriate excess chronic inflammation also increases the risk of cancer and increase the progression and spread:

The innate inflammation response against perceived and actual pathogens triggers proinflammatory cytokines, via NF-kappaB, which are involved in the up regulation of inflammatory pathways. This promotes the infiltration of natural killer (NK) and other white cells into the tissues, where they then hunt for perceived pathogens and further drive the inflammatory process and stimulate acquired immune pathways. Pro-inflammatory cytokines and include: Interleukin-1 (IL-1), IL-1β, IL-6, IL-12, IL-18; tumour necrosis factor (TNF), gamma-interferon (IFN-gamma), granulocyte-macrophage colony stimulating factor. Once the threat has gone the body then releases anti-inflammatory cytokines which switch 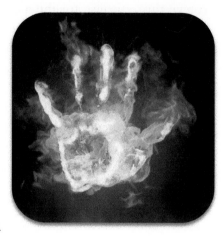 off the innate processes and these include IL4, IL-10, IL-13; IFN-alpha and transforming growth factor-beta.

This repeated overstimulation of the innate immune system by the factors listed below leads to premature ailing of the function of natural killer (NK) and T lymphocytes on a 'per cell' basis. This reduces the ability of the body to fight genuine infections. The immune feedback mechanisms then try to maintain immunosenescence by increasing production of inflammatory biomarkers, which in turn increase NK cells and T cells levels but at a cost of higher levels of pro-inflammatory cytokines and lower anti-inflammatory cytokines which cause many of the ongoing symptoms and increase the risk of degenerative diseases:

Inflammatory linked symptoms:	Inflammatory linked diseases:
• Depression	• Cancer
• Fatigue	• Amyloid
• Joint pains	• Dementia & Alzheimer's
• Premature skin wrinkles	• Arthritis
• Abdominal bloating	• Macular degeneration
• Excess bowel gas	• High cholesterol
• Mental fog	• Heart disease & Stroke
• Breast pain	• Parkinson's disease
• Prostatitis	• Type two diabetes
• Muscle aches post exercise	• Premature ageing

In terms of cancer, chronic inflammation is associated with increased free radical formation, increasing oxidative stress and DNA damage. It affects epigenetic expression of the genes we have been born with – promoting cancer genes and blocking suppressor genes. It interferes with DNA repair and reduces immune surveillance. Finally, inflammatory cytokines promote cancer growth and spread by causing cells to divide faster, undergo further mutagenesis, grow new blood vessels, invade and metastasise. A diagram summarising chronic inflammation's multiple effects on cancer is illustrated below:

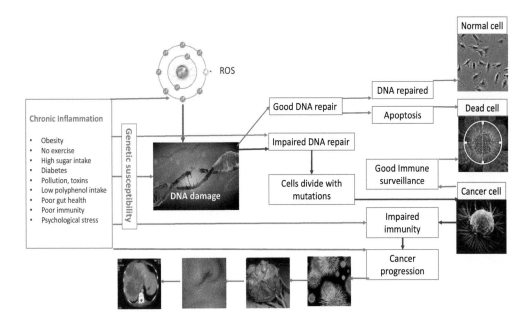

Several **lifestyle and environmental factors** act together with the body's genetic profile and chronological age to influence the immunity and level of chronic inflammation. While elderly individuals are by no means immunodeficient, they often do not respond as efficiently to new or previously encountered antigens. This is why the elderly have increased vulnerability to pneumonia, urinary tract infections, influenza or reactivation of varicella-zoster, causing

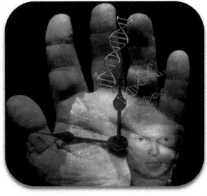

shingles. Although we cannot turn back time, we can influence the rate and consequences of ageing. In fact, a recent study showed that individuals who lead a healthy active lifestyle had better immunity, lower inflammation and longer telomeres than those who did not. The telomere is the biological clock at the end of each chromosome. The shorter the telomere, the biologically older an individual is. This shows us that the ageing process is strongly linked to excess inflammation. The rest of this chapter will highlight the factors which either promote or reduce inflammation.

Pro-inflammatory factors	Anti-inflammatory factors
• Chronic infection	• Regular exercise
• Dental caries	• Having a healthy waistline
• Chronic irritation	• Good gut health
• Smoking & toxic chemicals	• Probiotic bacteria
• Processed sugar	• Higher polyphenol intake
• Obesity	• Healthy omega fat intake
• Food intolerances	• Treating chronic infections
• Rancid oxidized fats	• Vaccinations
• Vitamin & mineral deficiencies	• Psychological wellbeing

The effects on chronic inflammation have been already been covered, within the sections above, for obesity, fats, mineral and vitamin deficiencies, poor gut health, polyphenols, exercise and processed sugar. Other factors are summarised below:

Chronic infections: Bacteria, fungus, viruses and parasites can trigger chronic low-grade infections if they are not immediately killed by the body's defences and are allowed to form colonies on and in our organs. Ongoing, untreated, periodontal disease around the gums and teeth, is linked to increased bowel cancer risk and this, in part, may be due to chronic inflammatory factors. Overgrowth of candida and other fungal infections have not been linked directly to cancers, but they do trigger inflammatory markers in the rest of the body. This is one explanation why obesity is linked to higher inflammation markers. Chronic local infections such as H.pylori in the stomach, flukes in the liver and parasites in the bladder can trigger hyperplasia (thicker layers of tissue) in the surrounding cells, leading to dysplasia (cell change in character), the first stages of cancer (atypia) and then eventually cancer itself. A local infection can stimulate both local and whole body inflammatory processes to remain "switched on" a common example would be dental caries especially if associated with chronic gum disease.

Chronic irritation: Minor repeated trauma over long periods of time can predispose susceptible cells to cancerous transformation. The best established example of chronic irritation leading to cancer relates to acid reflux from the stomach causing Barrett's oesophagus eventually causing adenocarcinoma Kidney, gall bladder and bladder stones increase the risk of cancer in these organs. Non-digestible agents such as asbestos, coal, and silica dust lead to chronic

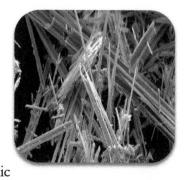

inflammation in the lung and cancers such as mesothelioma. In animal studies, skin cancer is induced by administration of carcinogens such as benzoyl peroxide, which induce inflammation. Intraperitoneal introduction of mineral oils or plastic discs into mice have been shown to promote the formation of a type of cancer called plasmacytoma. In women, a possible association has been discovered between textured breast implants and the development of a type of cancer called breast-implant associated anaplastic large cell lymphoma. Research suggests this disease is usually found near the breast implant within the surrounding scar tissue, not the breast itself. The lifetime risk of developing this from an implant is estimated to be from one in 4,000 to one in 30,000. Fortunately, early surgical removal of the implants and the cancer is usually effective. Patients with either chronic ulcerative colitis or Crohn's disease have a six-fold increased risk of colorectal carcinoma, especially if present for more than 8 years.

Smoking and pro-inflammatory carcinogens: Carcinogens in smoke cause cancer in many different ways, but one significant factor is their ability to promote chronic inflammation. Carcinogens in our diet also have this effect, the most common being acrylamides, generated through high-temperature cooking of carbohydrates; polycyclic or aromatic hydrocarbons from smoked, burnt, grilled or barbecued foods; and nitrosamines from meats, heated fats and rancid oils.

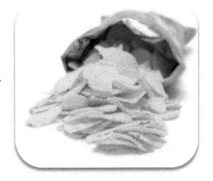

Exposure to cold; There are a lot of myths and hearsay related to immunity and the risks of catching infections, most of which have no substantiation. Take, for example, the widely held but incorrect assumption that wrapping up warm will protect you from catching a cold. The common cold does have seasonal spikes in colder months, but nobody knows exactly why. The most likely answer is that in winter we spend most of our time

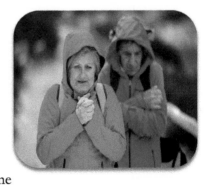

huddled inside in the warmth with other people and all their bugs. On the contrary, there is some evidence that hot then cold showers or saunas, followed by adequate cooling down can actually help stimulate a healthy immunity and reduce the chance of catching a cold. What's more, when a person takes a cold shower, brown fat is activated, resulting in an increase in energy and calories burned to keep your body warm. Taking a hot and cold shower is very much a test of mental strength, especially in the winter months when all you want to do is stay in the warm forever.

Tips to improve immunity and reduce chronic inflammation

- If you smoke – stop
- If overweight – try to slim down
- Aim for a waist size <34 inches
- Avoid chronic dental inflammation
- Keep teeth and gums clean
- Keep skin creases clean and fungal free
- Keep nails clean and fungal free – consider Polybalm
- Cut out refined sugars e.g. added sugar in tea, sweets, sugary drinks
- Reduce high glycaemic index foods - e.g. white bread and rice
- Avoid burnt meats, burnt toast, roasted snack bars
- Avoid fats and oils which have been repeatedly heated
- Avoid rancid oils and "off" nuts
- Increase intake of fresh nuts
- Increase berries, fruit, vegetables and pulses
- Consider a healthy, whole food purified, polyphenol-rich supplement
- Increase omega 3 fat intake e.g. Oily fish, algae, seaweed, shellfish
- Consider an omega 3 supplement if blood levels are low
- Increase healthy bacteria intake e.g. miso soup, live yoghurt, kimchi
- Consider a healthy probiotic bacteria supplement
- Optimise vitamin and mineral intake with a healthy diet
- Take mineral and vitamin supplements only to correct low levels
- Sunbathe sensibly and take vitamin D supplements in the winter
- Avoid sedentary behaviour on a daily basis
- Perform moderate to intense exercise for at least 3 hours a week
- Take hot then very cold showers regularly

Chapter 19

Energy modifying diets after cancer

There are thousands of diets which have sea-sawed in popularity over the years. Most diets are aimed at weight loss or lowering blood sugars and cholesterol, but in recent years there's been an increasing trend towards adopting diets which help fight cancer or reduce symptoms.

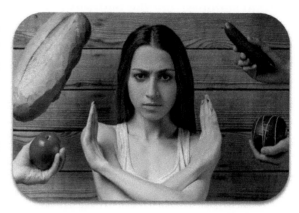

Energy restriction (ER) is a good way to control weight and has potential anti-cancer benefits. Lab studies have shown that, even without weight loss, energy restriction lowers IGF and leptin levels, improves insulin sensitivity and adiponectin levels, and reduces chronic inflammation. The three types of ER are continuous energy restriction (CER), intermittent energy restriction (IER) and intermittent fasting (IF). Studies have not demonstrated an advantage of one type over another. To understand how these diets may help, it is necessary to explain the normal processes of how cells feed themselves – known as cellular respiration. This is a little complicated, so some readers may wish to skip to the diet section.

How do cells generate energy (cellular respiration)?

Our bodies primarily use sugars broken down from carbohydrates for energy, but if sugar levels drop in the bloodstream, cells use fats (ketone) and, if needed, proteins. Biochemical pathways are responsible for forming the packets of energy called adenosine triphosphate (ATP), derived from adenosine diphosphate ADP, and reduced nicotinamide adenine dinucleotide (NADH), derived from NAD+. When either ATP or NADH are broken down, energy is released:

- ATP = ADP + energy
- NADH = NAD^+ + energy

The energy used by human cells requires the metabolism of 50 to 75kg of ATP daily, so a typical human will use up his or her body weight of ATP each day. The process of producing these energy-storing molecules is called cellular respiration. The three phases of cellular respiration are:

- Glycolysis (using sugars)
- Citric acid (Krebs) cycle
- Oxidative phosphorylation (OXOPHOS)

Diagram summarising the pathways of energy production

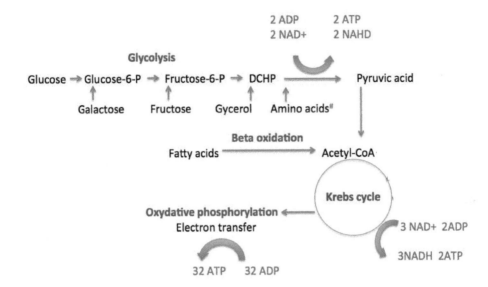

Glycolysis

Glycolysis is the metabolic pathway which converts glucose, galactose (from milk), fructose (from fruit) and glycerol (from triglyceride fats) into pyruvic acid. The pyruvic acid generated enters the next stage of cellular respiration, known as the Krebs cycle. Glycolysis is an oxygen-independent metabolic pathway, meaning it does not require molecular oxygen for any of its reactions. When molecular oxygen is present under normal breathing conditions (aerobic respiration), pyruvic acid enters the Krebs Cycle. If no oxygen is available (sprint training or hypoxia due to respiratory illnesses), the process is said to be anaerobic, in which case pyruvic acid is fermented into lactate (lactic acid). Lactic acid can be used as an energy source by the heart, but it is generally converted back to pyruvic acid when oxygen becomes available again.

Citric acid cycle (Krebs cycle)

When oxygen is present, acetyl-CoA is produced from pyruvate molecules created by glycolysis. Acetyl-CoA then enters the Krebs cycle inside a structure called the mitochondria and is oxidised to form carbon dioxide and water while at the same time producing NADH from NAD^+.

Oxidative phosphorylation (OXPHOS)

Oxidative phosphorylation also occurs in the mitochondria and requires a great deal of oxygen being transported to the cells from the lungs. Oxidative phosphorylation is made up of two closely connected components, the electron transport chain and chemiosmosis. In the electron transport chain, NADH moves from outside to inside the mitochondria, where it donates an electron to the electron transport chain. The electron transport chain consists of a group of proteins (and some lipids) that work together to pass electrons "down the line", forming an electrochemical gradient producing 32 ATP's which provide energy for many cellular functions.

Many diets try to modify these energy production processes by altering the sugars, carbohydrates, proteins and fats in the diet. This is now explained in more detail:

Utilising sugars and carbohydrates for energy: The sugars in the blood are derived from the breakdown of ingested carbohydrates such as bread, potatoes and pasta. When blood sugar levels drop, a hormone called glucagon converts sugar stores in the liver (glycogen) into glucose. When sugar levels rise, after a meal for example, insulin stimulates the conversion of glucose back to glycogen. Lactose in milk is broken down to glucose and galactose by lactase. Both these sugars also enter the glycolysis pathway directly. As the diagram above shows, fructose from fruit enters directly a little further along. Glycerol is released when triglycerides are broken down to free fatty acids (FFA), and this can also enter the glycolysis pathway directly – this is one way triglycerides are used for energy.

Sugars are the body's preferred primary source of energy, but fats, proteins and ketones can easily be used instead when blood sugar levels fall. Prolonged periods without food triggers the use of proteins for energy. This is commonly seen in severely ill patients who have had trouble eating or absorbing food for some time – a state called cachexia. Ketones (see below) can be used by cells outside the liver. The heart can even use lactic acid as an energy source.

Fats as energy sources: Fats (lipids) are stored in adipose tissue, usually as triglycerides. They are composed of glycerol and fatty acids which can be broken down in a process known as lipogenesis. Eating excess calories leads to more fats being made and stored between muscles and under the skin. Conversely, when we eat less, levels of both blood glucose and insulin fall, while production of a hormone called glucagon increases. This stimulates the release of triglycerides from the adipose stores and its breakdown into glycerol and free fatty acids (FFA). Glycerol then enters glycolysis to produce pyruvic acid which, if oxygen is present, then enters the Krebs cycle. Fatty acids are changed, via a series of reactions called beta-oxidation, into ketones. In the liver, ketones cannot be used for energy, as liver cells do not have the enzyme succinyl-CoA required for this reaction. Instead, ketones are released into circulation and cells outside the liver are able to convert them into acetyl-CoA, which also enter the Krebs Cycle to produce energy. The enzyme carnitine is important in this process, as it is also increased by glucagon and enhances the utilisation of FFA by increasing their transport into the mitochondria of cells, where the conversion to ketones then acetyl-CoA occurs.

Cells can happily utilise sugar or fatty acid throughout the day, depending on the timing of meals and the amount of sugar in the bloodstream. Obviously, if an individual never lets their blood glucose levels drop by snacking constantly, fatty acids are used less, fat stores are not metabolised and obesity sets in.

Proteins as energy sources: When proteins are eaten, the body breaks them down into individual amino acids before they can be used by the cells. Most of the time, amino acids are recycled and used to make new proteins, rather than being oxidised for fuel. However, if there are more amino acids than the body needs, or if cells are starving, some amino acids will be broken down for energy. In order to enter cellular respiration, most amino acids must first have their amino group removed in a process called deamination. A toxic by-product of this step is ammonia, which the liver converts to urea and uric acid by adding carbon dioxide before it is then filtered and excreted by the kidneys. Once the amino acids have been deaminated, some glucogenic products can enter glycolysis, while others called alpha-keto amino acids are degraded directly into acetyl-CoA and ketone bodies to enter the Krebs cycle. Some intact amino acids, such as glutamine, are also important for the maintenance of the Krebs cycle, and thus help regulate energy production.

Ketones as energy sources: As you have just read, ketones are produced when the body burns fats or proteins to produce energy molecules. They are also produced when there is not enough insulin to help your body use sugar for energy, such as during an uncontrolled type 1-diabetic crisis. As mentioned above, fatty acids are changed via a series of reactions called beta-oxidation into ketones, then acetyl-CoA molecules, which enter the Krebs cycle to produce energy molecules. The three most well-known ketones are Acetone, B-hydroxybutyrate and acetoacetate.

To understand why ketones are found in the bloodstream, it is important to note that liver cells lack the enzyme (Succinyl CoA transferase) which converts ketones to acetyl-CoA which enters the Krebs cycle. Instead ketones are released into the bloodstream, enabling them to feed other tissues such as the brain, muscles and heart. In these tissues (which have the enzyme) the ketones are then converted back to acetyl-CoA which then enters the Krebs cycle to produce energy. This mechanism has survival advantages because it allows vital organs such as the brain and heart to keep being fed even when sugar levels have dropped in starvation

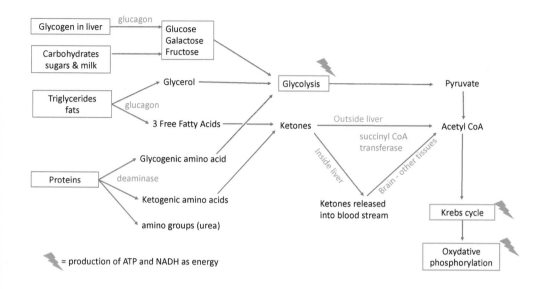

Diagram labels:
- Glycogen in liver
- Carbohydrates sugars & milk
- Triglycerides fats
- Proteins
- glucagon → Glucose / Galactose / Fructose
- Glycerol
- glucagon
- 3 Free Fatty Acids
- Glycogenic amino acid
- deaminase
- Ketogenic amino acids
- amino groups (urea)
- Glycolysis → Pyruvate
- Ketones
- Outside liver
- succinyl CoA transferase
- Acetyl CoA
- Inside liver
- Brain - other tissues
- Ketones released into blood stream
- Krebs cycle
- Oxydative phosphorylation
- ⚡ = production of ATP and NADH as energy

Triggers to use different parts of cellular respiration

Depending on the blood sugar levels, degree of oxygenation and rate of proliferation required, normal cells fluctuate between using either sugars or fatty acids. In normal conditions, 70% of the energy is supplied by OXPHOS. In the presence of low blood sugars but plenty of oxygen, cells slow glycolysis in favour of oxidative phosphorylation (OXPHOS), which can also use ketones from fats and proteins. However, in conditions of low oxygen (hypoxia) but where plenty of sugar is available, such as within many tumours, glycolysis becomes enhanced to compensate for the weakened function of OXPHOS.

Interestingly, normal cells which require rapid proliferation, such as those involved in healing scars, also favour glycolysis because while it only produces 2 ATP molecules, it is a much faster pathway and energy is provided instantly. Therefore, glycolysis and OXPHOS cooperate to maintain the cellular energetic balance. Rapidly proliferating cancer cells have also learnt to use aerobic glycolysis and have a unique ability to suck up sugar from the blood, even when levels are relatively low.

The ketogenic diet aims to exclude high-carbohydrate foods including some fruits and vegetables, bread, pasta, grains and sugar, while increasing the consumption of foods high in fat such as nuts, cream, and butter. The Atkins diet restricts carbohydrates to approximately 40–60 g per day, with the

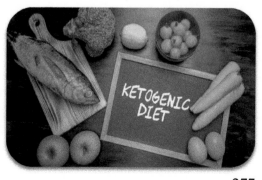

types of carbohydrates consumed restricted to those that have a glycaemic index lower than 50. The ketogenic diet aims to reduce all carbohydrates and favours medium chain triglycerides (MCT), such as coconut oil. These have fatty acids which are easily converted to ketones, then to acetyl-CoA outside the liver, which is used for energy in the Krebs cycle or converted to ketones in the liver and released into the bloodstream. This also means that, as less overall MCT fats are needed to trigger a ketogenic effect, a greater proportion of carbohydrates and proteins can be consumed, allowing a greater variety of food choices.

A ketogenic diet will lower blood sugar within three days and, by this point, the brain will be deriving 30% of its energy from ketones. After forty days this reaches as high as 70%, but it should be noted that the brain will always retain some need for glucose. It is worth highlighting that the ketogenic effect, or ketosis, is not the same as ketoacidosis, which occurs either with very high sugars and insulin deficiency, as in type-one diabetes, or in severe starvation. Nevertheless, regular users of the ketogenic diet are encouraged to monitor ketone body levels in their urine, and there are various commercial monitors available to help achieve this.

At first glance, it appears that cancer cells are more dependent on glycolysis for their energy. This was initially observed by Otto Warburg in the 1920s, and it was first thought to be an Achilles heel for the cancer cells and a target for drugs and nutritional strategies, including the ketogenic diet. Warburg hypothesised that the preference for glycolysis was caused by an impairment in mitochondrial function (the location for the Krebs cycle and OXPHOS apparatus) forcing cells to use glycolysis instead. So, in theory, if blood sugar drops, cancer cells have less energy and normal cells can switch to fat and ketone utilisation. The Warburg effect was apparently supported by an early laboratory experiment, which reported that proliferation of cancer cells was marginally reduced when glycolysis activity was blocked artificially, suggesting that fat and ketones, which by-pass glycolysis and enter the Krebs cycle directly, were not sufficient to meet all the requirements of cancer growth. However, this hypothesis has been challenged by recent investigations, which found that the function of mitochondrial OXPHOS in cancers is intact. Cancer cells are actually able to exhibit greater plasticity than normal tissues, so can change their metabolic preference to adapt to micro-environmental changes as and when they please. If glucose levels drop significantly through starvation, the pathways within mitochondrial (Krebs cycle and OXPHOS) are simply enhanced, so fatty acids and ketones can be metabolized in greater amounts. In cancer cells, since the glycolytic contribution (from sugar) to total energy (ATP) production does not generally exceed 60%, the rest of the energy production still comes from fats and ketones via the Krebs cycle and OXPHOS. In the presence of hypoxia, however, the contribution of energy production from OXPHOS is reduced to below 30%, so there is an even greater dependence on glycolysis. This also confirms that the preference of cancer cells to use glycolysis is primarily triggered by hypoxia rather than a defect in mitochondria.

Another theory behind the ketogenic diet relates to reactive oxygen species (ROS) and oxidative stress. It has been widely reported that cancer cells prefer glycolysis because it produces less damaging ROS. Warburg hypothesised that cancer cells are more vulnerable to oxidative stress than normal cells. In this case, forcing cancer cells to use OXPHOS instead of glycolysis, via diets which are high in fats and low in carbohydrates, would selectively cause increased metabolic oxidative stress in cancer cells. This hypothesis, however, is also not true, as recent research has shown that most cancer cells have learnt to develop resistance to oxidative damage by decoding oxidative-stress signals and converting them into pro-survival signals, promoting growth even in highly oxidative environments.

It appears, therefore, that much of the scientific theory underpinning the supposed benefits of the ketogenic diet is fundamentally flawed. That does not mean, however, that a diet of reduced sugars and carbohydrates and higher fats does not have significant health benefits. Avoidance of higher glycaemic index foods reduces IGF, insulin levels, helps restore insulin resistance and lowers markers of chronic inflammation, all of which have significant effects on cancer initiation and progression. That said, apart from isolated case reports showing some tumour shrinking, adequately powered studies in humans have yet to be published.

In terms of other conditions, it has been shown to significantly help children with epilepsy and it's is now recommended in many medical guidelines to support drug therapies. In adults, a ketogenic diet lowers blood markers of diabetes (haemoglobin A1c), helps diabetic control and reduces the risk of type 2 diabetes. As well as helping with weight loss, in animal and some limited human studies, the ketogenic diet has demonstrated tumour-slowing effects.

In summary, the theory behind the ketogenic diet is fundamentally flawed, and while the diet still has some healthy components, there are also pitfalls. Weight loss is an advantage for those who are overweight but is problematic for those off their food, with advanced disease or absorption problems. There is some evidence of a benefit in childhood epilepsy and reducing inflammation and diabetes risk in adults. The ketogenic diet excludes some fruits and veg which are rich sources of vitamins, minerals, polyphenols and fibre. It favours animal proteins and does not exclude carcinogenic cooking methods. It can cause constipation, raised cholesterol, kidney stones and stunted growth in children.

An optimal anti-cancer diet?

Dietary changes should be palatable, affordable, practical and designed for the long-term. After a cancer diagnosis, the diet must be sufficiently flexible to meet the individual needs of the patient, all of which could change depending on the stages of treatments, type and extent of disease. Some of the diets mentioned above, particularly the intermittent fasting ones, are beneficial

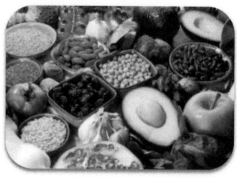

but difficult to maintain, especially if individuals have an active social, work or family life.

While it is important to watch what you are eating and have a good grasp on what is healthy and what is not, foods should still be enjoyable and sociable. Nobody should be afraid of food, and the occasional digression from a dietary plan is normal and to be expected. It is wise to remember the famous words of Oscar Wilde: "We live to eat not eat to live".

The philosophy and rationale for the best anti-cancer diet has been explained in the various sections of this book, but to recap, the salient elements include:

- Low in sugar & processed carbs
- Low in processed grains
- Low in carcinogens
- Not overeating
- Not snacking between meals
- Meat eaten <3 times a week
- Avoiding unhealthy fats
- Low to moderate alcohol intake
- Oily fish 3 times a week
- Regular overnight fasting
- High in low GI foods
- Moderate regular soy intake

- High in plant fats and fibre
- High in legumes
- High in probiotics bacteria
- High in prebiotic foods
- High in polyphenols
- High in other phytochemicals
- Adequate vitamins
- Adequate essential minerals
- Mixed nuts every day
- High in vegetables and fruit
- High in turmeric, green tea
- High in broccoli, pomegranate

It's important to have varied diet, which is why blog.cancernet.co.uk posts some really tasty healthy ideas every month in partnership with nutritionists and healthy chefs from across the world. These posts feature a film on how they are made and also explain why the food is healthy and where to buy the ingredients. Here are some examples:

For breakfast, it's really important to avoid processed carbs or sugar as the negative impact is greater on an empty stomach. Slow release carbs will provide energy through the morning, reducing the need to snack. Try banana, raspberries, grapes, walnuts, almonds, red peanuts, milled linseeds and puffed rice with organic sugar-free soy milk.

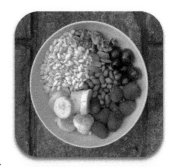

For a main meal, use plenty of herbs, spices and healthy extra virgin cold pressed olive oil. This dish has a mix of wild and white rice, onions, peas, mushrooms, massaged kale, sauerkraut (probiotic) and artichoke (prebiotics). Tuna and mackerel, mixed salad leaves, avocado, radish, red peppers, tomato, spinach and rocket are also included.

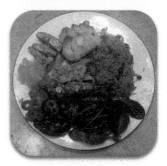

For a dessert, it's possible to make really tasty health desserts with no added sugars. This dessert is made with chia seeds, dates, coconut, banana, papaya and almond milk.

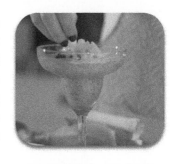

The relative quantities of different foods on the plate depends on varying factors between individuals at different stages in the cancer journey. More protein is needed to build up muscle, increase albumin levels or avoid cachexia. More carbohydrates and fats are needed to gain weight or if taking part in regular exercise. Fibre in vegetables and flaxseed is important to those with constipation but may need to be reduced if they have a shortened bowel or diarrhoea.

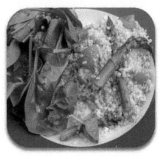

Try to be more adventurous with relatively new foods to the UK such as quinoa, which is an excellent source of protein, complex carbs, fibre and polyphenols. Mixed with asparagus, tomatoes and red pesto, it's delicious and includes virtually all the essential nutrients. Although it's important not to get stressed over combining the correct amount of foods with each meal, a simple guide would be as follows:

One half: Non-starchy vegetables such as asparagus, mushrooms, broccoli, avocado, peppers, carrots, radish, seaweed, onion, tomato, celery, cucumber, kale, cabbage, artichoke, Sauerkraut, multiple salad leaves
Quarter: Fibre-rich whole food carbohydrates such as quinoa, wild rice, polenta, oatcakes, whole potato, sweet potato, wholemeal bread, wholemeal pasta
Quarter: Healthy protein such as oily fish, other seafood, lake fish, seaweed, beans, lentils, tofu, nuts, seeds, lean meat

Fasting with chemo and other cancer treatments

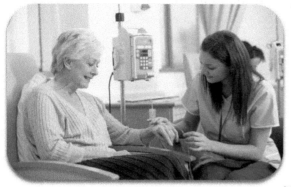

The effect of fasting on chemotherapy has been evaluated in a number of small laboratory studies involving mice and dogs. Most reported that fasting for 24 hours, before and after chemotherapy, reduced side effects such as organ damage, toxic features, immunosuppression, reduced body weight and chemotherapy-induced death. Moreover, it appeared to enhance the effectiveness of chemotherapy by suppressing tumour growth and spread. The reason for this benefit is thought to be because when normal cells are deprived of glucose and nutrients after short-term fasting, they down-regulate cell growth, diverting energy from growth to maintenance and ultimately slowing their proliferation, protecting them from chemotherapy. Conversely, dividing cancer cells continue to expend energy while starving, making them more susceptible to chemotherapy because they are still dividing rapidly, especially if dose intensity is maintained or even increased. Some researchers have termed this phenomenon "Differential Stress Resistance (DSR)" and harnessing it could, in theory, help chemo outcomes.

The results of radiotherapy were likewise improved in mice with mammary tumours fed an alternate day fasting regimen. The authors hypothesised this was due to enhanced oxidative stress and DNA damage within cancer cells during short-term fasting. Biological treatments including the tyrosine kinase inhibitors (TKIs), such as erlotinib, gefitinib and lapatinib, slow cancer cell growth by inhibiting grow signalling pathways. Laboratory studies, involving mice with implanted cancers, have shown that combining short-term fasting with TKI's significantly enhanced their effect.

Human studies: While these lab studies are interesting, convincing clinical evidence is lacking. In one uncontrolled case report involving 10 patients, those who fasted for a day before chemo, and up to 24 hours afterwards, reported greater tolerance to treatment and less fatigue, weakness, and nausea. Authors commented that fasting did not appear to prevent chemo-induced tumour shrinkage or affect tumour markers, although it is not possible to make this conclusion definitive with such a small group. There were complaints during fasting of minor dizziness, hunger and headaches, as well as slight weight loss which was quickly recovered. Another study evaluated the safety of fasting (<200 kcal calories/day) in twenty patients receiving platinum-based regimens 48 hours pre and 24 hours post-chemotherapy. They were instructed to consume only non-calorific beverages such as water. There were no grade 3 toxicities attributed to fasting and laboratory studies revealed no evidence of malnutrition. The researchers excluded patients with more than 10% recent weight loss, a body mass index of less than 20.5 and diabetes mellitus. Another small study from Holland involved a group of 13 women being instructed to either follow a standard diet or fast the day before and after chemotherapy. There was no difference in nausea, other symptoms, white blood cells levels or infection rates, but platelets and red cells (haemoglobin) were statistically higher in the fasting group. They also measured levels of γ-H2AX phosphorylation in blood lymphocytes, a protein which indicates the presence of DNA damage and is thought to serve as a marker for chemotherapy toxicity in healthy cells. After seven days this was significantly lower in the fasting group, suggesting that fasting may promote the recovery of chemotherapy-induced DNA damage in cells.

Effects of dexamethasone (steroids): Due to their anti-sickness capabilities and effectiveness at curtailing hypersensitivity reactions, corticosteroids are often administered before and after chemo. The metabolic effects of steroids, however, are likely to significantly affect the influence of fasting as they raise blood glucose and insulin levels. Most of the studies summarised above do not mention steroids, but many of the subjects taking part would have had them prescribed, particularly those containing taxanes. Perhaps clinical studies of fasting should investigate chemo regimens which do not require steroids.

Fasting mimicking

Given the nutritional concerns most patients with cancer there is increasing interest in manoeuvres which may trigger similar biochemical pathways, particularly those which decrease blood sugar, reduce tumour-associated inflammation or increase metabolic stress in cancer cells. Several alternative measures have been considered, including exercise, but studies so far of 'fasting mimickers' which are now discussed:

Everolimus is an mTOR inhibitor, licenced for ER^+ advanced breast cancer, which has been shown in mice to mimicking the anticancer effects of fasting by sensitising certain cells to chemo and radiation therapy. In humans, a number of phase I and II clinical trials are aiming to determine the effect of combining everolimus with chemo for various cancer types including breast, sarcoma, pancreas and myeloma.

Metformin is a biguanide commonly used to reduce glucose and insulin levels in T2D by restoring insulin sensitivity and inhibiting gluconeogenesis. Metformin suppresses tumour development and growth in experimental cell lines. Humans with treated cancer who have been taking metformin, as opposed to other diabetic drugs, have significantly lower relapse rates. Several phase II trials evaluating the potential efficacy of combining metformin with chemotherapy are currently underway.

Hydroxycitrate is an over-the-counter weight loss drug which encourages acetyl-CoA to enter the Krebs cycle. Its effectiveness for weight loss has been questioned, and it does not affect systemic glucose or insulin levels. One small lab study showed enhanced anticancer effects when combining it with chemo, although this was not confirmed in subsequent trials. Despite this weak data clinical studies are underway, but it's best to avoid in the meantime.

Polyphenols: There have been some concerns that polyphenols may interfere with oncology treatments via their antioxidant properties. However, they also slow glucose absorption and reduce insulin resistance and excess inflammation, much like short-term calorie restriction. This results in direct anticancer properties by inhibiting cell proliferation, de-differentiation, cell adhesion and metastasis, enhancing apoptosis. Lab studies have actually reported that polyphenols reduce damage to normal tissues by enhancing repair. It is hardly surprising that several studies have actually found that polyphenols enhance the cytotoxic effects 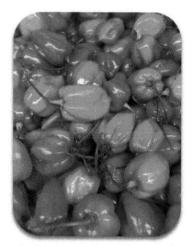 of chemotherapy. Curcumin has been shown to significantly improve the efficacy of docetaxel, with one laboratory study involving prostate cell lines demonstrating that a combined treatment of curcumin and docetaxel inhibited proliferation far more effectively than when docetaxel was used alone. Curcumin has also been found to enhance the effectiveness of cisplatin by helping to reduce cell proliferation in an in vitro laryngeal carcinoma cancer stem cell model, while another study highlighted how it can help to overcome cisplatin resistance. Beetroot extract has been shown to both help promote apoptosis of breast cancer cells after exposure of the cells to doxorubicin, while also protecting normal cardiomyocytes (heart muscle cells) from the toxic effects of doxorubicin. Resveratrol, found in grapes, berries and red wine, has also been under consideration as a CR mimetic, and several in vitro and in vivo studies have indicated that resveratrol can enhance anti-cancer treatments.

Not all laboratory studies, however, have shown such positive effects on chemo. One cell line study suggested resveratrol interfered with paclitaxel, while another suggested high levels of turmeric may have blocked apoptosis. Moreover, while many human studies have been encouraging, data is still relatively limited and more trials need to be conducted for us to develop a more complete understanding of their role during chemotherapy to improve outcome and reduce side effects.

Patient stories

Individual anecdotes are fascinating, thought-provoking and, although they have little scientific credibility on their own, often provide motivational human stories and inspiration for future research studies. Indeed, the amazing response of Mr B to broccoli soup was the initial reason why this ingredient was explored and included in the Pomi-T study by the scientific committee. The danger with anecdotal cases of 'wonder cures' in the media is that they often do not tell the whole story.

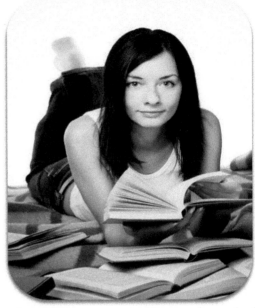

Some stories have lacked a solid diagnosis of cancer in the first place. At least once or twice a year, I am sent a patient with apparent widespread terminal cancer which instead turns out to be any one of a number of different conditions such as a chronic infection causing lymph node enlargement, or osteoporosis causing dramatic changes to the appearance of bone scans. One memorable case involved a young Indian lady who had previously had breast cancer and was preparing for the worse after being informed that the cancer had spread to her bones. On closer inspection, she turned out to have osteomalacia caused by a severe vitamin D deficiency and was successfully treated with vitamin and mineral replacement.

Although spontaneous remission certainly does exist, newspaper reports highlighting supposed miracles neglect to mention conventional therapies being used simultaneously. For example, a report of a UK woman with a brain tumour who had a response to cannabis failed to mention that she was also receiving chemo. Another report of a lady with breast cancer who made a remarkable recovery against all the odds did not credit the conventional hormone therapies she was being treated with.

Most of the amazing responses to lifestyle changes go largely unnoticed. Of particular note are the increasing proportion of men with low-grade prostate cancer who, after changes to their lifestyle, are no longer having to endure surgery or radiotherapy and the toxicities associated with these treatments. Likewise, countless men and women with metastatic disease are living substantially longer than expected due to comprehensive nutritional changes. Lifestyle programmes have also been identified as influential in preventing numerous patients with aggressive, advanced disease from relapsing after initial treatments, despite considerable odds being stacked against them.

The cases highlighted below all had confirmed cases of cancer and featured no hidden confounding factors or treatments. As they have been managed in a mainstream oncology unit, responses have been verified with clinical examination and an array of scans and blood tests.

Mrs A was a 52-year-old lady who had advanced cancer of the ovary. Following a

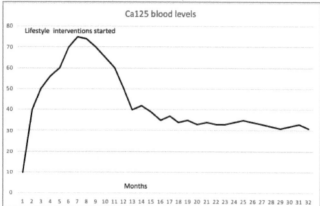

combination of surgery, chemotherapy and radiotherapy, all measurable disease disappeared from the scans. Unfortunately, a year later a blood test (a tumour marker called CA125) showed signs of cancer reactivating. Despite recommencing further chemotherapy, the CA125 count continued to rise, and chemotherapy was stopped. She then decided to embark on an intense dietary programme which involved significantly boosting polyphenol-rich food intake. The cancer count rose for one more month, then fell for three months and stabilised for a further twenty-one. In this instance, despite the cancer being resistant to all chemotherapy options, the dietary change had given her almost two years of further control and an excellent quality life.

Mr B was a very healthy, active 73-year-old man diagnosed with early low-grade prostate cancer. After considering the treatment options, he entered into an active surveillance programme, a useful manoeuvre to assess the tempo of disease. Over the next four months, his PSA levels increased from 9.6 to 13.1, suggesting progression. As a result, it was recommended he undergo a course of radiotherapy, a treatment which, given in

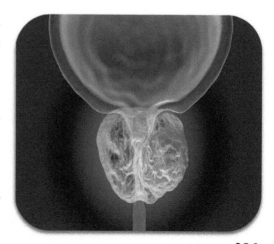

286

conjunction with hormone therapy, may well have left him permanently impotent. At his oncology appointment, seeing his wife's distress and still not keen himself to rush into radical treatment, he decided to try a new dietary approach which involved increasing intake of nuts and polyphenol-rich foods. Three months later his PSA levels dropped to 10.1, six months later they were at 6.5, and to his delight four years later they were less than 5. At the same time, his symptoms had improved, while there was no evidence of change on examination of pelvic MRI scans. However, after five years his PSA levels started climbing again, with MRI suggesting cancer progression. Again, he was offered radiotherapy but decided instead to renew lifestyle and nutritional strategies which he had neglected in the preceding months. He started exercising before breakfast, lost one stone in weight (he was a little overweight), cut out processed sugar and entered the polyphenol-rich supplement Pomi-T trial. Within three months his PSA levels had dropped to 8 and two years later were less than 4. More reassuringly, the size of the prostate cancer seen on his last MRI had decreased. As a bonus, his cholesterol, fasting blood sugar and blood pressure all dropped to the normal range, allowing him to stop all other medication.

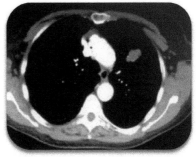

Mrs C was a fit 70 years old lady who developed bowel cancer. Unfortunately, 3 years later it appeared in her lung and in some lymph node areas. The metastasise were confirmed by a biopsy and PET scan but they could not all be removed completely by surgery or destroyed by targeted radiotherapy. Despite her metastatic disease she had no symptoms so was

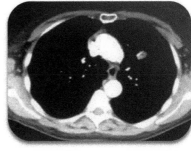

understandably reluctant to embark on a course of palliative chemotherapy, with its associated toxictities. Instead, she shed her excess weight, exercised every day, cut out carcinogenic foods and processed sugar and ate a high polyphenol diet. A scan six months later showed no change and four years later she is still asymptomatic and the main lung nodule, seen on the adjoining x-rays, are now clearly smaller.

Mr C was a 64-year-old man with prostate cancer who, despite initially receiving successful radiotherapy, began relapsing. He was disappointed to see his PSA levels starting to rise significantly. Although bone and CT scans did not identify bulky disease, PSA levels above 8 ng/l suggest likely reactivation of cancer. He was offered hormone therapy but instead chose to have a lifestyle intervention aided by formal nutritional testing which showed he had low levels of antioxidant enzymes, low zinc and low vitamin D. He increased his polyphenol intake with new dietary measures and two tablets of Pomi-T, 25mg of Zinc and 1000iu of vitamin D daily, while he also ate more fish oil and started regular exercise. His PSA levels dropped to 4 within three months and then 2 within a year. Levels remain low three years later, and he continues to be symptom-free.

Mrs D had a three-month history of colicky indigestion and tiredness. Further investigations found a large cancer which, despite removal via a lengthy operation, had unfortunately spread to 20 out of 21 lymph nodes. Moreover, there was evidence of spread to the surface of the bowel and within the abdominal fat, making relapse within the abdomen or elsewhere inevitable. She started chemotherapy but unfortunately had to stop after only two of eight cycles due to side effects. To try and offset progression for as long as possible, she accepted an exercise referral and lost two stone in weight. She also had nutritional testing and was found to have excess vitamin A and selenium due to the taking of a regular supplement, alongside low levels of omega 3 and vitamin D, which she decided to remedy by improving her intake of fish oils and crushed linseeds, alongside increasing her exposure to sunlight. In the last four years, she has cut all processed sugars from her diet and takes a probiotic supplement to counteract symptoms related to a shortened gut. Despite only having two cycles of chemotherapy she did have troublesome pins and needles in here fingers and toes, so began taking CBD (cannabis oils) which helped resolve these issues and made exercise more comfortable. She remains alive and well 8 years later, and it's highly likely that her ongoing lifestyle has helped her remain in remission from a disease which otherwise was definitely going to progress rapidly

Mr E was a man in his 60s with prostate cancer which had spread to the lymph nodes in his pelvis and abdomen and had led to PSA levels exceeding 500ng/l. He was treated for six years with hormones, repeated radiotherapy and chemotherapy, but despite this initial success his disease continued to progress, with his PSA levels rising to 50. Without any change to his medical management, his wife started making him a rich broccoli soup every morning. To everyone's delight, his PSA levels dropped

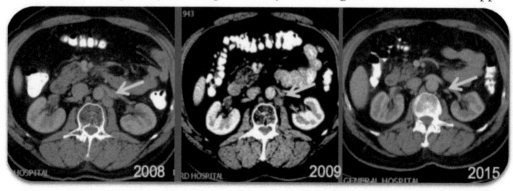

to 20 within four months, and over the next seven years, they fell to less than 4, and the nodal disease resolved, as seen on the CT scans below an amazing result considering he was given less than six months to live.

Eight years later his cancer spread to his bones and, despite localised radiotherapy, bone hardening drugs and six cycles of chemotherapy, the cancer continued to progress. He then started taking a polyphenol supplement and extra turmeric capsules and began responding again to chemotherapy (despite a significantly lower dose being used). At the time of writing this edition, he is still going strong two years later on a very low dose of regular chemotherapy (a metronomic regimen).

Miss F had initially successful treatment but developed metastasis in the lining of the lung six years later. She was given a hormone tablet which kept her disease under control for a further five years. She then suffered a fit (seizure), and subsequent investigations revealed that her cancer had spread to the brain. Her prognosis at that time, even with palliative chemo and radiotherapy, gave her less than 3 months. As her disease was incurable and wanting to avoid unpleasant side effects, she understandably declined further chemotherapy or radiotherapy. Instead, she embarked on a number of radical lifestyle changes which included:

- Stopping smoking
- Cutting out processed sugars and processed carbohydrates
- Beginning the day with a 20-minute brisk walk
- Including vegetable juice and two Pomi-T capsules with breakfast
- Removing all processed meat from her diet
- Eating oily fish three times a week
- Taking an organic CBD-rich oil twice a day
- Taking probiotics two weeks on and two weeks off
- Taking vitamin D and zinc after discovering a significant deficiency

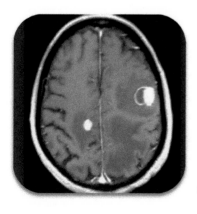

A year later, a repeat CT showed her metastases had not changed. For the next three years, she remained well without symptoms. Over this period, she avoided chemo and radiotherapy and her lifestyle initiatives

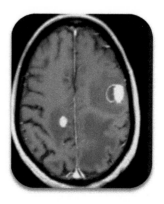

extended her good quality life considerably. At this point she developed symptomatic progression requiring medical intervention from which she responded well initially.

Mr G was a 51 year old man with metastatic melanoma. He was given the biological targeted agent ipilimumab but developed severe life threatening diarrhoea. After a prolonged recovery, with the melanoma beginning to progress again, re-exposure of ipilimumab was commence but this this the man decided to embark on a significant dietary and lifestyle change first as prehabilitation and during the treatment. This involved avoiding processed meats and carbohydrate, stopping all processed sugar, alcohol and reducing milk. Eating unrefined grains, polyphenol rich fruit and vegetables and some oily fish. This time he tolerated full dose with no diarrhoea and his melanoma metastasises responded promptly and his response is ongoing

This is a great example how the interaction of gut and general health are so important to both tolerability and effectiveness of the new biological treatments. Numerous ongoing studies are confirming similar benefits when the population of bad (firmicutes) species are replaced with good (bacteroidetes) bacterial species using a combination of prebiotic polyphenols and probiotic bacterial supplements.

Chapter 20

Conclusions
Final comments

Hopefully, this book has provided the requisite information and explanation to motivate and guide readers towards appropriate and fulfilling lifestyle strategies. Although this information is based solely on bona fide published evidence, it must be emphasised that not everyone will benefit from the measures advocated in this book. Although a healthy lifestyle will improve the chances of a better outcome, it does not guarantee it. Even the most motivated of individuals may suffer a relapse of their disease or see their cancers continue to grow, despite their best efforts.

Some people will not have the resources to make significant changes, while others will not want to embark on a major disruption to their daily lives, even if they understand the risks of not doing so. This is entirely up to them - it is their choice, and they should not be made to feel guilty. There may be many good reasons why someone, with cancer or otherwise, chooses to live as they do. In practical terms, ability or willingness to change depends on individual circumstances and pre-diagnosis attitudes to lifestyle. The cancer itself, surgery or the cancer treatments may have caused physical disability, fatigue, weight gain, reduced self-esteem and body image worries. Many people see lifestyle changes as insurmountable hurdles, so it is important that they are able to ask for help from hospital specialist nurses, the family doctor, physiotherapists and exercise professionals. With supervised support, it's easier to relearn exercise and dietary patterns. Recruiting friends and relatives into a healthy change programme will ensure a higher level of motivation and commitment. Most people are keen to help, so what better way to make them feel more involved!

In terms of timing, many people may put thoughts of exercise or nutrition in the back of your mind until treatments have finished. There is, however, strong evidence that lifestyle strategies should be considered as early as possible, as they can reduce the chance of serious complications both after surgery and during active cancer treatments. It's even encouraged to embark on formal programmes before surgery in order to reduce the immediate post-operative risks (prehabilitation).

Enacting lifestyle changes can provide many people with a feeling of empowerment and self-control. Several studies have demonstrated that patients who believe they have been involved in their own treatment management, have a significantly enhanced sense of well-being compared to those who feel their treatments have been dictated to them by paternalistic doctors. Furthermore, patients who embark on a self-help lifestyle change are often better at distracting their minds from more sombre thoughts.

Exercise, particularly group classes, are a good reason to leave the house, meet people and make friends. Diets with reduced saturated fats, less meat and more fruit and vegetables, reduce cholesterol and blood pressure and prevent the need for statins and blood pressure lowering medication. A healthy lifestyle has a positive influence on digestion, reducing the need for anti-acids and laxatives, both of which cost the NHS millions of pounds each year.

Keeping fit means more energy and stamina to play and interact with children and grandchildren, while it also opens up opportunities to participate in sport and social interaction with friends. It keeps the mind clear to enjoy intellectual pursuits and can improve the ability to enjoy a loving and sensual relationship.

In conclusion: Despite the rapid advances in scientific knowledge, there is still a huge amount which is not known about the interaction between medical treatments and lifestyle interventions. Vast amounts of money and resources are now being invested by prestigious scientific bodies into understanding the interaction between lifestyle and improved responses to new biological therapies. Looking to the future, medical systems will, in all likelihood, be used to chart intricate maps of biological pathways in both the cancer and host. Computer-generated individual therapies will then be able to restore these defects with a complex array of targeted drugs. Lifestyle strategies which enhance their effect and reduce toxicities by improving immunity and reducing chronic inflammation are likely to have an even greater role.

Good luck!

Background information about cancer

This section describes the fundaments of cancer, how it starts, grows and spreads. It is rather technical in parts and if you are someone who does not need to look under the bonnet of the car in order to drive, it may not interest you. For others, including myself, this level of understanding provides strong rationale and motivation to live a healthy lifestyle and recommend it to others.

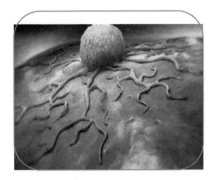

What is Cancer?

For a disease which affects one in two of the population, there still often remains confusion amongst patients and their families regarding the terminology used by doctors and nurses when describing cancers. Malignancy, masses, growths, neoplasms, lesions, tumours, cysts, hot spots, shadows, nodules are all used to describe abnormality which could be cancer. In most cases, a biopsy is needed to tell the medical team what an abnormality is, so the doctors may be reluctant to use the c-word until it's proven to be benign or malignant. For clarification, masses of cells that grow abnormally but don't invade and metastasise are called benign tumours. For the rest of this chapter, we will concentrate on malignant tumours (cancer) and focus on the differences between them and normal cells.

Normal cells follow their genetic instructions to grow to their desired size, space themselves evenly, stick to their original site and respect their neighbours. They obey instructions from the regulatory systems of the body. They grow at a controlled pace and die when they are supposed to in order to make room for new healthy cells.

Cancer cells grow as fast as they can, don't die when they ought to, clamber on top of each other and quickly run out of space in the organ of origin. They not only expand the organ they started in but infiltrate and invade their neighbouring structures, causing considerable damage. This invasion is one of the hallmarks of cancer. The other ways cancers can make room for themselves is to lose their stickiness to the organ of origin and break off and metastasise to other parts of the body and start growing there.

Cancers are named after the organs where they originated rather than where they end up. Each organ is capable of developing several different types of cancers depending on the type of tissue they start from. It is also possible that usual normal cell population within one tissue can change (called metaplasia), such as in response to chronic irritation from acid in the lower oesophagus (Barrett's oesophagus) or a stone in the bladder. These irritated cells grow faster than they should, piling cells on top of each other in a process called hyperplasia. Eventually, this rapid growth leads to more spontaneous mutations, disorganised growth or dysplasia, and from there to an established cancer. The more common types of cancers include adenocarcinomas from glands; squamous cell carcinomas from the skin or lining of tubes; leukaemia from blood, lymphoma from the immune systems and sarcoma from the muscles, bone and joints.

Even though cancers have common characteristics, their growth rate, pattern of spread and response to different treatments can vary considerably. Even cancers from the same origin can behave very differently depending on their grade and which genetic receptors are activated. Pathologists now spend a great deal of time profiling cancers in order to guide oncologists on the best choice of surgery, radiotherapy, chemotherapy, hormone and biological therapies. This is why the management of patients with the same cancer can vary enormously.

How do cancers start?

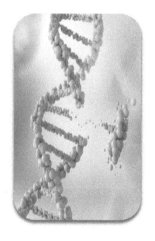

Within each cell lies a nucleus, containing strips of material called DNA. To be precise, 46 strips, each containing millions of packages of information called genes. These genes are the templates for all the functions of the body. In particular, they contain the codes or instructions for the development of organs and structures to an exact size, telling cells when to grow, when to stop and when to die to make room for healthy new cells.

That's why our skin is a certain thickness, the hairs on our arms stop growing at a precise length and when we cut ourselves, skin is able to grow at an alarming rate but stop when it is healed. These growth signalling and check point are controlled by genes which have evolved over millennia and countless generations to produce the humans we know today. Over this time, however, our genes have picked up considerable amounts of genetic debris from non-fatal mutations generated through spontaneous damage or infections, particularly from viruses. This genetic debris, if it goes wrong, can cause our normal cells to become cancerous. With this in mind, it may not be a surprise then that one in two of us will get cancer at one stage in our lives. Perhaps instead of asking **"why me?"** when we develop cancer, we should be asking **"why not me?"** when we don't.

Some of this debris includes strips of genes that interfere with controlled growth, but are kept from doing harm by other genes which lie next to them on the same strip of DNA. These *good* genes, called tumour suppressor genes, have the essential function of guarding the body against the *bad* cancer genes, called promotor oncogenes. When either one or both strands of DNA are damaged by chemicals or x-rays, the normal sequence of genes, separating (translocating) the suppressor genes from the promoter genes or placing oncogenes next to genes, causing overexpression of their function, dysfunctional growth and ultimately the first steps to cancer.

The first evidence of translocated DNA causing cancer was discovered in Philadelphia in 1959. Scientists showed that a type of leukaemia called Chronic Myeloid Leukaemia (CML) had a translocation of a strip of DNA between chromosome 9 and chromosome 22. This became known as The Philadelphia Chromosome. Drugs have subsequently been developed which successfully target this defect and are now keeping people with CML alive and well for many years. Numerous other promoter oncogenes have been discovered which, when activated, promote the development, abnormal growth and spread of many cancers. Targeting the function of these oncogenes has resulted in successful anti-cancer biological therapies, most famously transtuzumab (Herceptin) targeting HER-2 amplified breast cancers. Many others targeting melanoma, other leukaemias and bowel cancer have been discovered, and the race is on to develop biological agents for every cancer.

Some people are fortunate to be born with their cancer genes locked in tightly by very stable suppressor genes, resulting in very robust DNA. Put another way they have been dealt good genetic cards – always easier to win! Others have DNA which can be easily damaged or have defective repair mechanisms that make the development of cancer almost inevitable. Most people are somewhere in between these two extremes, but whichever risk group you are in, a healthy lifestyle can reduce the odds of cancer forming by half, delay the age of diagnosis or lead to less aggressive more easily treatable types. Studies of identical twins provide insight into the relative influence of nurture over nature. Due to the common genes they share, there is an increased likelihood that the twin of a person diagnosed with cancer will suffer from the same disease. Recent studies of breast cancer in twinned women from Scandinavia found that heritability accounted for 30% of cases, with environmental factors accounting for 70% of cancer incidence. This means that the most important contributor to the causation of breast cancer is environmental not the genes we are born with. The pathwaths required for a normal cell to transform into a malignant (cancer) cell are now described:

Initial DNA damage

The illustration below shows how DNA can be damaged by reactive oxygenated species (ROS) formed by dietary carcinogens and other hazards. These ROS can be formed spontaneously when the cell makes energy. DNA also sustains spontaneous breaks during normal cell division. Some carcinogenic hazards such as ionizing radiation and UV light can directly damage DNA. The susceptibility of DNA to carcinogens and damage from free radicals is strongly influenced by the genes we are born with (somatic genes) and other environmental factors which alter the expression of these genes - a phenomenon called **epigenetics**:

Epigenetics explains why, even if an individual has an increased genetic risk of cancer, the severity of the syndrome could change from one person to another. This is called penetrance and is often affected by outside factors in a process called epigenetics. This describes a series of processes which can alter the expression of both the genes we were born with (germline) and those acquired by cancers (somatic). Expression or penetrance of a gene refers to influence it has on the function of the cell. If a gene is highly expressed, it has a strong influence on the biochemical function of the cell and, if this involves abnormal growth, this could lead to cancer. The expression of a gene can be influenced, or even silenced, by other neighbouring genes, the time of day and different lifestyle choices. Complex epigenetics processes which regulate how the gene is presented to the messenger RNA, which then form the proteins which signal growth or metabolism, are outside the scope of this book. Put simply, epigenetics alters the supportive components of DNA which are responsible for the winding and unravelling of the helix. If the gene is hidden from the RNA by tightly woven DNA, it is difficult for the RNA to reach it. One of the main mechanism, the lifestyle factors highlighted in this book influences the development and spread of cancer is via its influence on epigenetics.

Diagram to summaries how DNA can be damaged (directly and indirectly)

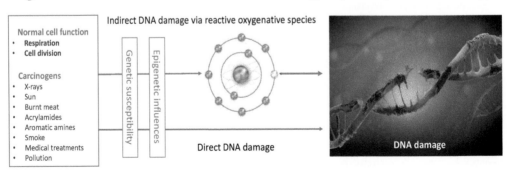

296

Oxidative stress

Living creatures have developed a series of complex biological defenses within each cell which protect and repair DNA, preventing the formation of mutations that could lead to cell death, premature ageing or cancer. These defenses are not actually part of the immune system, which occurs outside the cell. It has been estimated that each cell incurs on average over 5000 potentially harmful beaks in DNA every day, so it's important we look after our intracellular defences. Oxidative stress is a name given to a state of excessive formation of harmful reactive oxygen species (ROS) which overwhelm the anti-oxidant mechanism that normally controls them. This occurs either by overexposure to hazards which damage DNA or by deficiencies in the anti-oxidant defense apparatus. Although we need some ROS for the normal functioning of our cells, the reality is that, with a western lifestyle, we have far too many.

Factors which increase oxidative stress: Most people are aware that environmental, cosmic and ingested carcinogens can damage DNA either directly, or via the formation of highly energetic ROS. However, the reality is most ROS are generated within the cell by normal cellular respiration (energy production). The electrons that escape the energy making process combine with oxygen to form a very nasty molecule called superoxide radical ($O2^{\bullet}-$) or combine with water to form hydrogen peroxide ($\bullet OH$). As these have an unstable electron in their outer electron orbital, they damage intracellular structures by donating single electrons or literally stealing electrons from them. Free radicals can also be generated from lipids called lipidperoxides and proteins called reactive nitrogen species (RNS). Once formed, these nasty free radicals whiz through the cell, damaging everything in their path, including DNA, leading to mutations. If these mutations affect genes which regulate growth, this could lead to cancer. If these mutations affect other important biological pathways, they can lead to a host of age-related diseases including heart disease, arthritis, diabetes, Alzheimer's disease, Parkinson's disease, cataracts and macular degeneration.

Factors such as obesity, strenuous or unaccustomed exercise, and chronic inflammation increase the cells' need for energy and, in doing so, increase ROS production. In these situations, it's vital to have adequate levels of the building blocks for the antioxidant enzymes such as essential minerals, vitamins and polyphenols. These antioxidant enzymes can mop up ROS by donating or absorbing aberrant electrons. The three most well-known groups of antioxidant enzymes are:

Superoxide Dismutase: SOD helps reduce the superoxide radical ($O2^{\bullet}-$) to form hydrogen peroxide (H_2O_2), which is then detoxified by the enzyme catalase into water and oxygen. SODs contain metal ion cofactors that, depending on the isozyme, can be copper, zinc, copper, manganese or iron. Deficiencies in these metals will impair the formation of SOD. Some people have genetic defects which impair SOD formation, making them particularly susceptible to increased oxidative stress.

Glutathione is an important water-soluble, sulfur and selenium containing antioxidants, synthesized from amino acids. It breaks down (•OH), organic hydroperoxides and lipid peroxides, and has various forms such as glutathione reductase, glutathione peroxidases and glutathione "S"-transferases. There are high levels of these enzymes in the liver, where they deal with environmental pollutants including xenobiotics, such as dioxins and polychlorinated biphenyl, food additives, hydrocarbons, and pesticides. Exposure of the liver to these substances stimulates the production and utilisation of more glutathione. Glutathione then conjugates and neutralises these toxins, rendering them less likely to damage cells. Research suggests that glutathione and vitamin C work interactively to neutralise free radicals.

Catalases are enzymes that catalyse the conversion of H_2O_2 to water and oxygen, using iron or manganese cofactors. They are found in all living organisms exposed to oxygen including bacteria, plants and animals. They are a very important enzyme in protecting the cell from ROS, One molecule can convert a million H_2O_2 to water and oxygen each second.

Diagram summarising the factors which affect oxidative stress

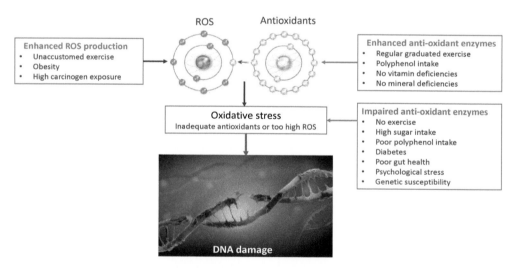

Factors which reduce oxidative stress In response to oxidative damage, our cells generate anti-oxidant enzymes and use certain antioxidant vitamins to protect themselves. Numerous compounds have antioxidant properties, either because they have direct free radical scavenging properties or they support pathways which do. The more notable chemicals and factors are:

Coenzyme Q_{10} This fat-soluble, sulfur-containing chemical, common to all animals and bacteria, contains 10 isoforms vital for electron transfer within the energy production pathway of the cell. Organs with the highest energy requirements such as the heart, liver and kidney have the highest levels. Coenzyme Q10 shares a biological pathway with cholesterol, and its formation can be inhibited by blood pressure drugs, beta blockers and statins. It is well reported that statin can lower blood Coenzyme Q10 levels. Dietary sources of coenzyme Q10 include heart, liver and kidney, but it is also found in reasonable quantities in soybeans, sesame seeds, parsley, peanuts, red mullet and other dark fish, good quality grapeseed and olives. CoQ_{10} supplements, including an important isoform called ubiquinol, are commonly seen adorning the shelves of health food shops, yet in 2004 a "secret shopper" analysis showed that many did not contain the quantity identified on the label. An adequately prepared supplement was studied in 2013 and did reduce cardiovascular events in people with heart failure. However, a substantially larger study found no convincing evidence to support its use for heart failure, high blood pressure, and statin-induced muscle and joint pains. Other studies have reported it helped some migraine suffers and increased sperm count. In terms of cancer, the few small studies that have been conducted were poorly designed and underpowered, so it remains unclear if the reported benefits were caused by the CoQ_{10} or by something else. The National Cancer Institute and The American Cancer Society have concluded that the evidence of an anti-cancer effect is poor and, as CoQ_{10} could potentially reduce the effectiveness of chemotherapy, should be avoided during cancer treatments.

Alpha lipoic acid (ALA) This anti-oxidant and its reduced form, dihydrolipoic acid (DHLA), is unusual as it is both fat and water soluble. ALA is a naturally occurring sulfur-containing compound not to be confused with the short chain omega 3, alpha-linolenic acid. It acts as a cofactor for several important enzymes; It works with vitamin B to enhance the conversion of carbohydrates into energy, which is why some athletes use ALA pills to enhance performance. It protects cells by acting as a chelator of heavy metals such as mercury and arsenic, reducing their toxic effects. It can also bind with other sulfur-containing anti-oxidants such as glutathione, neutralising both the lipid and aqueous ROS produced by energy production. Well-designed studies looking at ALA pills are awaited, but in the mean-time, when exercising, it's certainly worth increasing intake of yeast, spinach, broccoli, potatoes, parsley or, if not a vegetarian, liver or kidney, both of which contain ALA.

Vitamins as antioxidants Vitamins have essential roles in multiple pathways throughout the body. Vitamin A, E and C have direct antioxidant properties, so are important components in balancing oxidative stress. Vitamin C protect cells from toxic products such as H_2O_2 by enabling DNA to 'sense' the damage by integrating with the iron imbedded in DNA. Which then signals DNA repair pathways. Vitamin E's direct antioxidant properties are due to its ability to donate a hydrogen atom (a proton plus electron) to ROS formed when fat undergoes oxidation. Vitamin A and carotenoids can quench oxygen, peroxyl and thiyl radicals directly particular in low oxygen environments such as cancers or some tissues after exercise. The chapter on vitamins explains that deficient levels can increase oxidative stress but because Vitamin A and E they are direct anti-oxidants, high levels however can also do harm because they can mop up too many ROS, some of which are needed for normal cell physiology including apoptosis.

Minerals as antioxidants Minerals, such as zinc, copper, selenium, iron and manganese are not direct antioxidants but are required for the formation of antioxidant. Their deficiency could lead to reduced antioxidant production and hence increased oxidative stress. Taking a higher than needed intake of minerals will, therefore, not increase intracellular defenses or immune immunity and, as discussed in part two, could actually have a negative impact on health.

Exercise as an antioxidant Exercise, particularly if strenuous, produces more ROS because more energy is required by the cell. In response to this transient increase in ROS, especially after regular training, an adaptive upregulation of antioxidant genes occurs which results in greater production of antioxidant enzymes. However, if exercise is unaccustomed or strenuous, there is a danger that exercise could do more harm than good. This is especially the case in the elderly, where this adaptive process is slower. It is therefore important to gradually increase the intensity and strength of exercise over time. Greater attention also needs to be given to avoid vitamin and mineral deficiencies and consume a higher intake of polyphenol-rich foods to ensure the building blocks for the antioxidant enzymes are readily available.

Polyphenols as antioxidants Some phytochemicals have anti-oxidant properties, but in the past, this aspect has been overstated. In fact, many people previously referred to them only as anti-oxidants, which diminishes the importance of their other biochemical properties. Fortunately, this misconception is being increasingly recognised although this term is still seen in many older websites. Phytochemicals protect DNA via their ability to up-regulate the nuclear factor, Nrf2, which switches on the genes that code for the anti-oxidant enzymes, such as super oxide dismutase and catalyse. This has already highlighted in the chapter above.

DNA repair

It has been estimated that 5000 DNA breaks occur in each cell every day, so without an efficient repair mechanism, living organisms would not be able to exist. The vast majority are repaired completely, or dealt with in ways to stop mutated cells dividing and passing on the genetic damage to subsequent cells. DNA damage leading to amplification of our own genes or mutated versions of our own genes could lead to a number of different scenarios:

- Cell cannot function so dies immediately
- Damage is fully repaired and subsequent growth is normal
- Damage can't be repaired, so cell commits "suicide" (apoptosis)
- Cells not repaired fully - cells functional but can't divide (senescence)
- Cells not repaired - cells function but divide dysfunctionally

Damaged cells which are able to continue growing dysfunctionally are the seeds of cancer. Some people are born with defects in their DNA repair pathways making them more susceptible to cancer. Cancers themselves have also developed ingenious mechanisms to bypass or suppress DNA repair. The diagram below shows the consequences of good and impaired DNA repair

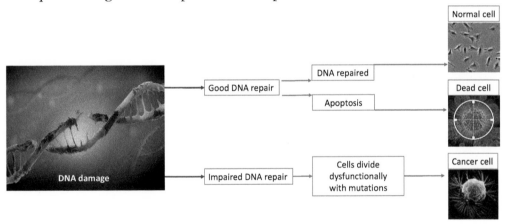

How do cancers progress and spread?

Cancer cells have done well so far to escape DNA repair mechanisms, avoid immune surveillance and corrupt numerous biochemical mechanisms to harness available energy and nutrients in order to feed themselves. However, in order for individual cells or clusters of cells to grow into fully formed life-threatening cancer, they have to develop some clever but nasty tricks, including the ability to:

Rapid growth (proliferation)
Cancer cells have a much higher growth rate than normal cells, so require a lot of energy, which is one reason why they light up on a glucose-PET scan. There are a number of reasons why cancer cells are able to grow so fast:

301

Cancer cells generate their own growth signals; Normal cells require growth signals before they can move from a dormant state into an active proliferative state. These signals are transmitted into the cell via receptors on the cell surface. Normal cells can't grow without these signals, which is why they don't grow when put on a petri dish in a lab. Cancer cells, on the other hand, grow and proliferate on their own on a petri dish (and in the body) because they have learnt to generate their own growth signals – this is called growth signal autonomy. Many of the genes which promote cancer act by mimicking normal growth signalling via chemicals called tyrosine kinase. New targeted anti-cancer drugs have been developed called tyrosine kinase inhibitors which aim the reinstate this control.

Over-riding checkpoint anti-growth signals: Normal cells stop growing when they need to in response to checkpoint signals which tell them to switch off. Cancer cells have learnt to be insensitive to anti-growth signals, so they continue to grow despite overcrowding themselves and their neighbours.

Loss of hormonal control: Via a process called de-differentiation, cancer cells, although starting off similar to those in the organ of origin, soon start evolving into more aggressive forms. These undifferentiated cells lose the receptors (antennae) which pick up signals from hormones and allow them to grow unchecked and become resistant to hormonal therapies.

Loss of circadian rhythm: Normal cells slow down at night, helping them repair genetic damage and preserve energy. Some cancers have learnt to switch off the normal circadian biochemical clock, so they can grow 24/7. Drugs are now being developed to help restore circadian rhythm in cancers, while melatonin is increasingly being touted as playing a possible role in helping slow cancer growth.

Immortality

The ability of tumour cells to expand in number is determined not only by the rate of cell proliferation but also by the rate of cell attrition (shedding or death). In stark contrast to normal cells, which only divide a finite number of times before they enter into a permanent state of growth arrest or simply die, cancer cells divide and proliferate forever, or at least until the host dies, they run out of oxygen, treatment kills them or lifestyle measures stop them. There are a number of explanations for this, but the three most well-known are:

Damage to the DNA policeman: A widely known protein, which protects DNA is p53 - nicknamed the DNA policeman. If a cell is partially damaged, p53 slows the cell cycle and allows DNA repair to take place. If repair is not possible, it does not allow the cell to divide with damaged DNA which could eventually cause cancer. Instead, it triggers pathways to tell the cell to commit suicide – this is called programmed cell death or apoptosis. Some people are born with a defect in this policeman gene (known as Li-Fraumeni syndrome). As you can imagine, they usually develop multiple cancers at a very early age in life. Acquired defects in p53 have been identified in over 50% of cancers. This allows cells to pass through the various stages of the cell cycle rapidly – too fast for apoptosis pathways to be triggered, allowing cells to dividing with partially defective DNA, leading to further mutations.

Resistance to programmed cell death (apoptosis): Even if p53, is functioning well, so is able to send a signal to the cell to commit suicide, the suicide apparatus may not functional in some cancer cells (apoptosis resistance) and the cell carries on growing and dividing.

Telomere protection: A lynchpin to the immortality of malignant cells is the ability to maintain the length of a small strip of nuclear proteins at the end of each DNA called the telomeres. Telomeres become shorter each time a cell divides, acting as a kind of cellular clock ticking down a cell's age. Eventually, the cell enters a permanently arrested state called senescence. To escape this inevitable demise, about 90% of human tumours are able to boost levels of an enzyme called telomerase, which adds nuclear proteins to telomeres, thus turning the clock backwards.

Recruitment of more blood vessels (angiogenesis)

Chemicals called vascular epithelial growth factors (VEGF) signal the local blood vessels to grow into the rapidly expanding tumours in order to supply the energy and nutrients they need. The oxygen and nutrients supplied by the vasculature are crucial for cell function and survival. A number of cancer drugs have been developed such as Avastin, which target angiogenesis-initiating signals including vascular endothelial growth factor (VEGF), stopping cancers from growing too big.

Loss of adhesion, invasion and metastasis

Cancers soon run out of space, so in order for them to make more room for themselves, they invade adjacent organs and metastasise to other parts of the body. The first stage of expansion is to lose the glue that keeps normal cells in place - *loss of adhesion*. The molecules responsible for this glue are called cell adhesion molecules. In normal tissues, they are responsible for wound healing and tissue repair. Cancer cells have learnt to block the adhesion molecule function, so are able to move around more freely, allowing them to reach the next stage of the process - *migration*. Migration occurs when cells release chemicals which break down the extracellular matrix proteins and fibroblasts - barriers to their spread. They can either spread directly into tissues or migrate along nerves, lymphatic and blood vessels in an amoeboid manner.

Sometimes they migrate, initially, just within the gland of origin, such as the breast ductal system. In this case, they are called carcinoma in situ. However, if they have managed to breach the basement membrane of the organs or glands, they are called invasive cancers and have the capacity to spread to distant sites in the body via the bloodstream - *metastasis*.

Thriving in adverse environments

Rapid turnover of cancer cells with damaged DNA and impaired repair processes potentially makes them more susceptible to damage from ROS, which could damage them further and potentially kill them. ROS can be generated from continued carcinogen exposure, or formed naturally as a byproduct of energy production. Cancer cells have learnt two adaptions in order to reduce intracellular ROS. First, they have a higher priority to use glucose which is utilised in glycolysis rather than fat and ketones which utilised in Oxidative phosphorylation which produces more ROS Secondly, cancer cells have developed resistance to oxidative damage by decoding oxidative-stress signals and converting them into pro-survival signals, thereby actually promoting growth even in highly oxidative environments.

Diagram summarising of the pathways from normal cell to established cancer

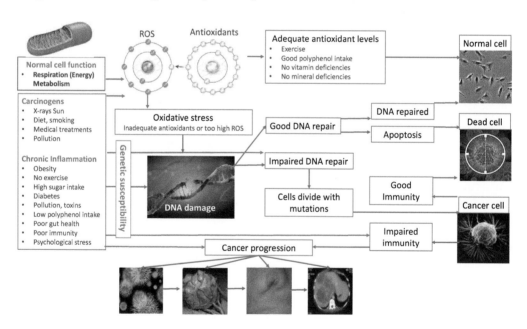

About the authors

Prof Robert Thomas MRCP MD FRCR trained at the Royal Marsden, Royal Free and Mount Vernon Hospitals, London. A period of full-time lab and clinical research followed at the Institute of Cancer, National Hospital for Nervous Diseases and Duke University, North Carolina. He is now clinical teacher at Cambridge University, a visiting professor in Sports Science at Coventry 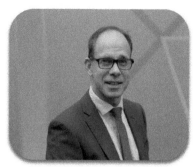 and Bedford Universities, Research Lead at the Primrose Oncology Unit, and a Consultant Oncologist at Bedford and Addenbrooke's Hospitals.

Current medical interests include the treatment of breast, colon and prostate cancers with medical therapies and radiotherapy. He has an academic interest in lifestyle, functional medicine and survivorship and has published over 100 peer-reviewed scientific papers and countless book chapters.

As both an oncologist and sports scientist, he is able to bridge the gap between the two specialisations. He lectures in sports science at Bedford and Coventry Universities and has chaired sessions on exercise and cancer at numerous international medical conferences. Working with both The Wight Foundation and Macmillan Cancer Support, he wrote the national standards for the 'Skills Active' Level 4 cancer rehabilitation course for exercise professionals.

He is a patron of two cancer support charities, has run several marathons to help raise money and talks regularly at fundraising events. He regularly contributes to information materials for several charities. He helped write the evidence base for the National Survivorship Programme and now leads the Macmillan National Exercise Expert Advisory Committee.

He has previously been awarded Hospital Doctor Magazine 'Hospital Doctor of the Year' and the British Oncology Association 'Oncologist of the Year', while he has also won the NHS Communication Prize and the Royal College Frank Ellis Medal. He edits the CancernetUK newsletter, blog and social media updates, all of which can be found at:

Twitter:@cancernetuk

Blog.cancernet.co.uk

Facebook: cancernetuk

Contributing authors

This book wouldn't have been possible without the generous input from experts who have given their time and shared their skills, knowledge and experience:

Dr Daniel Bailey
Seniors lecture Bedford Uni
Nutrition & Exercise

Simon Blackburn
Patient advocate

Frances R. Dawson
cambridgecancerhelp.org

Dr Rob Lawson
Chairman of the British Society
Lifestyle Medicine (bslm.org.uk)

Rhiannon Lewis
Clinical Aromatherapy - ijca.net

Mary Ann Howard
The Royal Horticultural Society
rhs.org.uk

Gillian Horton
Post breast cancer attire.
colleens.com.au

Janet Hickman
cambridgecancerhelp.org

Jennifer Lenhart
Royal London Hospital
Harleystreetchildrenshopital.com

Anna Bowzyk Al-Naeeb
Consultant Oncologist
Bedford and Cambridge

Simon Maguire
Mindfulness counsellor
cambridgecancerhelp.org

Šarūnas Narbutas
President of Lithuanian Cancer
cmladvocates.net

Dr Karl Neff
Consultant Endocrinologist
King's College Hospital Trust

Lisa Punt
Cambridge (maggiescentres.org

Dan Thomas
London School of Economics

Rowan Sanderson
themodernsensei.com

Julie Woodgate
woodgatemarketing.com

Catherine Woodward
Consultant Oncology
Cambridge-hypnosis.co.uk

Dr Catherine Zollman
pennybrohn.org.uk

Dr Ashwin Mehta
Director Integrative Medicine,
Memorial Healthcare System
mhs.net

Other recommended resources

Macmillan cancer support provides information and support on treatment options and side effects after cancer. It funds a network of nurses who offer advice and care. They welcome contact with patients and carers from shortly after diagnosis right up to palliative care. (**Macmillan.org.uk**)

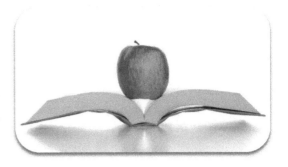

Cancernet-UK has over 500 pages related to cancer management and therapies. It describes common risks and side effects, as well as providing advice on how to help cope with them. It has links to services which are often required by individuals with cancer such as travel insurance, support groups and clinical trials. It outlines the lifestyle, exercise and nutritional measures which can be taken to improve chances of survival (**cancernet.co.uk**).

Social media: The cancernetUK Facebook, Twitter and Instagram accounts are an ideal way to be updated regularly with stories, recipe tips, news of events, lectures and research publications. These can all be accessed via **Cancernet.co.uk**.

The Cancernet blog: Topical are posted once a month, in response to a published article or frequently asked question. It has editors from experts in their field with topics so far include the benefits of fasting, the advantages of organic foods, the effects of cycling and prostate cancer the risks of processed sugar. It also has contains a series of informative, entertaining films which show how to make wholesome and nutritious meals that follow the advice given in this book. There are over 30 so far, including a sugar-free summer pudding, a vegetarian bodybuilder shake, gluten-free pizza, scrambled tofu, a seaweed salad and a turmeric latte (**Blog.cancernet.co.uk**).

The British Society of Lifestyle Medicine is a multidisciplinary group of professionals who aim to establish Lifestyle Medicine as central to health and wellbeing. They promote the prevention of avoidable lifestyle-related diseases by advocating realistic treatment and by influencing healthcare and health policy. They raise awareness of Lifestyle Medicine principles and provide leadership, education and support for healthcare practitioners (**bslm.org.uk**).

The cancer risk micro-nutritional blood analysis: This is a service which is ordered online and measures over 50 essential nutrients which are important for the biological processes which help fight cancer and other diseases. As well as the results, participants receive a report providing specific dietary advice relevant to their individual results. This may include eating more of some types of foods, avoiding others and, if necessary, taking specific supplements to target a particular mineral, vitamin or polyphenol deficiency (**cancernet.co.uk/nutritional-tests.htm**).

Keep-healthy is an online resource which provides substantiated lifestyle advice to help prevent or reduce the effect of common disease such as high BP, arthritis, hot flushes, weight gain, high cholesterol and fatigue. This website also provides information and links to practical products which have particular relevance to lifestyle and functional medicine including; high-grade, evidence-based nutritional supplements such as multi-strain probiotic bacteria; organic CBD (cannabis) oil; natural anti-inflammatory creams for muscle and joint pains; herbal supplements to enhance exercise performance and improve joint health (**keep-healthy.com**)

Pomi-T.co.uk is an online resource which outlines the UK National Cancer Research Institute's Pomi-T study. It provides links to the full published papers, as well as information on the product itself.

Polybalm.com is an online resource providing practical advice on how to prevent distressing nail damage during chemotherapy. It includes information from the UK National Cancer Research polybalm study, alongside links to the product itself.

Penny Brohn UK is a charity which offers a combination of physical, emotional, psychological and spiritual support that is designed to provide holistic help for anyone affected by cancer. It offers supervised group and individual sessions where people affected by cancer can learn how to eat well, stay physically active, manage their thoughts, emotions and relationships, and use a range of evidence-informed complementary therapies, all of which can help support their physical health and help them cope with the impacts of cancer and cancer treatments (**pennybrohn.org.uk**).

Maggie's cancer care centres are located in the grounds of large hospitals throughout the UK and internationally. Within each centre, a small, professional team provide emotional, practical and social support to anyone living with cancer and their family and friends. The centres are warm, welcoming and uniquely designed to foster a sense of well-being. The support offered is free, and no appointment is needed. Simply drop in for a cup of tea, meet the team and find out more about the support offered (**maggiescentres.org**).

Disclaimer

This book is for educational interest and guidance only. The lifestyle advice is aimed to complement the established management of malignant disease. It should not be considered as offering alternative medical advice. Never disregard medical advice or delay in seeking it because of something you have read in this book. The advice provided in this book is not intended as a substitute for consulting a licensed medical professional. Check with a family doctor or specialist physician if you suspect you are ill or believe you may have one of the problems discussed in this book, as many problems and disease states may be serious and even life-threatening.

Also note that while the information was up to date at the time of initial publication, medical information changes rapidly, so it is possible that some information may be out of date or even possibly inaccurate and erroneous at the time of reading. If you find information on our site that you believe is in error, please let us know by emailing health-education@clara.co.uk. The author makes no representations or warranties with respect to any information offered or provided through this book regarding treatment, action, or application of medication. The author or his affiliates will not be liable for any direct, indirect, consequential, special, exemplary, or other damages.